Multidisciplinary Approach to Head and Neck Cancer

Editor

MAIE A. ST. JOHN

OTOLARYNGOLOGIC CLINICS OF NORTH AMERICA

www.oto.theclinics.com

Consulting Editor
SUJANA S. CHANDRASEKHAR

August 2017 • Volume 50 • Number 4

ELSEVIER

1600 John F. Kennedy Boulevard • Suite 1800 • Philadelphia, Pennsylvania, 19103-2899

http://www.oto.theclinics.com

OTOLARYNGOLOGIC CLINICS OF NORTH AMERICA Volume 50, Number 4
August 2017 ISSN 0030-6665, ISBN-13: 978-0-323-53249-5

Editor: Jessica McCool
Developmental Editor: Alison Swety

Otolaryngologic Clinics of North America (ISSN 0030-6665) is published bimonthly by Elsevier, Inc., 360 Park Avenue South, New York, NY 10010-1710. Months of issue are February, April, June, August, October, and December. Business and Editorial Offices: 1600 John F. Kennedy Blvd., Suite 1800, Philadelphia, PA 19103-2899. Customer Service Office: 6277 Sea Harbor Drive, Orlando, FL 32887-4800. Periodicals postage paid at New York, NY and additional mailing offices. Subscription prices are $381.00 per year (US individuals), $803.00 per year (US institutions), $100.00 per year (US student/resident), $500.00 per year (Canadian individuals), $1017.00 per year (Canadian institutions), $556.00 per year (international individuals), $1017.00 per year (international institutions), $270.00 per year (international & Canadian student/resident). Foreign air speed delivery is included in all *Clinics'* subscription prices. All prices are subject to change without notice. **POSTMASTER:** Send address changes to *Otolaryngologic Clinics of North America*, Elsevier Health Sciences Division, Subscription Customer Service, 3251 Riverport Lane, Maryland Heights, MO 63043. **Telephone: 1-800-654-2452 (U.S. and Canada); 314-447-8871 (outside U.S. and Canada). Fax: 314-447-8029. E-mail: journalscustomerservice-usa@elsevier.com (for print support); journalsonlinesupport-usa@elsevier.com (for online support).**

Reprints. For copies of 100 or more of articles in this publication, please contact the Commercial Reprints Department, Elsevier Inc., 360 Park Avenue South, New York, NY 10010-1710. Tel.: 212-633-3874; Fax: 212-633-3820; E-mail: reprints@elsevier.com.

Otolaryngologic Clinics of North America is also published in Spanish by McGraw-Hill Interamericana Editores S.A., P.O. Box 5-237, 06500 Mexico D.F., Mexico.

Otolaryngologic Clinics of North America is covered in *MEDLINE/PubMed (Index Medicus), Current Contents/Clinical Medicine, Excerpta Medica, BIOSIS, Science Citation Index,* and *ISI/BIOMED*.

PROGRAM OBJECTIVE

The goal of the *Otolaryngologic Clinics of North America* is to provide information on the latest trends in patient management, the newest advances; and provide a sound basis for choosing treatment options in the field of otolaryngology.

LEARNING OBJECTIVES

Upon completion of this activity, participants will be able to:

1. Review the roles of the patient and practitioner in the management of head and neck cancer.
2. Discuss radiation and surgical approaches to head and neck cancer.
3. Recognize outcomes in head and neck cancer.

ACCREDITATION

The Elsevier Office of Continuing Medical Education (EOCME) is accredited by the Accreditation Council for Continuing Medical Education (ACCME) to provide continuing medical education for physicians.

The EOCME designates this enduring material for a maximum of 15 *AMA PRA Category 1 Credit*(s)™. Physicians should claim only the credit commensurate with the extent of their participation in the activity.

All other healthcare professionals requesting continuing education credit for this enduring material will be issued a certificate of participation.

DISCLOSURE OF CONFLICTS OF INTEREST

The EOCME assesses conflict of interest with its instructors, faculty, planners, and other individuals who are in a position to control the content of CME activities. All relevant conflicts of interest that are identified are thoroughly vetted by EOCME for fair balance, scientific objectivity, and patient care recommendations. EOCME is committed to providing its learners with CME activities that promote improvements or quality in healthcare and not a specific proprietary business or a commercial interest.

The planning committee, staff, authors and editors listed below have identified no financial relationships or relationships to products or devices they or their spouse/life partner have with commercial interest related to the content of this CME activity:

Elliot Abemayor, MD, PhD; Emily Beers, MD; Phillip J. Beron, MD; Carol R. Bradford, MD; Margaret Brandwein-Weber, MD; Sujana S. Chandrasekhar, MD; Allen M. Chen, MD; Dinesh Chhetri, MD; Robert K. Chin, MD, PhD; Barbara Ebersole, MA, CCC-SLP; Andrew Erman, MS, CCC-SLP; Anjali Fortna; Shabnam Ghazizadeh, MD; John V. Hedge, MD; Thomas Heineman, MD; Rebecca C. Hoesli, MD; Jakun W. Ing, MD, MPH; Prashant Natarajan Iyer, BE (Chem), MTPC, SCPM; Ryan S. Jackson, MD; Nausheen Jamal, MD; Jonas T. Johnson, MD, FACS; Young J. Kim, MD, PhD, FACS; Edward C. Kuan, MD, MBA; Quang Luu, MD; Amy Lewis Madnick, MSW, LCSW; Jon Mallen-St. Clair, MD; Kelly M. Malloy, MD, FACS; Jessica McCool; Elizabeth Grace Morasso, MSW, LCSW; Vishad Nabili, MD; Marci Lee Nilson, PhD, RN; Anna M. Pou, MD, FACS; Banafsheh Salehi, MD; Ali R. Sepahdari, MD; Aditya V. Shetty, MD; Andrew G. Shuman, MD; Maie A. St. John, MD, PhD, FACS; Oscar E. Streeter Jr, MD; Jeyanthi Surendrakumar; Alison Swety; Daniel Wang, MD; Randal S. Weber, MD, FACS; Richard O. Wein, MD, FACS; Amy Williams; Charlene Williams, PhD.

The planning committee, staff, authors and editors listed below have identified financial relationships or relationships to products or devices they or their spouse/life partner have with commercial interest related to the content of this CME activity:

Jill Gilbert, MD is a consultant/advisor for Genzyme Corporation, and has research support from Az; Merck & Co., Inc; Bristol Myers-Squibb Company; Pfizer Inc.; and Novartis AG.

Cecelia E. Schmalbach, MD, MSc, FACS receives royalties from AO North America.

Deborah J. Wong, MD, PhD is a consultant/advisor for Bristol Myers-Squibb Company, and has research support from Bristol Myers-Squibb Company; Merck & Co., Inc; ARMO Biosciences; Kura Oncology, Inc; AstraZeneca; BioMed Valley Discoveries, Inc; and F. Hoffmann-La Roche AG.

UNAPPROVED/OFF-LABEL USE DISCLOSURE

The EOCME requires CME faculty to disclose to the participants:

1. When products or procedures being discussed are off-label, unlabelled, experimental, and/or investigational (not US Food and Drug Administration [FDA] approved); and
2. Any limitations on the information presented, such as data that are preliminary or that represent ongoing research, interim analyses, and/or unsupported opinions. Faculty may discuss information about pharmaceutical agents that is outside of FDA-approved labelling. This information is intended solely for CME

and is not intended to promote off-label use of these medications. If you have any questions, contact the medical affairs department of the manufacturer for the most recent prescribing information.

TO ENROLL

To enroll in the *Otolaryngologic Clinics of North America* Continuing Medical Education program, call customer service at 1-800-654-2452 or sign up online at http://www.theclinics.com/home/cme. The CME program is available to subscribers for an additional annual fee of USD 260.

METHOD OF PARTICIPATION

In order to claim credit, participants must complete the following:
1. Complete enrolment as indicated above.
2. Read the activity.
3. Complete the CME Test and Evaluation. Participants must achieve a score of 70% on the test. All CME Tests and Evaluations must be completed online.

CME INQUIRIES/SPECIAL NEEDS

For all CME inquiries or special needs, please contact elsevierCME@elsevier.com.

Contributors

CONSULTING EDITOR

SUJANA S. CHANDRASEKHAR, MD
Director, New York Otology, Department of Otolaryngology–Head and Neck Surgery, Hofstra-Northwell School of Medicine, Icahn School of Medicine at Mount Sinai, New York, New York

EDITOR

MAIE A. ST. JOHN, MD, PhD, FACS
Samuel and Della Pearlman Chair in Head and Neck Surgery, Co-Director, UCLA Head and Neck Cancer Program, Jonsson Comprehensive Cancer Center, University of California, Los Angeles, David Geffen School of Medicine, Los Angeles, California

AUTHORS

ELLIOT ABEMAYOR, MD, PhD
Professor of Head and Neck Surgery, Co-Director, UCLA Head and Neck Cancer Program, Department of Head and Neck Surgery, Ronald Reagan University of California, Los Angeles Medical Center, Los Angeles, California

EMILY BEERS, MD
Assistant Clinical Professor, Section of Palliative Care, Department of Plastic Surgery, Pittsburgh, Pennsylvania

PHILLIP J. BERON, MD
Associate Professor, Department of Radiation Oncology, Ronald Reagan University of California, Los Angeles Medical Center, Los Angeles, California

CAROL R. BRADFORD, MD
Department of Otolaryngology–Head and Neck Surgery, Comprehensive Cancer Center, University of Michigan Medical School, Ann Arbor, Michigan

MARGARET BRANDWEIN-WEBER, MD
Professor of Pathology, Site Chair, Pathology, Mount Sinai Health System, Icahn School of Medicine, New York, New York

ALLEN M. CHEN, MD
Department of Radiation Oncology, University of California, Los Angeles, David Geffen School of Medicine, Los Angeles, California

DINESH CHHETRI, MD
Professor, Department of Head and Neck Surgery, University of California, Los Angeles, California

ROBERT K. CHIN, MD, PhD
Department of Radiation Oncology, University of California, Los Angeles, David Geffen School of Medicine, Los Angeles, California

BARBARA EBERSOLE, MA, CCC-SLP
Clinical Instructor, Department of Otolaryngology–Head and Neck Surgery, Lewis Katz School of Medicine, Temple University, Department of Speech Pathology, Fox Chase Cancer Center, Philadelphia, Pennsylvania

ANDREW ERMAN, MS, CCC-SLP
Speech Pathology Clinic Director, Department of Audiology and Speech, University of California, Los Angeles, California

SHABNAM GHAZIZADEH, MD
Resident Physician, Department of Head and Neck Surgery, Ronald Reagan University of California, Los Angeles Medical Center, Los Angeles, California

JILL GILBERT, MD
Professor of Medicine, Department of Medicine, Division of Hematology and Oncology, Vanderbilt–Ingram Cancer Center, Vanderbilt University Medical Center, Nashville, Tennessee

JOHN V. HEGDE, MD
Department of Radiation Oncology, University of California, Los Angeles, David Geffen School of Medicine, Los Angeles, California

THOMAS HEINEMAN, MD
Department of Otolaryngology–Head and Neck Surgery, University of California, Los Angeles, David Geffen School of Medicine, Los Angeles, California

REBECCA C. HOESLI, MD
Ruth L. Kirschstein Institutional National Research Service Award Research Fellow, Department of Otolaryngology–Head and Neck Surgery, Comprehensive Cancer Center, University of Michigan Medical School, Ann Arbor, Michigan

JAKUN W. ING, MD, MPH
Health Sciences Assistant Clinical Professor, UCLA Comprehensive Pain Center Director, Inpatient Chronic Pain Service, Ronald Reagan University of California, Los Angeles Medical Center, UCLA Department of Anesthesiology and Perioperative Management, University of California, Los Angeles, Los Angeles, California

PRASHANT NATARAJAN IYER, BE (Chem), MTPC, SCPM
Product Director, Healthcare Solutions, Oracle Corporation, Pleasanton, California

RYAN S. JACKSON, MD
Assistant Professor, Head and Neck Oncology and Microvascular Reconstructive Surgery, Department of Otolaryngology–Head and Neck Surgery, Washington University School of Medicine, St Louis, Missouri

NAUSHEEN JAMAL, MD
Assistant Professor, Department of Otolaryngology–Head and Neck Surgery, Lewis Katz School of Medicine, Temple University, Assistant Professor, Department of Surgical Oncology, Fox Chase Cancer Center, Philadelphia, Pennsylvania

JONAS T. JOHNSON, MD, FACS
The Eugene N. Myers, M.D., Professor and Chairman of Otolaryngology, Professor and Chairman, Department of Otolaryngology, Professor, Department of Radiation Oncology, University of Pittsburgh School of Medicine, Professor, Department of Oral and Maxillofacial Surgery, University of Pittsburgh School of Dental Medicine, Pittsburgh, Pennsylvania

YOUNG J. KIM, MD, PhD, FACS
Barry and Amy Baker Endowed Chair, Co-Leader, Translational Research and Interventional Oncology, Director, Head and Neck Oncologic Research, Department of Otolaryngology, Vanderbilt–Ingram Cancer Center, Cancer Biology, PMI, Biochemisty, Vanderbilt University Medical Center, Nashville, Tennessee

EDWARD C. KUAN, MD, MBA
Resident Physician, Department of Head and Neck Surgery, Ronald Reagan University of California, Los Angeles Medical Center, Los Angeles, California

MARCI LEE NILSEN, PhD, RN
Assistant Professor, Department of Acute and Tertiary Care, School of Nursing, University of Pittsburgh, Pittsburgh, Pennsylvania

QUANG LUU, MD
Associate Professor, Division of Facial Plastic and Reconstructive Surgery, Department of Head and Neck Surgery, Ronald Reagan University of California, Los Angeles Medical Center, Los Angeles, California

AMY LEWIS MADNICK, MSW, LCSW
Clinical Social Worker, Department of Care Coordination and Clinical Social Work, Ronald Reagan University of California, Los Angeles Medical Center, Los Angeles, California

JON MALLEN-ST. CLAIR, MD
Bryan Hemming Endowed Fellow in Head and Neck Cancer, University of California San Francisco, San Francisco, California

KELLY M. MALLOY, MD, FACS
Associate Professor, Department of Otolaryngology–Head and Neck Surgery, University of Michigan Medical School, Ann Arbor, Michigan

ELIZABETH GRACE MORASSO, MSW, LCSW
Clinical Social Worker, Department of Radiation Oncology, Ronald Reagan University of California, Los Angeles Medical Center, Los Angeles, California

VISHAD NABILI, MD
Associate Professor, Residency Program Director, Division of Facial Plastic and Reconstructive Surgery, Department of Head and Neck Surgery, Ronald Reagan University of California, Los Angeles Medical Center, Los Angeles, California

ANNA M. POU, MD, FACS
Professor and Administrative Vice Chair, Department of Otolaryngology–Head and Neck Surgery, Louisiana State University Health Sciences Center, New Orleans, New Orleans, Louisiana

BANAFSHEH SALEHI, MD
Department of Radiology, Scripps Clinic Medical Group, University of California, Los Angeles, Los Angeles, California

CECELIA E. SCHMALBACH, MD, MSc, FACS
Professor of Otolaryngology–Head and Neck Surgery, Vice Chair, Clinical Affairs, Division Chief, Head and Neck Surgery, Indiana University School of Medicine, Indianapolis, Indiana

ALI R. SEPAHDARI, MD
Department of Radiology, Scripps Clinic Medical Group, University of California, Los Angeles, Los Angeles, California

ADITYA V. SHETTY, MD
Fellow Physician, Division of Hematology-Oncology, Ronald Reagan University of California, Los Angeles Medical Center, Santa Monica, Los Angeles, California

ANDREW G. SHUMAN, MD
Department of Otolaryngology–Head and Neck Surgery, Comprehensive Cancer Center, University of Michigan Medical School, Ann Arbor, Michigan

MAIE A. ST. JOHN, MD, PhD, FACS
Samuel and Della Pearlman Chair in Head and Neck Surgery, Co-Director, UCLA Head and Neck Cancer Program, Jonsson Comprehensive Cancer Center, University of California, Los Angeles, David Geffen School of Medicine, Los Angeles, California

OSCAR E. STREETER Jr, MD
Medical Director, The Center for Thermal Oncology, Santa Monica, California

DANIEL WANG, MD
Clinical Fellow, Department of Medicine, Division of Hematology and Oncology, Vanderbilt–Ingram Cancer Center, Vanderbilt University Medical Center, Nashville, Tennessee

RANDAL S. WEBER, MD, FACS
Professor, Chairman, Associate Division Head of Surgery, Department of Head and Neck Surgery, University of Texas MD Anderson Cancer Center, Houston, Texas

RICHARD O. WEIN, MD, FACS
Associate Professor, Department of Otolaryngology–Head and Neck Surgery, Tufts Medical Center, Boston, Massachusetts

CHARLENE WILLIAMS, PhD
Clinical and Health Psychologist, Head and Neck Cancer Program, Department of Head and Neck Surgery, University of California Los Angeles, Los Angeles, California

DEBORAH J. WONG, MD, PhD
Assistant Clinical Professor of Medicine, Division of Hematology-Oncology, Ronald Reagan University of California, Los Angeles Medical Center, Santa Monica, Los Angeles, California

Contents

therapy after transoral robotic surgery. Additionally, recent studies of modern proton therapy are reviewed.

Oscar E. Streeter Jr, Phillip J. Beron, and Prashant Natarajan Iyer

Precision medicine is the application of genotypic and Omics biomarkers to determine the most appropriate, outcome-driven therapy for individual patients. To determine the best choice of therapy, institutions use significant information technology–enabled data from imaging, electronic medical records, sensors in the clinic/hospitals, and wearable sensors to determine treatment response. With genomic profiling, targets to affect a disease course are continuing to be developed. As clonal mutational prevalence continues to be understood, information can be communicated to patients to inform them that resistance is common, requiring collection of more genetic mutations from patients with further biopsies or blood collection.

Aditya V. Shetty and Deborah J. Wong

In patients with locally advanced squamous cell cancer of the head and neck, a multimodality treatment approach is recommended. The addition of platinum-based systemic therapy concurrently with radiation has been shown to be superior to radiation alone and is considered standard therapy for locally advanced disease. No study has shown superiority of induction therapy followed by chemoradiotherapy versus chemoradiotherapy alone. In the adjuvant setting only patients with nodal extracapsular extension or positive margins seem to benefit from chemoradiotherapy versus radiotherapy alone. In the recurrent or metastatic setting, systemic treatment with chemotherapy is palliative. A subset of patients treated with PD-1 immunotherapy may achieve durable responses.

Rebecca C. Hoesli, Andrew G. Shuman, and Carol R. Bradford

The diagnosis and treatment of head and neck cancer is extremely complex. As a result, multiple medical providers are involved in a patient's care, and the multidisciplinary tumor boards provide a forum whereby they can share and discuss the intricacies of each individual patient's case. When recommendations are presented to the patient and decisions are to be finalized, the patient should benefit from the collective wisdom of a team of providers to achieve and implement a patient-centric and clinically sound consensus.

Jakun W. Ing

Pain is a significant morbidity resulting from head and neck cancer. Pain may also be the result of the treatments directed against head and neck cancer. An experienced practitioner may manage this pain by understanding the multifactorial mechanisms of pain and the various pharmacotherapies available. Pain should be managed with multiple medications in a

Psychosocial Distress and Distress Screening in Multidisciplinary Head and Neck Cancer Treatment   807

Charlene Williams

Psychosocial distress screening (DS) for cancer and head and neck cancer (HNC) patients is rapidly becoming the standard of care. DS is of particular importance for patients with HNC, given their heightened incidence of distress, depression, anxiety, suicide, quality of life impacts, and negative medical outcomes. In the absence of DS, distress is frequently missed in oncology settings. However, when identified, distress is highly responsive to treatment, with cognitive behavioral and behavioral medicine interventions demonstrating evidence of efficacy. Multidisciplinary HNC teams are uniquely positioned to implement effective DS programs and treatment tailored to HNC patients' psychological and medical vulnerabilities.

Changes at the Dinner Table and Beyond: Nourishing Our Patients Throughout the Trajectory of Their Cancer Journey   825

Amy Lewis Madnick and Elizabeth Grace Morasso

Patients with head and neck cancers (HNC) can experience significant distress from presentation of symptoms to surveillance/survivorship and end-of-life. It is of value to all members of the HNC team to practice patient-centered care in assessment and interventions with patients and their support systems to achieve the best possible outcome given patient health status. Early assessment and referral to ancillary support provide a strong foundation across the illness trajectory. Specific attention should be given to the psychosocial implications of changes in physiologic functioning. Support around these changes involves a strong multidisciplinary team familiar with the biopsychosocial effects of HNC and its treatment.

Maximizing Functional Outcomes in Head and Neck Cancer Survivors: Assessment and Rehabilitation   837

Nausheen Jamal, Barbara Ebersole, Andrew Erman, and Dinesh Chhetri

With increases in survivorship for patients with head and neck cancer, attention is turning to quality-of-life issues for survivors. Care for these patients is multifaceted. Dysphagia and issues of voice/speech, airway obstruction, neck and shoulder dysfunction, lymphedema, and pain control are important to address. Rehabilitation interventions are patient-specific and aim to prevent, restore, compensate, and palliate symptoms and sequelae of treatment for optimal functioning. Central to providing comprehensive interdisciplinary care are the head and neck surgeon, laryngologist, and speech-language pathologist. Routine functional assessment, long-term follow-up, and regular communication and coordination among these specialists helps maximize quality of life in this challenging patient population.

Survivorship: Morbidity, Mortality, Malignancy   853

Kelly M. Malloy and Anna M. Pou

Survivorship encompasses the entire therapeutic, psychosocial, functional, and financial experience of living with and through a cancer diagnosis. The period of survivorship starts on the day of the cancer diagnosis and lasts until the end of the survivor's life, regardless of the cause of death. The National Cancer Institute's Office of Cancer Survivorship expands the term "survivor" to include, importantly, caregivers, family, and friends close to the survivor who also live through this period.

Recurrent and/or metastatic head and neck cancer portends a poor prognosis with traditional treatments, but current immunotherapy with immune checkpoint inhibitors has the potential to improve these clinical outcomes. This review focuses on the major breakthroughs that have led to the current understanding of immunotherapy in head and neck cancer as well as the future direction of the field. Ultimately, this understanding will guide clinicians on the selection of patients with head and neck cancer and practical considerations before starting immunotherapy.

OTOLARYNGOLOGIC CLINICS OF NORTH AMERICA

RELATED INTEREST

Hematology/Oncology Clinics
December 2015 (Vol. 29, Issue 6)
Head and Neck Cancer
A. Dimitrios Colevas, *Editor*
Available at: http://www.hemonc.theclinics.com

THE CLINICS ARE AVAILABLE ONLINE!
Access your subscription at:
www.theclinics.com

Foreword

More than Just Mitoses: Complete Care of the Patient with Head and Neck Cancer

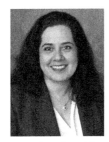

Sujana S. Chandrasekhar, MD
Consulting Editor

Dr Maie St John has put together a most comprehensive, readable "monograph" on care of the patient with head and neck cancer, in this issue of *Otolaryngologic Clinics of North America*.

Cancer care has evolved from treatment of the cancer to treatment of the patient with cancer and their loved ones. Relying on the scientific knowledge about carcinoma as well as medical, surgical, and radiation treatment options gets the treating physician to a very good point in the patient's care. Adding scientific knowledge regarding nutrition, pain management, and psychosocial factors gets us beyond that very good point. The apex is reached when the patient and their family enter into shared decision making (SDM), and the multidisciplinary team is enabled to contribute fully to the discussion, thereby enabling absolutely scientific, holistic, patient-centered care.

By organizing this issue of *Otolaryngologic Clinics of North America* the way that she has, Dr St John has allowed the reader, physician, surgeon, nurse, ancillary care provider, to take the journey to patient-specific, comprehensive care of the individual with cancer, in a systematic fashion.

This issue begins with understanding why we should pursue multidisciplinary care, not just as a popular "buzz" word, but as an actual, thoughtful shift toward ideal patient care. SDM is also a term that is often used but poorly understood. The techniques for SDM are specific and involved and are explained well in the article in this issue by Beers and colleagues. Without the input from our colleagues in Radiology and Pathology, we cannot even begin to grasp the full effect that the cancer is and could be having on the patient. The articles in this issue by Sepahdari and Banafsheh Salehi and Brandwein-Weber indicate the importance of avoiding "silos" between specialists, in order to provide optimal patient counseling and care.

Otolaryngol Clin N Am 50 (2017) xv–xvi
http://dx.doi.org/10.1016/j.otc.2017.06.001
0030-6665/17/© 2017 Published by Elsevier Inc.

Otolaryngologists–head and neck surgeons are surgeons. Innovations in surgical techniques, both for resection and for reconstruction, have made the days of horrible disfigurement and social isolation a part of history. Ditto for advances in radiation oncology, genomics, and systemic treatment, including immunotherapy. Even understanding this paragraph may require a multidisciplinary team of readers!

The patient benefits from all of the scientific and surgical advances above, but what the patient and their family experience used to be left to the wayside. Paying attention to depression and anxiety, to pain, to nutrition, and to functional restoration takes the very old field of head and neck cancer management to an extraordinary level. Empowering the patient and their family, who know that all of the physicians, surgeons, and scientists are working in concert for their best outcomes, empowers the multidisciplinary team to continue to push forward.

I congratulate Dr St John as Guest Editor and all of the authors who have written so beautifully and have thought so completely about the care of the individual with head and neck cancer. I hope that you enjoy reading this issue of *Otolaryngologic Clinics of North America* as much as I have.

Sujana S. Chandrasekhar, MD
New York Otology
Departments of Otolaryngology–Head and Neck Surgery
Hofstra-Northwell School of Medicine
Icahn School of Medicine at Mount Sinai
1421 Third Avenue, 4th Floor
New York, NY 10028, USA

E-mail address:
ssc@nyotology.com

Preface

Multidisciplinary Approach to Head and Neck Cancer

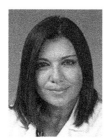

Maie A. St. John, MD, PhD, FACS
Editor

The complexity of cancer care in the twenty-first century mandates the input of a spectrum of health care providers to achieve the best possible outcome. Head and neck cancer in particular occurs in an anatomical region unmatched in the number of physiological functions potentially affected with disease and treatment, including respiration, physical appearance, vocalization, gustation, olfaction, and alimentation. Further complicating treatment is the wide range of tumor types and tumor locations in head and neck cancer, all of which taken separately are relatively rare cancers. Each patient also has their unique opinion as to what they would like to prioritize in their treatment plan (ie, survival, quality of life, length of intervention.). Patients come to us seeking knowledge, direction, and refuge. They come from every social class, every age group, every corner of the planet. They come to us "speaking innumerable languages," and we must be able to communicate effectively on every front. The care of the patient with head and neck cancer is no longer solely resecting a tumor, or offering the latest in immunotherapy. *The care of the patient with head and neck cancer is the art of caring for the whole patient*: multimodal surgical and medical management, aesthetic considerations, nutrition, pain management, and psychosocial support.

A medical "village" functions best when it unites for a common goal of optimal oncologic results while reducing functional deficits and minimizing suffering. This issue of *Otolaryngologic Clinics of North America* will highlight the team approach to head and neck cancer care, commonly referred to as multidisciplinary teams (MDTs), including the wide range of members and their roles in diagnosis, tumor board, treatment, and surveillance.

With the exponential increase in medical complexity over the past several decades, the need for increased communication, coordination, and shared decision making between medical specialties resulted in the formation of MDTs. The MDT as a functional unit of cancer care delivery has been adopted worldwide for nearly all tumor types.

Otolaryngol Clin N Am 50 (2017) xvii–xviii
http://dx.doi.org/10.1016/j.otc.2017.06.002
0030-6665/17/© 2017 Published by Elsevier Inc.

For patients, separate appointments and "noncoordinated care" add challenges to an already stressful diagnosis. Let us look at the most common scenario that occurs at most clinics and academic institutions: a patient is given a diagnosis of head and neck cancer and is then given at least three different appointments (ie, Head and Neck Surgeon, Medical Oncologist, and Radiation Oncologist). The patient then has to take time off to come to each appointment, and when they see each physician, there may be confusion as to which treatment option to pursue. The patient may feel like each physician does not really know what was offered by the other specialists they saw. They may leave each appointment feeling more anxious and confused about their options. In addition, most patients are not seen by Nutritionists, Head and Neck Mind and Body Psychologists, or Pain Specialists even though the vast majority of patients with head and neck cancer are not receiving adequate nutrition; their pain is not well controlled, and they do not have the psychosocial support they need.

It was out of witnessing such situations that our Multi-Disciplinary Head and Neck Cancer Program was born. We wanted to create a *patient-centric* multidisciplinary clinic to address all of the patient's needs in one clinic session. There is a one-hour high-level conference where each case is discussed in detail, all pathology are reviewed by expert Head and Neck Pathology Specialists, and all scans are reviewed by highly trained Head and Neck Radiologists. Robust conversation then ensues as to the options that will be available to the patient, and then a consensus comes to life.

After this meeting, all providers head to clinic where the patient is then seen by a Surgeon, a Medical Oncologist, a Radiation Oncologist, a Head and Neck Mind and Body Psychologist, a Nutritionist, and a Pain Specialist. Treatment options and the consensus recommendation are then presented directly to the patient. The patient and their family can then ask about the risks, benefits, outcomes, and side effects of each treatment modality. We also feel that a crucial component of the MDT beyond pre–meeting organization, case presentation, and treatment decision is *real-time direct conversation with the patient*. This discussion with multiple providers in real time allows a consensus to come to life and gives the patient confidence in their treatment plan. The involvement of the team members must also include involvement of the patient.

At its foundation, the MDTs function to present a unified *patient-centric* voice in the plan of therapy in the heterogeneous and multifaceted disease process that is head and neck cancer. In this issue, we detail the pearls we have learned caring for patients and working together as a team. As anyone who cares for patients with cancer can attest: "If you take care of cancer, sometimes you win and sometimes you lose; if you take care of the patient, you always win."

Maie A. St. John, MD, PhD, FACS
UCLA Head and Neck Cancer Program
Jonsson Comprehensive Cancer Center
David Geffen School of Medicine at UCLA
10833 Le Conte Avenue, CHS 62–132
Los Angeles, CA 90095, USA

E-mail address:
mstjohn@mednet.ucla.edu

It Takes a Village: The Importance of Multidisciplinary Care

 CrossMark

Thomas Heineman, MD[a], Maie A. St. John, MD, PhD[b],
Richard O. Wein, MD[c],*, Randal S. Weber, MD[d]

KEYWORDS

- Integrated patient care unit • Multidisciplinary teams • Tumor board

KEY POINTS

- Multidisciplinary teams are the functional unit of cancer care.
- Integrated patient care units optimize the ability to deliver efficient, value-driven care.

The complexity of cancer care in the 21st century mandates the input of a spectrum of health care providers to achieve the best possible outcomes. Complex disease management is best delivered by a defined team of physicians organized into an integrated patient care unit (IPU). The IPU is the optimal organizational structure to deliver evidence-based, efficient, and value-driven care.

As an entity, head and neck cancer represents a wide variety of anatomic tumor subsites with varied biologic properties and etiologies. The care philosophy and typical comorbidities for a patient with early stage laryngeal care can be dramatically different than that for a patient with an advanced stage Epstein-Barr virus–positive nasopharyngeal carcinoma or an intermediate stage human papilloma virus–positive tongue base cancer. The importance of a dynamic multidisciplinary tumor board cannot be underemphasized. It has the capacity to minimize duplication associated with patient assessment (eg, imaging), expand the capacity for collaborative research, support enrollment in clinical trials, and allow for a unified voice in a patient's care plan.

Disclosure Statement: There are no conflicts of interests for any of the authors relative to the production of this article.
[a] Department of Otolaryngology–Head and Neck Surgery, David Geffen School of Medicine at UCLA, Los Angeles, CA 90095, USA; [b] UCLA Head and Neck Cancer Program, Jonsson Comprehensive Cancer Center, David Geffen School of Medicine at UCLA, Los Angeles, CA 90095, USA; [c] Department of Otolaryngology–Head and Neck Surgery, Tufts Medical Center, 800 Washington Street, Box 850, Boston, MA 02111, USA; [d] Department of Head and Neck Surgery, University of Texas MD Anderson Cancer Center, Houston, TX 77030, USA
* Corresponding author.
E-mail address: rwein@tuftsmedicalcenter.org

Otolaryngol Clin N Am 50 (2017) 679–687
http://dx.doi.org/10.1016/j.otc.2017.03.005
0030-6665/17/© 2017 Elsevier Inc. All rights reserved.

As care has become more patient centric, we have learned that each patient is unique in their outcome priorities with respect to survival, quality of life, duration of treatment, and side effects. Patients come to us seeking knowledge, direction, and refuge. They come from every social class, and every age group. Thus, they come to us "speaking innumerable languages" and we must be able to communicate effectively on every front. The care of the patient with head and neck cancer is no longer involves solely resecting a tumor or offering the latest in immunotherapy. The care of the patient with head and neck cancer is the art of caring for the whole patient: multimodal care involving surgery, systemic therapy, radiation, medical management of comorbidities, aesthetic considerations, nutrition, pain management, and psychosocial support.

As referenced in the title proverb, a medical "village" or IPU functions best when it unites for a common goal of optimal oncologic results while reducing functional deficits and minimizing suffering. This article highlights the team approach to head and neck cancer care, multidisciplinary teams (MDTs) that come together as an IPU to provide coordinated care for the patient with head and neck cancer from diagnosis, tumor board discussion, and treatment recommendations through therapy, recovery, and posttreatment surveillance. At its foundation, the MDTs function to present a unified voice in the plan of therapy in the heterogeneous and multifaceted disease process that is head and neck cancer. As anyone who cares for cancer patients can attest, "If you take care of cancer, sometimes you win and sometimes you lose; if you take care of the patient, you always win."

MEMBERS OF THE MULTIDISCIPLINARY TEAM

The diagnosis of head and neck cancer most often occurs outside of the head and neck surgery clinic. Patients are commonly referred from primary care physicians and dentists who discover lesions on physical examination. Radiologists may detect suspicious masses incidentally on imaging for other reasons. Head and neck surgeons often make the final diagnosis of cancer through appropriate history taking, physical examination, diagnostic evaluation, and ultimately staging of disease.

The tumor board is a multispecialty group of experts in their respective disciplines who meet at scheduled intervals to discuss each individual patient. **Fig. 1** presents the large number of potential roles involved in head and neck cancer care.[1] The core members are head and neck surgeons, radiation oncologists, medical oncologists, head and neck radiologists, and pathologists. The "leader" of the team is frequently the head and neck surgeon, because most patients are evaluated and diagnosed by these specialists initially.[2] For decades, radiation therapy has been typically used in the adjuvant setting after surgery, but with the advent of refined techniques of photon and particle beam therapy (protons) based therapy, such as intensity-modulated radiation therapy, radiation has assumed a primary treatment modality role for several indications. Radiation in combination with chemotherapy as a means of treatment escalation has gained widespread use in organ-sparing approaches. Selecting the right treatment, for the right indications, and for the right patient with the goal of maximizing survival and preservation of function is the essence of multidisciplinary care.

For a tumor board to function smoothly, participation from disciplines beyond medical oncology, radiation oncology, and otolaryngology–head and neck surgery is necessary. Ensuring punctual scheduling of pretreatment interventions, such as dental extractions and gastrostomy tube placement for selected patients, is critical to facilitate the timely administration of integrated care of the whole patient.

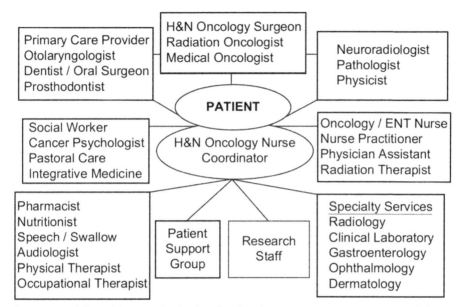

Fig. 1. Potential specialists involved in head and neck cancer care. ENT, ear, nose, and throat; H&N, head and neck. (*From* Weiderholt PA, Connor NP, Hartig GK, et al. Bridging gaps in multidisciplinary head and neck cancer care: nursing coordination and case management. Int J Radiation Oncology Biol Phys 2007;69:S88–91; with permission.)

having representatives from dentistry, oral–maxillofacial surgery, and oral medicine participating in a tumor board can facilitate each phase in the care of a patient with head and cancer and help to avoid, if not address early, the potential long-term complications that can come with multimodality care. Nutrition medicine and speech–language pathology also serve important roles in this process and should be active members of any tumor board. These services have the capacity to minimize a patient's weight loss and need for a break in therapy during radiation or chemoradiation therapy while also improving wound healing and the patient's functional recovery.

Most institutions require "in-house" pathology review of biopsies performed before referral to the treating institution. Verification of the diagnosis is critical to correct diagnostic errors that are not infrequent for rare tumors of salivary gland or soft tissue origin. After surgery, pathologists may determine genetic and histologic characteristics of the surgical specimen that may change the treatment paradigm, including extracapsular spread and perineural invasion. Although most often involved in initial diagnosis, radiologists play a key role in tumor boards with the increasing sensitivity and specificity of imaging modalities.

An emerging player in multidisciplinary cancer teams is the pain or palliative care specialist. Regardless of their tumor site or stage, almost all patients with head and neck cancer present with pain that is not controlled optimally. The palliative care team can play a crucial role in maximizing patient comfort before, during, and after treatment. Because patients with head and neck cancer are often malnourished before treatment and may continue to lose weight during treatment, the intervention of nutritionists can also prevent malnutrition and dehydration. Tumor boards at larger institutions may also include nuclear medicine physicians, molecular biologists, and health psychologists in the MDT.

The work of a multidisciplinary tumor board should not end after diagnosis and treatment have been rendered, but should have a role in the collaborative management of the aftercare of our patients. The framework of the tumor board should facilitate a platform where active discussions concerning a patient's posttreatment monitoring for recurrence and attention to the long-term side effects of care (physical, functional, or psychoemotional) can also be discussed.

IMPORTANCE OF THE TEAM APPROACH

MDTs as a functional unit of cancer care delivery has been adopted worldwide for nearly all tumor types. The implementation of MDTs has been at an exponential rate. In 1994, fewer than 20% of cancer patients in England were managed by MDTs. By 2004, this number had increased to 80%.[3]

For patients, separate appointments and "noncoordinated care" adds challenges to an already stressful diagnosis. Let us look at the common scenario that can occur outside of the IPU: a patient is given a diagnosis of head and neck cancer and is then given at least 3 different appointments (ie, head and neck surgeon, medical oncologist, and radiation oncologist). The patient then has to take time off to come to each appointment and when they see each physician, there may be confusion as to which treatment option to pursue. The patient may feel like each physician does not really know what the other specialists they saw offered, or how the treatment plans fit together. They may leave each appointment feeling more anxious and confused about their options.

The shortcomings of the nonintegrated approach make the need for an organized structure of care delivery and imperative for head and neck cancer management. Variation of this concept is institutional specific, but the goals are the same: rapid and efficient patient-centric evaluation, diagnosis and treatment. Some MTD IPUs have a patient-centric multidisciplinary clinic where the providers are colocated to address all of the patient's needs in 1 clinic session. There is a 1-hour, high-level conference and each case is discussed in detail, all pathology reviewed by expert head and neck pathology specialists, and all scans reviewed by highly trained head and neck radiologists. Robust conversation then ensues as to of the options that will be available to the patient and then a consensus comes to life. Other programs have sequential but clustered evaluation by specialists and diagnostic evaluations. Subsequently, when the consultations and diagnostic studies are complete, the patient is presented at the MTD. Patients are not present for the discussion but are subsequently informed of the treatment recommendations by a member of the team, usually the head and neck surgeon.

At the core, MDTs were built to improve coordination and continuity of care across medical specialties by fostering communication and shared decision making.[4] Published data support the benefit of the MDTs by demonstrating improved clinical decision making as well as clinical outcomes.[5] Kelly and colleagues[6] performed a study examining head and neck cancer care patterns at a hospital in Australia before and after the implementation of an MDT. In the study, 113 patients were examined (48 before MDT and 68 after MDT). They measured several clinical quality indicators that were used to evaluate individual patient treatments, including whether pretreatment dental and nutrition evaluations were performed, the attainment of PET imaging when indicated, the use of chemoradiation therapy in stage III or IV disease, and extracapsular spread, as well as the time interval from surgery to radiation therapy. After the implementation of an MDT, clinical quality indicator scores improved in all categories ($P < .05$).

The organization of MDTs varies between institutions but optimally has 3 main components: premeeting organization, case presentation, and treatment consensus, which is then communicated clearly to the patient.[7] The premeeting organization is the formal process on how patients are selected for presentation. After patients have been identified, an agenda is created and circulated before the meeting. During the meeting, the case presentation is best when efficient and concise. An MDT director may act as a moderator to ensure equal participation, respect for discussion, and facilitate efficiency. The treatment plan is decided on, with responsibilities of what are the next steps for each provider.

There are several factors that have been analyzed as keys to maximizing MDT quality.[8] The MDT is best when dedicated preparation time is built into a contributor's schedule. Offering team and leadership skills training for the group allows for an improved collaboration dynamic. When each specialty area understands the roles and limitations of others, the MDT best embodies the team approach to head and neck cancer care. In her presidential address to the American Head and Neck Society, Carol Bradford described the experience at the University of Michigan in the multidisciplinary care of patients with head and neck cancer. She highlighted "trust, commitment to excellence, respect, open-mindedness, recognizing a diversity of talent, and a common belief in making a difference," as pillars of the MDT.[9]

The crucial component of the MDT, beyond premeeting organization, case presentation, and treatment plan, is real-time direct conversation with the patient. This discussion with multiple providers in real time allows a consensus to come to life, and gives the patient confidence and personal direction in their treatment plan.

The potential of MDTs, as outlined by Bradley, can be "to harmonize and improve cancer care through improved documentation of imaging and pathology cancer stage and prognosis, the evaluation of available treatment, surgery, radiotherapy, chemotherapy and novel therapies, involvement of team members in audit of outcomes and active participation in clinical research."[10] We support this initiative and also want to emphasize that involvement of the team members must also include involvement of the patient.

IMPROVED COMMUNICATION OF IMAGING, PATHOLOGY, AND CANCER STAGING

MDTs have been shown to have a positive effect on clinical staging.[10] With proper staging, outcomes are improved because patients are given disease-appropriate treatment without the undue morbidity from overly aggressive therapy. Petty and Vetto[11] examined the influence of MDTs on cancer care, noting that recommendations were made that influenced diagnosis in 16% of cases.

EVALUATION OF AVAILABLE TREATMENTS

The broad scope of the MDT allows it to provide the highest quality patient care, including individualized treatment tailored to a patient's priorities and unique disease, effective care based on current evidence based medicine, and timely care with avoidance of long wait periods for diagnosis and treatment, as well as resource efficient care, minimizing redundant tests and appointments.[12] An important aspect of the treatment discussions at MDTs involves the balance of quality of life versus survival. Although used primarily in research settings, patient-generated metrics such as symptom score, perception of functional status, and general health before and after treatment are an essential part of selecting the appropriate therapy for the individual patient.[13]

In a study assessing the adoption of a multidisciplinary care approach for patients with head and neck cancer within a United States Veteran's Administration hospital system, timeliness and access to care were actually improved after transition to a more collaborative approach. Significant improvements were noted in the time to first visit after initial consult and the time from biopsy to the initiation of treatment. The use of a multidisciplinary approach led to an increase in the number of pretreatment consultations (1:4) from allied services.[14]

An example of a treatment dilemma that may present at MDT is a patient with early stage laryngeal cancer. Radiation therapy and surgery may provide nearly equivalent outcomes, but in collaboration with the treatment team, the patient must evaluate how the side effects and benefits of each therapy in terms of impact on voice, quality of life during treatment, availability for several weeks of radiation therapy, and so on affects their ultimate decision. Head and neck–mind and body psychologists are able to facilitate and support these discussions: allowing patients to put forth their priorities. Head and neck–mind and body psychologists can then ensure that effective communication has occurred between the patient and the treating physician, thus, maximizing the patients capacity to make an informed choice in their therapy.

AUDIT OF OUTCOMES

MDTs can function as a forum, similar to surgical morbidity and mortality conference, to discuss areas of success or improvement. Outcomes should be tracked with successes and failures monitored and associated feedback provided to the team members. An example of a key feedback relationship is that between the radiologist and the surgeon when operative findings vary from preoperative radiographic interpretations. Liao and colleagues,[15] in a study that compared 1616 patients undergoing treatment for an advanced stage oral cavity squamous cell carcinoma, used the participation of a multidisciplinary care team as the variable that was investigated relative to survival. Patients that were cared for by a group that used a multidisciplinary care team approach achieved significantly improved 5-year overall and disease-specific survivals than those individuals not managed in this fashion. Additionally, the rates of completion of adjuvant radiation therapy were significantly improved in the group using a multidisciplinary care approach.

An example of how effective cross-disciplinary communication can facilitate improvement in a patient's result can be seen with the concept of treatment package time. This refers to the time from the initiation of care (day of surgery) to the completion of adjuvant therapy. Rosenthal and colleagues[16] showed that, for patients with a total treatment package time of less than 100 days, 2-year locoregional control and survival rates were statistically improved when compared with those with a package time of greater than 100 days. This finding speaks to how delays in care can impact the beneficial relationship of pairing surgery with adjuvant care in a short time frame. Postoperative complications leading to extended durations of hospital stay and delays in initiating radiation, issues with obtaining dental care/extractions, delays in getting a percutaneous endoscopic gastrostomy (PEG), or unplanned breaks in radiation therapy all have the potential to expand treatment package time and impact a patient's resultant survival.

CLINICAL RESEARCH

Clinical research is an important component of MDTs. Cancer care is changing at an incredible rate, yet there remain many unanswered questions and suboptimal outcomes. Because many different providers are involved in MDTs, patients treated in MDTs are more likely to be included in clinical trials that advance the field of head and neck cancer, have the capacity to improve individual patient outcomes, and may provide therapy for patients who have failed standard of care modalities. Inclusion in clinical trials may be optimized with the involvement of a clinical trial coordinator.

PATIENT COORDINATOR OR NAVIGATOR

A relatively new development in multidisciplinary head and neck cancer teams is role of patient coordinator or navigator.[17] He or she makes every patient feel that they are cared for and supported at every level. In the complexity of cancer care, patients and families may feel increasingly lost, powerless, and unsure of where to seek information related to the varying complex treatment options. This situation is particularly pertinent to head and neck cancer, with concerns of changes in speaking and breathing abilities, nutritional difficulties, work-related issues, and body image. In the "maze" of health care, the role of patient navigation has emerged to guide patients from diagnosis to treatment to recovery. Fillion and colleagues[17] studied 2 cohorts of patients with head and neck cancer—those with and those without a cancer navigator. Not surprisingly, the cohort with a patient navigator had higher satisfaction and a shorter duration of hospitalization. The coordinator is an essential part of the MDT, functioning as a liaison to allow improved patient input in decision making that has the capacity to positively impact treatment package time.

NATIONAL GUIDELINES

Multidisciplinary tumor boards also enable the team to use National Cancer care frameworks, such as the National Comprehensive Cancer Network (NCCN) guidelines, to improve standardization and quality of care. Familiarity with NCCN guidelines and use in a multidisciplinary setting has the capacity to minimize the use of imaging, such as PET-computed tomography scans for routine surveillance, in the asymptomatic patient when it is unnecessary.[18] A retrospective review validated the benefit of using the NCCN guidelines by demonstrating an improved overall survival in patients with head and neck cancer who were treated with a guideline-compliant multidisciplinary approach.[19]

Contrary to this perspective, Sharma and colleagues[20] demonstrated that Medicare patients with advanced stage head and neck cancer at high-volume hospitals, not specifically seeking guidance or compliance with NCCN recommendations, could obtain superior survival statistics over low-volume hospitals that were practicing NCCN-compliant care plans in this population. Other authors have expressed concern about the ability of selected populations, such as individuals with a heavy smoking history, to tolerate the toxicity of the treatment paradigms set forth within the NCCN guidelines.[21,22] Familiarity with the NCCN guidelines allows the team to understand the national recommendations and to adjust these for individual patients as specific circumstances may dictate.

THE CANCER MOONSHOT PROJECT

The "Cancer Moonshot" project, initially present by President Barack Obama in the in the State of the Union address in January of 2016 and spearheaded by Vice President Joe Biden, has sought to facilitate greater collaboration across the entire cancer care community. The ultimate goal of the program is to double the rate of progress in cancer research and discovery over the next 5 years. The Cancer Moonshot Summit, held on June 28, 2016, at Howard University, was subsequently broadcast to 270 nationwide community gatherings in an attempt to initiate the discussion and networking across disciplines. In September 2016, a Blue Ribbon Panel presented 10 research recommendations to the National Cancer Advisory Board that were considered transformative and would facilitate achieving the goals set forth by the Cancer Moonshot. Some of the recommendations include expanding prevention and early detection efforts, developing a 3-dimensional cancer atlas, increasing the mining of patient data to improve future outcomes, creating a clinical trial network focused on immunotherapy, and building a national cancer data ecosystem.

SUMMARY

In a system where we are now measured in relative value units, we need a rekindling of why we took the Hippocratic oath. As cancer care specialists, we are dedicated to providing compassionate care for our patients that will hopefully cure their disease and alleviate their suffering. No single provider or specialist has all the expertise needed to attain these goals. The team approach in head and neck cancer care functions to unite a wide range of medical specialties into a unified voice to provide optimal care for the patient. When all members participate in generating and executing a plan of therapy, patients stand the best chance of overcoming a potentially devastating disease. If we focus on taking care of our patients, everything else takes care of itself.

REFERENCES

1. Weiderholt PA, Connor NP, Hartig GK, et al. Bridging gaps in multidisciplinary head and neck cancer care: nursing coordination and case management. Int J Radiat Oncol Biol Phys 2007;69:S88–91.
2. Varkey P, Liu YT, Tan NC. Multidisciplinary treatment of head and neck cancer. Semin Plast Surg 2010;34:331–3.
3. Griffith C, Turner J. United Kingdom National Health Service, cancer services collaborative "Improvement Partnership", redesign of cancer services: a national approach. Eur J Surg Oncol 2004;30:1–86.
4. Bradley P. Multidisciplinary clinical approach to the management of head and neck cancer. Eur Arch Otorhinolaryngol 2012;269:2451–4.
5. Blazeby JM, Wilson L, Metcalfe C, et al. Analysis of clinical decision-making in a multi-disciplinary cancer teams. Ann Oncol 2006;17:457–60.
6. Kelly SL, Jackson JE, Hickey BE, et al. Multidisciplinary clinic care improves adherence to best practice in head and neck cancer. Am J Otolaryngol 2013; 34:57–60.
7. Ruhstaller T, Roe H, Thurlimann B, et al. The multidisciplinary meeting: an indispensable aid to communication between different specialties. Eur J Cancer 2006; 42:2459–62.
8. Lamb B, Brown K, Nagpal K, et al. Team decision making by cancer care multidisciplinary teams: a systematic review. Ann Surg Oncol 2011;18:2116–25.
9. Bradford CR. The care of the head and neck cancer patient is a team sport. JAMA Otolaryngol Head Neck Surg 2013;139:337–9.
10. Nguyen NP, Vos P, Lee H, et al. Impact of tumor board recommendations on treatment outcome for locally advanced head and neck cancer. Oncology 2008;75: 186–91.
11. Petty JK, Vetto JT. Beyond doughnuts: tumor board recommendations influence patient care. J Cancer Educ 2002;17:97–100.
12. Weber RS. Improving quality of head and neck cancer care. Arch Otolaryngol Head Neck Surg 2007;133:188–92.

13. Morton R. Toward comprehensive multidisciplinary care of head and neck cancer patients: quality of life versus survival. Otolaryngol Head Neck Surg 2012;147: 404–6.
14. Patil RD, Meinzen-Derr JK, Hendricks BL, et al. Improving access and timeliness of care for veterans with head and neck squamous cell carcinoma: a multidisciplinary team's approach. Laryngoscope 2016;126(3):627–31.
15. Liao CT, Kang CJ, Lee LY, et al. Association between multidisciplinary team care approach and survival rates in patients with oral cavity squamous cell carcinoma. Head Neck 2016;38(Suppl 1):E1544–53.
16. Rosenthal DI, Liu L, Lee JH, et al. Importance of the treatment package time in surgery and postoperative radiation therapy for squamous carcinoma of the head and neck. Head Neck 2002;24(2):115–26.
17. Fillion L, Derres MD, Cook S, et al. Professional patient navigation in head and neck cancer. Semin Oncol Nurs 2009;25:212–21.
18. Roman BR, Patel SG, Wang MB, et al. Guideline familiarity predicts variation in self-reported use of routine surveillance PET/CT by physicians who treat head and neck cancer. J Natl Compr Canc Netw 2015;13(1):69–77.
19. Lewis CM, Nurgalieva Z, Sturgis EM, et al. Improving patient outcomes through multidisciplinary treatment planning conference. Head Neck 2016;38(Suppl 1): E1820–5.
20. Sharma A, Schwartz SM, Méndez E. Hospital volume is associated with survival but not multimodality therapy in Medicare patients with advanced head and neck cancer. Cancer 2013;119(10):1845–52.
21. Sandulache VC, Hamblin J, Lai S, et al. Oropharyngeal squamous cell carcinoma in the veteran population: association with traditional carcinogen exposure and poor clinical outcomes. Head Neck 2015;37(9):1246–53.
22. Lyon J. Cancer moonshot stalls on launch pad. JAMA 2016;316(10):1035.

The Role of Patients
Shared Decision-Making

Emily Beers, MD[a], Marci Lee Nilsen, PhD, RN[b], Jonas T. Johnson, MD[c,d,e,*]

KEYWORDS

- Shared decision-making • Autonomy • Bioethics • Patient-centered care
- Head and neck cancer • Physician-patient communication

KEY POINTS

- Treatment priorities between patients and clinicians may not be congruent.
- Most patients want to be offered choices.
- Treatment options need to be explained.
- Risks and benefits should be outlined and realistic.
- Clinical practice guidelines may facilitate these discussions.
- Decision aids, specifically patient education materials, support informed choices.
- Patient preferences vary.

INTRODUCTION

Most patients with squamous cell carcinoma of the head and neck present with advanced disease (stage III or IV).[1,2] They will face many decisions about their treatment, which can be very difficult for patients and their families. For many patients, the effects of their cancer and its treatment will persist for years and impact basic function of everyday life, such as swallowing, speech, and cosmesis. The Institute of Medicine now recognizes that shared decision-making (SDM) is a central component to patient-centered care and is essential to improving quality of care, especially in oncology.[3] Sharing in this process with patients helps ensure that they are educated and informed while incorporating their values and preferences into the decision process.

The authors have nothing to disclose.
[a] Section of Palliative Care, Department of Plastic Surgery, 3600 Forbes Avenue, Suite 405, Pittsburgh, PA 15213, USA; [b] Department of Acute and Tertiary Care, School of Nursing, University of Pittsburgh, 318A Victoria Building, 3500 Victoria Street, Pittsburgh, PA 15261, USA; [c] Department of Otolaryngology, University of Pittsburgh School of Medicine, Pittsburgh, PA, USA; [d] Department of Radiation Oncology, University of Pittsburgh School of Medicine, Pittsburgh, PA, USA; [e] Department of Oral and Maxillofacial Surgery, University of Pittsburgh School of Dental Medicine, Pittsburgh, PA, USA
* Corresponding author. Department of Oral and Maxillofacial Surgery, University of Pittsburgh School of Dental Medicine, Pittsburgh, PA.
E-mail address: johnsonjt@upmc.edu

Otolaryngol Clin N Am 50 (2017) 689–708
http://dx.doi.org/10.1016/j.otc.2017.03.006
0030-6665/17/© 2017 Elsevier Inc. All rights reserved.

EVOLUTION OF DECISION-MAKING MODELS

The American Medical Association's 1847 original *Code of Medical Ethics* advised doctors that "the obedience of a patient to the prescriptions of his physician should be prompt and implicit. The patient should never permit his own crude opinions as to their fitness to influence his attention to them."[4] This antique, authoritarian model of patients as passive recipients of doctor's orders is fortunately becoming a thing of the past. Despite that slow fade, however, the normative values of that paradigm that reigned for millennia have not entirely vanished. The increased emphasis on patient autonomy has in general been good; however, autonomy is itself a complex concept that has great bearing on the physician-patient relationship.

In the paternalistic extreme, the physician provided a plan that patients obeyed, removing agency from patients and giving all of the power to the physician. This model spanned from the time of Hippocrates to the 1970s. In that decade, massive culture shifts in America forever changed the roles of women, minorities, and society's view of authority. This change created a reactionary backlash to the paternalistic past on many fronts, and medical case law evolved in parallel. The 1972 case of *Canterbury v Spence* transformed our health culture by drastically changing standards for informed consent. Until that point, informed consent for a treatment included a discussion that met the standard of community disclosure, that is, whatever the most physicians in a community would say about such treatment. *Canterbury v Spence* detailed a patient who was advised to have a laminectomy for back pain; in his case the surgeon did not disclose the 1% risk of paralysis for fear that it would cause the patient to reject the beneficial treatment. When the patient suffered paralysis (either from surgery or a postoperative fall), the court ruled that the lack of disclosure was a failure on the physician's part. The court challenged the concept of *community standard* on grounds that it incentivizes physicians to protect themselves by limiting standard disclosure, which is not a practice aligned with patients' best interests.[5] In that ruling they noted "…the test for determining whether a particular peril must be divulged is its materiality to the patient's decision: all risks potentially affecting the decision must be unmasked."[6] This ruling resulted in legal codification of a physician's duty to fully inform, from which all current standards of informed consent have developed.

Bioethics also had a rapid evolution in that time, and the wave of antipaternalism caused some to advocate for a cultural reversal of power in the patient-physician dyad: in this version, patients dictated their preferences for treatment, and the physician's role was simply to execute a logical plan that honored those preferences. This version was the first stirring of patient-centered medicine, a model in which "the object of our studies is…therapy: not an isolated or specialized medical skill, but the doctor's whole professional activity regardless of whether he is a specialist or general practitioner."[7] As the pendulum swung from paternalism to physician as passive executor of medical possibility, the current standard has settled somewhere in the middle of those two margins.

In modern SDM, the physician provides the medical facts and treatment options, patients provide their values, and together they form a plan that best matches the facts to the values.[8] Although this model is far superior to either of the extremes, troubles remain with the way it is implemented. Firstly, this model presumes facts and values can remain completely separate. When physicians are giving facts, the data show that it is rare that they can provide these in completely value-neutral manner. In an analysis of 1057 audiotaped conversations of medical and surgical outpatients containing 3552 clinical decisions, only 9.0% of basic and 0.5% of complex decisions made met the criteria for informed decision-making.[9] That is, when we deliver information to patients we are not just conveying facts but overlaying a complex set of our own values and symbolism about what is important.[10,11] Much of current practice in SDM evolved from the principles of informed consent. Unfortunately, modern informed consent has become only more informed over time, as evidenced by medication package inserts and exhaustive forms designed to protect the physician from liability. When *Canterbury v Spence* ruled that all risks must be disclosed, we accelerated disclosure without proportional increase in patient knowledge.

Secondly, this still deprives the physician of much input: patients' values are always seen as foremost; in the era of health care consumers, we are generally taught that the customer is always right. As drug companies, insurance providers, and clinicians all battle in the era of cost-containment, every side is scrambling to represent themselves as patients' biggest advocate.[12] Although it is crucial to be our patients' best supporter, it is unfair to expect doctors to act as impartial fact-delivery agents without their own moral systems and values to uphold. Additionally, patients who are ill are often suffering from fear, anxiety, and uncertainty amid an ocean of freely available, and sometimes inaccurate or misleading, medical information. They should not be expected to analyze this in such a state and claim sole responsibility as preference-agent whom the doctor obeys.

In their pioneering 1979 book *Principles of Biomedical Ethics*, Beauchamp and Childress[13] outlined the 4 main principles of medical ethics: autonomy, beneficence, nonmaleficence, and justice. Beneficence and nonmaleficence relate heavily to a physician's performance/nonperformance of various treatments for a condition, and justice is frequently a broader principle of recognizing and overcoming health care disparities. Autonomy, however, is the elemental core in a patient-provider relationship. In modern medicine, patients' right to self-determination is rightly considered sacrosanct. The cutting edge of truly SDM is that it fully supports patients' autonomy while not neglecting the physician's autonomy either. Both parties are seen as able to provide facts and values. In complex treatment decisions, physicians have an obligation to explore the patients' values while presenting the facts. The things that constitute value in life vary significantly from person to person: one may think it is imperative to be able to perform high-level cognitive tasks, whereas another may find value in simply being present and aware for one's family. When physicians make a recommendation, we automatically incorporate our own system of values about quality of life based on our experiences, which is not a bad thing but something we must remain aware of. For patients to benefit from our expertise, we must guide them; but in order to do that best, we must explore their values and goals to give us both a road map and sense of direction.

COMPONENTS OF SHARED DECISION-MAKING

The increasing emphasis on patient involvement in treatment decisions represents a new approach to improving the quality of care we provide to our patients. Although research supports that SDM can improve patient satisfaction, treatment adherence, and well-being when faced with long-term decisions specific to chronic illness,[14] evidence is beginning to emerge regarding the benefits of SDM in oncologic care.[15]

In order to understand how to begin to implement SDM into clinical practice, it is important to understand the components or steps that are involved. There are essentially 4 steps to SDM: (1) informing patients that a decision needs to be made, (2) explaining the treatment options, (3) identifying patients' values and goals while supporting the deliberation, and (4) making the decision and arranging the follow-up (**Box 1**).[16–18]

Box 1
The essential components of shared decision-making

Four steps

1. Inform

2. Explain

3. Identify

4. Make

In order to help illustrate the components of SDM, the authors would like to present the following case study:

Ms F is a 70-year-old woman. She has a history of multiple head and neck cancers and has undergone several surgical procedures over the past 15 years, including a partial glossectomy, partial maxillectomy, and resection of the buccal mucosa squamous cell carcinoma. Ms F returned to the authors' head and neck clinic as a routine follow-up. In addition to her extensive head and neck cancer history, she has multiple comorbidities, including rheumatoid arthritis, diabetes, heart disease, macular degeneration, and advanced vasculopathy requiring bilateral below-the-knee amputations.

During her initial physical examination, an abrasion was noted on her chin. Ms F reported that she had fallen several days ago and was going to follow-up with her general practitioner about the abrasion. On further examination of her chin, Ms F was informed that this could potentially be another cancer and she agreed to have a biopsy done in the office. The authors acknowledged that if the biopsy proves that this cancer, it would be advanced cancer and we would need to discuss treatment options. In asking about her support system, she requested that her niece, who was the durable power of attorney, be present when the treatment options were discussed.

The pathology results confirmed that the lesion was invasive squamous cell carcinoma. A follow-up visit was scheduled with the patient, and a computed tomography (CT) scan was ordered. The CT scan demonstrated that lesion was extensive and included the floor of mouth with erosion through the mandible into and through the overlying skin. With her family present during the follow-up visit, all treatment options were outlined with the benefits and potential side effects.

When asked about her thoughts on the treatment options, Ms F acknowledged that surgery would be extensive with a lengthy recovery that could be very difficult for her, especially knowing that the result may not be curative. She was also aware that radiation with or without biochemotherapy was not likely to be curative and may present additional side effects. During the discussion, Ms F stated that her preference was to remain at home. With a life expectancy of 4 to 6 months without treatment, Ms F was referred to hospice agency that was identified by the patient and her family.

Step 1: Informing Patients

Clinical decisions regarding the treatment of head and neck cancer can be complex, and the best action may not always be clear. With current multimodality treatment, only 60% of patients with head and neck cancer will be alive at 5 years after diagnosis[19]; for some patients, surgical and nonsurgical options may provide similar survival outcomes.[20] Although preference for the degree of participation in medical decision-making may vary, most people want to be offered choices and be given an opportunity to voice their opinion.[21] Therefore, the first step is to inform patients that a decision needs to be made and seek their participation. As demonstrated in the case study, Ms F was informed via telephone that her results did demonstrate cancer and that treatment decisions needed to be made. She expressed her interest in having family present, and a follow-up appointment was set up.

Step 2: Explaining the Treatment Options

The treatment options need to be explained to patients in a neutral manner, including open and honest communication regarding their prognosis and treatment outcomes. Discussing the treatment options, including benefits and potential side effects of treatment, can help build a trusting relationship between the physician and patients. The risk and benefits need to be outlined for each treatment options in terms that are clear and meaningful for patients. It is also important to assess what patients already know because they may have existing knowledge from other sources (eg, Internet, word of mouth) and verify patients' understanding by asking them to explain what they perceive the treatment options to be. In terms of the authors' case study, all potential treatment options, including the options of no active treatment but instead palliative and supportive care, were presented.

Step 3: Identifying Patients' Values and Goals

Although discussion of patient preferences and goals can be incorporated into discussion of the treatment options, many patients may not have clear preferences at the onset of the discussion. It is important that physicians help guide patients in identifying their preference through asking open-ended questions that explore what matters to patients. When discussing pros and cons of treatment, it is imperative that we explore the relevance of the outcome to patients. When treatment priorities are compared between patients and clinicians, they are often not congruent.[22–26] Ms F was allowed time to express her thoughts on the treatment options. With her prior treatment history, Ms F was aware of the potential effect of the treatment options and the extent of recovery that would be involved with surgery. She acknowledged that being home and the avoidance of further toxicities of treatment were important to her.

Step 4: Making the Decision

Once we have established the treatment options and what outcomes are important to patients, the actual decision-making can occur. The physician should summarize what has been addressed and ask for patients' input or opinion. Depending on the patient and situation, patients may need time to think about the decision or may want to discuss it with their loved ones. If not, the physician and patients can agree on how to proceed. In this case, Ms F and family had an extended discussion in the treatment room before making a decision. The treatment team worked with Ms F and her family to find a hospice agency to help continue her care and symptom management.

STATE OF THE SCIENCE IN SHARED DECISION-MAKING
Multidisciplinary Team Management

Head and neck cancers represent a heterogeneous group of malignancies, which require multimodality therapies; therefore, a multidisciplinary teams (MDTs) approach has become the standard care. MDTs have been shown to have an impact on patient assessment and management.[27,28] Although overall there is limited evidence that MDT management improves cancer survival,[28,29] one report showed that for patients with stage IV head and neck cancer, there was an improvement in survival when managed by an MDT.[27]

The focus of MDT management, such as tumor boards, is to make individualized treatment decisions for patients based on their clinical presentation. Although treatment plans are patient specific, there is emerging evidence to support that this approach may not be patient centered. Instead, it may present a barrier to effective SDM as patients' values and preferences are not acknowledged during the MDT's treatment discussion; this has been described as health care "in absentia."[30–32] When patients' wishes and values are not fully identified or considered during the MDT meeting, a discordance between the MDT's recommendations and treatment implementation can occur.[33]

Clinical Practice Guidelines

Clinical practice guidelines (CPGs) are another way to help physicians structure discussions about treatment plans while incorporating the best possible evidence-based medicine. CPGs can be a jumping off point when evidence does not yet give us a clear direction,[30] such as whether to consider primary chemoradiotherapy for oral cavity carcinoma when surgery has been the historical standard of care.[34] The National Comprehensive Cancer Network (NCCN), American Society of Clinical Oncology, and European Society of Medical Oncology have all released CPGs to help providers guide patients in a world of an ever-expanding evidence base. Yet despite the development of consensus-based treatment guidelines for cancer, many physicians do not always routinely address the consensus topics in daily clinical practice.[35] In the case of patients with head and neck cancer, reduced compliance to the NCCN's guidelines has been shown to be correlated with lower overall survival.[36]

Decision Aids

One of the newest developments in the quest for better-informed patients in a busy clinic is the use of decision aids (DA), specifically formulated patient education materials designed to improve patient knowledge and support informed choices. DAs for both prevention and treatment decisions have just undergone their fifth Cochrane review, which shows that the evidence continues to mount in favor of their use. Quality evidence demonstrates DAs increase patient knowledge, reduce decisional conflict, stimulate a more active role in SDM, and improve accuracy of risk perceptions of treatments.[37] Unfortunately, in the oncology world, DAs tend to be more common for prevention and screening as opposed to treatment[38] and DAs specific to patients with head and neck cancer are surpassingly rare.[39] The International Patient Decision Aid Standards Collaboration has developed extensive criteria and guidelines to assist practitioners in formulating such materials, clear information delivery, methods to elicit patient values, providing structured guidance, peer review, and using plain language (eighth-grade reading level).[40,41] A successfully proven DA in oncology patients is the question prompt list (QPL).[42] The QPL is a booklet of questions about various dimensions of care designed to assist patients when their doctor asks if they have any questions and they may struggle to respond to all of the information. The University of Sydney has made this a printable booklet freely available online.[43] New Web-based DA platforms allow more rapid development of content that can be easily tailored to specific patient demographics.[44] The world of DAs in head and neck cancer is a largely unexplored frontier but one that has promise to improve communication without adding additional visit time.[45,46]

CHALLENGES
Patient Preferences Vary

Talking to patients about their desired role in decision-making is a critical part of treating physicians' role to help assure patient satisfaction with the process. Over the course of time, patients have tended to have an increasing preference for a more active role in treatment decisions[47–49]; however, there are many factors that influence patients' decision-making preferences. In general, most patients want to be offered choices and asked their opinion; none the less, a substantial portion may still prefer to leave final treatment decisions to the physician.[50–52] A critical part of the physician's duty is to ask about patients' decisional preferences, which creates higher levels of accord with patients' goals. When patient decision-making preferences are met or exceeded, patients have less conflict over the treatment decision, more satisfaction with their ultimate decision, more satisfaction with the consultant's communication, and perceived higher levels of their oncologist's use of SDM skills compared with patients who were less involved than they hoped to be.[53]

Patients tend to fall into 3 broad categories of decision-making preference: active, collaborative, and passive. Active patients wish to make the final decision about care after hearing the doctor's opinion; collaborative patients prefer to equally share responsibility for decision-making; passive patients wish the doctor to play the central role in choosing a treatment.[54] Although metrics somewhat vary, in general, approximately half of patients prefer a collaborative role, whereas the remainder are divided fairly evenly between preference for an active or passive role.[52,55–58] Patients who are younger, more educated, and of higher income tend to prefer an active decision-making role.[51,54,59,60] Patients who are older, nonwhite, and with lower socioeconomic status tend to have less satisfaction with decision information and are more likely to have knowledge gaps when providing informed consent.[61–65] Physicians must remain vigilant for their own racial bias, as those with implicit bias were rated as less supportive, spent less time per patient, and caused less patient confidence in and adherence to the treatment plan.[65] Studies have shown inconsistent results in terms of sex trends for SDM preferences, but it is worth noting that women are less likely to describe their role as active despite expressing a preference for an active role.[55]

There has been much focus recently on active patients' role, which is concordant with the trend away from paternalism. Despite this movement, however, incongruity between hoped-for and actual SDM outcomes persists. A meta-analysis of preferred versus actual decision-making roles in patients with cancer indicated a significant degree of discrepancy between the level of engagement patients preferred and what actually occurred.[66] Almost all patients in this review desired a higher level of engagement than transpired. In a separate sample of oncology patients, those who described physician-controlled decisions were *less likely* to report excellent quality of care, regardless of their stated decision-making preference.[67]

Even as we work toward increasing concordance between patient and physician decisional styles, there remains a substantial body of patients who still prefer passive decision-making left to the physician's judgment. Oncology patients who have a passive role tended to use less engagement in their coping strategies, that is, less active coping, planning, humor, or positive reframing. In addition, they have less resilience and higher levels of fatalism.[59] Cognitive coping style is also associated with patients' need for information, involvement, and satisfaction with SDM; importantly, even patients with an avoidant/blunting coping mechanism still desire significant amounts of information.[45,68]

Lack of Time and Training

Given the substantial evidence that exploring patient communication preferences and individually tailoring information delivery is critical for satisfied, informed patients, why does this not happen more consistently? Another pressing concern for head and neck cancer clinicians is the perceived lack of time or training to have such conversations. In busy surgery and oncology clinics, it can seem impossible to have the time to complete necessary documentation, much less for complicated discussions about difficult treatments decisions with no easy answers. This point is particularly true when conversations must involve shifting treatment focus to palliation or hospice care: we know clinicians often have these discussions poorly and too late.[69,70] Doctors ranging from trainees to senior clinicians often feel unprepared to have conversations that may include emotional reactions and address challenging treatment-related side effects.[70–72] Many providers fear that honest discussions with patients about difficult topics will take away their hope and reduce quality of life, but fortunately there is little evidence to support this fear.[72,73]

As we consider various treatment options for patients with head and neck cancer, clinicians must be aware of our tendency to err when discussing prognosis. We are systematically overoptimistic; the closer our relationship with patients, the more likely we are to overestimate survival[74]: the Lake Wobegon effect.[75] A recent meta-analysis indicated less than half of patients with advanced/terminal cancer understood their prognosis accurately.[76] Although most patients want to know specific information about prognosis, some remain more ambivalent.[69] The best way to avoid oversharing for those who find hope and data irreconcilable is to solicit preferences for level of detail early in the discussion and to allow some ambiguity if patients or caregivers eschew specifics.[77] Clinicians sometimes do this instinctively when giving bad news to soften the blow, such as saying: Average survival for people with this disease is 6 to 9 months; but you never know, it is different for everyone. Often when patients say they do not want to hear bad news, it is an emotional reaction; they frequently need time to process before they are ready to hear it. Some patients will want to know what to expect physically but will not want to know the specific time prognosis. The only thing we ethically must avoid is therapeutic privilege, wherein we decide to withhold specific information for fear the information itself will harm patients. Asking permission to disclose serious news is the best way to assure one does not give troubling news to patients. Having family present is also helpful, as they can often serve as a buffer and be available to hear news that patients may not be ready for.[78]

Although time is frequently a concern, satisfaction with treatment decisions can reliably be achieved in a 30-minute consultation for patients with advanced cancer.[56] Most clinicians worry about the more difficult discussions as being time consuming, but it is reassuring to consider that only a certain portion of patients per day will need the time resources potentially involved in more difficult discussions. Goldstein and colleagues[79] diagrammed the level of involvement in SDM required throughout patients' illness.

It is worth noting that the peak of the curve is where the benefits of SDM are most critical and the physician is potentially most involved. For many patients, the outcomes are much more predictable; in those cases, informational aids for the physician and patients are the tools to help have efficient, effective discussions.

Barriers to Transitioning to Palliative Care

When patients with advanced head and neck cancer are reaching the end of their curative treatment options, transitioning to a more palliative approach is warranted. Despite the continued expansion of the field, many barriers to the implementation of palliative care persist. A major barrier is the perception that palliative care is limited to the time when curative treatment is forgone.[80,81] In reality, palliative care has a goal of high-quality symptom management and care planning in advanced illness, both when aggressive curative treatment is being pursued and thereafter. Early palliative care intervention has been shown in multiple meta-analyses to improve symptom burden and reduce distress without detriment to caregivers[82–85] and reduce cost,[86,87] and randomized controlled trials have shown increased survival.[88,89] The literature in patients with head and neck cancer is far more limited. A recent review by Liao and colleagues[90] identified some common barriers to transitioning to palliative treatment in this group of patients, including physician's incorrect estimation of symptom impact, lack of investigation into patients' desire for family in SDM, lack of knowledge of financial impact of treatments, and physician emotion related to giving up hope. Patients with head and neck cancer often have substantial symptom burden at the end of life, but interestingly providers may *overestimate* the impact of these symptoms.[90,91] Given the anatomic communication difficulties that arise in these patients, it is even more imperative that we engage in a discussion of their preferences early in the treatment course. As disease progresses beyond the possibility of curative treatment, palliative and hospice care must eventually be discussed. Estimates have suggested that at least 20% of patients would qualify for hospice referral at the time of diagnosis.[92] Patients with head and neck cancer have a particularly challenging set of symptoms that test the limits of the hospice benefit.[93] Although hospice is an excellent care plan that can improve quality of life and reduce costs,[94,95] these are some of the most challenging hospice patients. Patients at risk of catastrophic bleeding or sudden airway collapse present the greatest challenge. Inpatient hospice is an excellent resource for this demographic, but the precipitous nature of the condition can make it hard to use these resources appropriately. The case that follows touches on some of the principles discussed:

Mr G initially presented at 23 years of age (1985) with a small cell carcinoma of the left maxilla while on active duty in the military. He was treated with conventional full-course radiation therapy and remained disease free until 2013 when he began to develop progressive dysplasia in the oropharynx. In January 2016, biopsy showed invasive squamous cancer (human papillomavirus negative). At that time, the area of involvement was circumferential in the oropharynx, with involvement of the base of tongue and all 4 walls. He declined surgery, further radiation, and chemotherapy at that time. In September 2016, he returned with stridor, at which time he initially declined tracheostomy. However, when told there were no good alternatives, he indicated he was not ready to die and tracheostomy and a percutaneous endoscopic gastrostomy (PEG) tube were performed.

How could the authors have improved this patient's care? He understood in January that he had untreatable, incurable cancer and yet returned to the emergency department 9 months later in distress. Introducing the topic of palliative surgery further upstream in the discussion can help obviate emergency department admissions for patients with no curative treatment available. When we know that patients are likely to have airway compromise or terminal dysphagia, open and honest discussion of the possibility of tracheostomy and PEG before they occur allows patients to consider them in a nondistressed state. It also important to remember that patients will almost always fluctuate in their level of acceptance of their illness. Although we tend to see denial and acceptance as binary states, patients tend to fluctuate between them and use each in various circumstances as a coping mechanism.[96]

Another major barrier to pursuing palliative treatment is intervention bias or the propensity to think that doing something is better than doing nothing. Intervention bias is a complex phenomenon involving portions of self-interest, confirmation, and publication biases.[97] Physicians wrap up their moral identities in the curing of disease and triumph over illness, and American physicians in particular are more apt to choose intervention over observation in a broad variety of circumstances.[98] This bias runs deep through the heart of our existence as professionals and is not easily reconciled. The financial incentives of the American health care system are deeply biased toward intervention; although we all strive to provide just, responsible care, it is impossible to eradicate this feature in the current health care environment. Increasing premiums and deductibles attempt to increase cost-sharing incentives for patients but in fact can lead to poorer compliance[99,100]: the model assumes that patients use health care services in the same way they do traditional consumer goods. Even our much-vaunted evidence-based medicine structure arises from a foundation of human researchers who spend lifetimes invested in their work and whose very sense of self is bound up in success of their work in a publication environment predisposed to report significant treatment results. Studies with positive results of the intervention can be 2 to 3 times more likely to be published,[101] and positive-outcome studies were more favorably reviewed and suggested for publication in the peer-review setting.[102] Intervention bias is a hydra-headed enemy that the treating clinician will confront in many arenas, and as we look back to the core of medical ethics we must remember that the irreducible principle of nonmaleficence dictates that before all other things we "first do no harm."[13]

Consequences of Treatment

There is a vast array of data published about head and neck cancer treatment complications and quality-of-life outcomes. Although dysphagia, xerostomia, dysphonia, mucositis, fistula, and fatigue can all plague these patients,[103] most of these symptoms have clinical algorithms for treatment. However, there is one silent symptom that is often underreported unless specifically queried by the physician: depression. Although patients generally feel comfortable talking about their physical symptoms, depression and anxiety often carry stigma.[104] In the context of SDM and improving our communication with patients, being attentive to depression in this group can substantially improve trust and influence treatment outcomes.

We know depression among the head and neck cancer population is a known concern. Some studies have shown a risk as high as 20% to 40%, with depression serving as a detriment to treatment adherence and functional outcome.[105–107] There are not enough data to definitively know if depression is linked to overall survival, but the high incidence of pretreatment and posttreatment depression should make clinicians watchful.[108,109] The most frightening complication of unrecognized or untreated depression is suicide, which has been shown to be present at a substantially higher incidence in this population. A general study of patients with cancer in Europe revealed that patients with head and neck cancer were at highest risk of cancer subtypes and were almost 5 times as likely to commit suicide as controls.[110] A more recent follow-up review of data from greater than 350,000 patients with head and neck cancer showed an overall suicide risk of 3 times, with laryngeal and oropharyngeal at 5 times, and patients with hypopharyngeal cancer at a stunning 14 times increase in risk.[111] There are multiple different depression screening instruments, many of which have been validated in the head and neck cancer population.[112] Although far from perfect, even asking patients the single question of whether they are depressed has a reasonable sensitivity and specificity in advanced illness.[113] In whatever fashion, the critical task of the clinician is to ask patients about depression and aggressively pursue treatment if it is discovered.

If I Do Not Offer Treatment, Will They Just Find Someone Who Will?

One thing many academic surgeons fear is the complexities of the second opinion. This role can come in many forms, from an elective office referral from a colleague to a patient being helicoptered to your facility after being told "they will fix you there" by the outside hospital emergency department. There is a small body of literature on the outcomes of second opinions in cancer care. The number of patients who seek a second opinion after cancer diagnosis can vary from 7% to 35%.[114] Patients who were female, more educated, or with more advanced disease at diagnosis were more likely to seek a second opinion.[115–117] Although many surgeons fear that if they do not operate someone else will, variance in treatment plan is less common than we may fear. In patients with head and neck cancer referred for a second opinion to a comprehensive center for MDT evaluation, the treatment plan was modified only 10% of the time.[118] Broader studies of general surgical oncology patients confirmed a 12% to 16% rate of treatment discrepancy and that, even when a second opinion was sought, 93% received surgery from the first surgeon consulted.[117,119] These data translate at the policy level: historically some states required mandatory surgical second opinions for elective Medicaid cases. Review of the policy revealed the low discrepancy of opinion and minimal change in cost to the system, leading to a program shift toward voluntary second opinions only.[120]

WHERE DO WE GO FROM HERE?
Improving Communication

The foundation of SDM is good communication. There is an epigram that best outlines the difficulty with such a simple-sounding task: "The single biggest problem with communication is the illusion that it has taken place."[121] Physicians, particularly surgeons, tend to think we are better communicators than either our colleagues or patients think.[122,123] Although head and neck clinicians will spend decades on medical education and advanced training to learn interventions, didactic sessions on communication skills are generally not thought to be of similar value. When talking about difficult topics, such as advanced cancer and possible end-of-life decision-making, patients prefer that physicians bring up the topic and expect they will do so.[124] When having difficult conversations, there are 2 critical skills that help these discussions go more smoothly: intelligent asking and responding to emotion.

The first is the *ask*. A widely used teaching model for physician communication is *ask-tell- ask*.[125] The first *ask* is an open-ended question about patients' understanding of the issue and, if there is bad news, permission to talk about a serious topic. For example, let us imagine you are a surgeon seeing a postoperative patient in clinic whose disease has progressed on adjuvant therapy, as you note from the most recent scans. A standard response to this is often something like the following: Unfortunately, I have some bad news. The CT shows that your disease has progressed despite the chemotherapy. This response is typically followed by a reassuring statement about the other treatment options available and how quickly we can get patients to the relevant specialist.[126] In the ask-tell-ask model, the surgeon begins by asking patients a question, such as the following: What brings you in today? or What have your other doctors been telling you about your cancer since the last time we spoke? The response to this question gives you critical information about patients' level of understanding of their disease. In this scenario, imagine the patient responds to the question of what brought he or she in today by saying the following: I don't remember exactly, I had the appointment on my calendar to have a checkup after surgery. This response reveals that the patient is not likely prepared to hear the bad news about disease progression. Knowing this, the next *ask* is for permission: Unfortunately, I have some bad news. Is it ok if we talk about what your most recent scans show? Asking for permission to talk about difficult topics serves 3 important purposes. First, it gives patients a warning shot that the conversation is about to become more serious. This warning helps patients reorient their expectations and prepare to discuss the news. Second, asking for permission gives patients authority to choose how they receive the news.

They may wish to proceed alone or may wish to have another person present to support them and help talk about options. Third, and perhaps most importantly, it gives them a measure of control in a situation that has suddenly become frightening and uncontrolled.[127] After delivering the news, at the close of the discussion, there is a final ask, which is to clarify understanding. Questions like the following can help guarantee that patients understood the information correctly: Does that make sense? Just so I'm sure I explained that well enough, could you tell me what you understand about what we discussed?

The second major hazard in clinical communication is emotion. Dealing with bad news brings up emotion in both patients and the physician.[128] Physicians are trained to deal with data and algorithms and procedures: emotion tends to feel disruptive and unpredictable. All people process information in both an emotional channel and a cognitive channel.[129] These two channels relate to each other in complex ways, and both are highly activated during the patient interview. When bad news about patients' cancer is conveyed, one must expect emotion and be able to respond. When delivering bad news, it is best to keep the news to a few short sentences and then pause, because emotional reactions happen almost instantaneously and irrespective of cognitive input.[130] The next reaction should be from patients; the physician tendency to fill uncomfortable-seeming silence with more clinical information should be avoided, as this activates the penchant of generating false optimism.[131–133] Another thing to remember is that highly emotional data can override the cognitive channel. When patients hear emotionally negative news, the negative affective experience can impair working memory.[134] This impairment leads to a decoupling of cognition after emotional stimulus and poorer recall of the very data we try to use to console our patients and ourselves. VitalTalk, an organization devoted to improving physician-patient communication, has created the acronym NURSE to give clinicians tools to help respond to emotion (**Table 1**).[135]

And lastly when dealing with emotion, it is important for clinicians to pay attention to body language. Maintaining eye contact and an open body posture (avoiding crossing

Table 1
Statements to help deal with and support emotion

NURSE Statements for Articulating Empathy		
	Example	Notes
Naming	It sounds like you are frustrated.	In general, turn down the intensity a notch when you name the emotion.
Understanding	This helps me understand what you are thinking.	Think of this as another kind of acknowledgment but stop short of suggesting you understand everything (you do not).
Respecting	I can see you have really been trying to follow our instructions.	Remember that praise also fits in here (eg, I think you have done a great job with this.).
Supporting	I will do my best to make sure you have what you need.	Making this kind of commitment is a powerful statement.
Exploring	Could you say more about what you mean when you say that…	Asking a focused question prevents this from seeming too obvious.

From VitalTalk. NURSE statements for articulating empathy. Available at: http://www.vitaltalk.org/sites/default/files/quick-guides/NURSEforVitaltalkV1.0.pdf. Accessed March 28, 2017; with permission.

arms or placing computer screens between you and patients) are shown to improve patient ratings of providers and foster empathy.[136,137]

The good news when considering all of the high-stakes components of patient communication and emotion is that training programs can help providers learn to manage this more expertly. Communication training interventions have been shown to improve confidence, increase response to emotion, increase patient engagement and trust,[138–141] and in some cases even improve Hospital Consumer Assessment of Healthcare Providers and Systems scores for doctor communication.[142] Fortunately, access to training programs is expanding as hospital systems and national organizations recognize the foundational nature of communication in our role as physicians.

SUMMARY

The evolution of SDM has been a gradual one, with a recent acceleration fueled by massive cultural changes and an exponentially expanding volume of scientific knowledge. Patients with head and neck cancer face a unique and steep set of challenges spanning physical, social, emotional, and cultural dimensions. As clinicians, we are obligated to provide the best care possible. Newer tools, such as DAs and multidisciplinary conferences, are first steps toward improving the breadth of our care; but there are still far more questions than answers about how to implement these best for patients with head and neck cancer. Increasing access to palliative care services and using them earlier in patients' trajectory will help improve symptom management, decrease cost, and increase the odds that patients' time is spent the way they desire. As providers, we will also have increasing access to continuing education opportunities to improve our communication skills, which will be critical to hone as more of our performance evaluation is linked to patient satisfaction. In total, the legal, ethical, and moral domains of SDM represent our most current understanding of "the pinnacle of patient-centered care."[143]

REFERENCES

1. Argiris A, Karamouzis MV, Raben D, et al. Head and neck cancer. Lancet 2008; 371(9625):1695–709.
2. Pulte D, Brenner H. Changes in survival in head and neck cancers in the late 20th and early 21st century: a period analysis. Oncologist 2010;15(9):994–1001.
3. Levit LA, IoM, Ganz PA, et al. Delivering high-quality cancer care: charting a new course for a system in crisis. Washington, DC: National Academies Press; 2013.
4. American Medical Association. Code of ethics of the American Medical Association, adopted 1847. Asa McFarland, Concord NH, 1850. Available at: https://collections.nlm.nih.gov/catalog/nlm:nlmuid-63310420R-bk. Accessed September 16, 2016.
5. Murray B. Informed consent: what must a physician disclose to a patient? Virtual Mentor 2012;14(7):563–6.
6. Canterbury v. Spence (464 F.2d 772) 1972.
7. Balint M. The doctor's therapeutic function. Lancet 1965;1(7397):1177–80.
8. Brock DW. The ideal of shared decision making between physicians and patients. Kennedy Inst Ethics J 1991;1(1):28–47.
9. Braddock CH 3rd, Edwards KA, Hasenberg NM, et al. Informed decision making in outpatient practice: time to get back to basics. JAMA 1999;282(24): 2313–20.
10. Metzl JM, Riba M. Understanding the symbolic value of medications: a brief review. Prim Psychiatry 2003;10(7):45–8.

11. Lentacker A. The symbolic economy of drugs. Soc Stud Sci 2016;46(1):140–56.
12. Tomes N. Patient empowerment and the dilemmas of late-modern medicalization. Lancet 2007;369(9562):698–700.
13. Beauchamp T, Childress J. Principles of biomedical ethics. Oxford University Press; 2012.
14. Joosten EAG, DeFuentes-Merillas L, de Weert GH, et al. Systematic review of the effects of shared decision-making on patient satisfaction, treatment adherence and health status. Psychother Psychosom 2008;77(4):219–26.
15. Kehl KL, Landrum M, Arora NK, et al. Association of actual and preferred decision roles with patient-reported quality of care: shared decision making in cancer care. JAMA Oncol 2015;1(1):50–8.
16. Kane HL, Halpern MT, Squiers LB, et al. Implementing and evaluating shared decision making in oncology practice. CA Cancer J Clinicians 2014;64(6):377–88.
17. Stiggelbout A, Pieterse A, De Haes J. Shared decision making: concepts, evidence, and practice. Patient Educ Couns 2015;98(10):1172–9.
18. Elwyn G, Frosch D, Thomson R, et al. Shared decision making: a model for clinical practice. J Gen Intern Med 2012;27(10):1361–7.
19. Surveillance Epidemiology and End Results (SEER) Program. SEER*Stat Database: incidence - SEER 18 Regs research data + Hurricane Katrina impacted Louisiana cases. 2016. Available at: http://seer.cancer.gov/canques/survival.html. Accessed September 2016.
20. Lin CC, Fedewa SA, Prickett KK, et al. Comparative effectiveness of surgical and nonsurgical therapy for advanced laryngeal cancer. Cancer 2016;122(18):2845–56.
21. Levinson W, Kao A, Kuby A, et al. Not all patients want to participate in decision making. A national study of public preferences. J Gen Intern Med 2005;20(6):531–5.
22. Mohide EA, Archibald SD, Tew M, et al. Postlaryngectomy quality-of-life dimensions identified by patients and health care professionals. Am J Surg 1992;164(6):619–22.
23. Jalukar V, Funk GF, Christensen AJ, et al. Health states following head and neck cancer treatment: patient, health-care professional, and public perspectives. Head Neck 1998;20(7):600–8.
24. Grossman SA, Sheidler VR, Swedeen K, et al. Correlation of patient and caregiver ratings of cancer pain. J Pain Symptom Manage 1991;6(2):53–7.
25. Otto RA, Lawrence V, Dobie RA, et al. Impact of a laryngectomy on quality of life: perspective of the patient versus that of the health care provider. Ann Otol Rhinol Laryngol 1997;106(8):693–9.
26. List MA, Rutherford JL, Stracks J, et al. Prioritizing treatment outcomes: head and neck cancer patients versus nonpatients. Head Neck 2004;26(2):163–70.
27. Friedland PL, Bozic B, Dewar J, et al. Impact of multidisciplinary team management in head and neck cancer patients. Br J Cancer 2011;104(8):1246–8.
28. Pillay B, Wootten AC, Crowe H, et al. The impact of multidisciplinary team meetings on patient assessment, management and outcomes in oncology settings: a systematic review of the literature. Cancer Treat Rev 2016;42:56–72.
29. Hong NJ, Wright FC, Gagliardi AR, et al. Examining the potential relationship between multidisciplinary cancer care and patient survival: an international literature review. J Surg Oncol 2010;102(2):125–34.
30. Hamilton D, Heaven B, Thomson R, et al. Multidisciplinary team decision-making in cancer and the absent patient: a qualitative study. BMJ Open 2016;6(7):e012559.

31. Thornton S. Time to review utility of multidisciplinary team meetings. BMJ 2015; 351:h5295.
32. Hahlweg P, Hoffmann J, Härter M, et al. In absentia: an exploratory study of how patients are considered in multidisciplinary cancer team meetings. PLoS One 2015;10(10):e0139921.
33. Blazeby J, Wilson L, Metcalfe C, et al. Analysis of clinical decision-making in multi-disciplinary cancer teams. Ann Oncol 2006;17(3):457–60.
34. Chinn SB, Myers JN. Oral cavity carcinoma: current management, controversies, and future directions. J Clin Oncol 2015;33(29):3269–76.
35. Kunneman M, Pieterse AH, Stiggelbout AM, et al. Which benefits and harms of preoperative radiotherapy should be addressed? A Delphi consensus study among rectal cancer patients and radiation oncologists. Radiother Oncol 2015;114(2):212–7.
36. Dronkers EA, Mes SW, Wieringa MH, et al. Noncompliance to guidelines in head and neck cancer treatment; associated factors for both patient and physician. BMC Cancer 2015;15:515.
37. Stacey D, Légaré F, Col NF, et al. Decision aids for people facing health treatment or screening decisions. Cochrane Database Syst Rev 2014;(1):CD001431.
38. Herrmann A, Mansfield E, Hall AE, et al. Willfully out of sight? A literature review on the effectiveness of cancer-related decision aids and implementation strategies. BMC Med Inform Decis Mak 2016;16:36.
39. Sawka AM, Straus S, Rodin G, et al. Thyroid cancer patient perceptions of radioactive iodine treatment choice: follow-up from a decision-aid randomized trial. Cancer 2015;121(20):3717–26.
40. Holmes-Rovner M. International Patient Decision Aid Standards (IPDAS): beyond decision aids to usual design of patient education materials. Health Expect 2007;10(2):103–7.
41. Elwyn G, O'Connor A, Stacey D, et al, The International Patient Decision Aids Standards (IPDAS) Collaboration. Developing a quality criteria framework for patient decision aids: online international Delphi consensus process. Br Med J 2006;333:417.
42. Clayton JM, Butow PN, Tattersall MH, et al. Randomized controlled trial of a prompt list to help advanced cancer patients and their caregivers to ask questions about prognosis and end-of-life care. J Clin Oncol 2007;25(6):715–23.
43. Available at: http://www.psych.usyd.edu.au/cemped/com_question_prompt.shtml.
44. Hoffman AS, Llewellyn-Thomas HA, Tosteson AN, et al. Launching a virtual decision lab: development and field-testing of a web-based patient decision support research platform. BMC Med Inform Decis Mak 2014;14:112.
45. Green MJ, Peterson SK, Baker MW, et al. Effect of a computer-based decision aid on knowledge, perceptions, and intentions about genetic testing for breast cancer susceptibility: a randomized controlled trial. JAMA 2004;292(4):442–52.
46. Green MJ, Peterson SK, Baker MW, et al. Use of an educational computer program before genetic counseling for breast cancer susceptibility: effects on duration and content of counseling sessions. Genet Med 2005;7(4):221–9.
47. Chewning B, Bylund CL, Shah B, et al. Patient preferences for shared decisions: a systematic review. Patient Educ Couns 2012;86(1):9–18.
48. Rood JA, van Zuuren FJ, Stam F, et al. Perceived need for information among patients with a haematological malignancy: associations with information satisfaction and treatment decision-making preferences. Hematol Oncol 2015;33(2): 85–98.

49. van den Brink-Muinen A, van Dulmen SM, de Haes HC, et al. Has patients' involvement in the decision-making process changed over time? Health Expect 2006;9(4):333–42.

50. Levinson W, Kao A, Kuby A, et al. Not all patients want to participate in decision making. J Gen Intern Med 2005;20:531–5.

51. Flynn KE, Smith MA, Vanness D. A typology of preferences for participation in healthcare decision making. Soc Sci Med 2006;63(5):1158–69.

52. Chawla N, Arora NK. Why do some patients prefer to leave decisions up to the doctor: lack of self-efficacy or a matter of trust? J Cancer Surviv 2013;7(4): 592–601.

53. Brown R, Butow P, Wilson-Genderson M, et al. Meeting the decision-making preferences of patients with breast cancer in oncology consultations: impact on decision-related outcomes. J Clin Oncol 2012;30:857–62.

54. Degner LF, Kristjanson LJ, Bowman D, et al. Information needs and decisional preferences in women with breast cancer. JAMA 1997;277(18):1485–92.

55. Singh JA, Sloan JA, Atherton PJ, et al. Preferred roles in treatment decision making among patients with cancer: a pooled analysis of studies using the Control Preferences Scale. Am J Manag Care 2010;16(9):688–96.

56. Hitz F, Ribi K, Li Q, et al. Predictors of satisfaction with treatment decision, decision-making preferences, and main treatment goals in patients with advanced cancer. Support Care Cancer 2013;21(11):3085–93.

57. Moth E, McLachlan SA, Veillard AS, et al. Patients' preferred and perceived roles in making decisions about adjuvant chemotherapy for non-small-cell lung cancer. Lung Cancer 2016;95:8–14.

58. Noguera A, Yennurajalingam S, Torres-Vigil I, et al. Decisional control preferences, disclosure of information preferences, and satisfaction among Hispanic patients with advanced cancer. J Pain Symptom Manage 2014;47(5):896–905.

59. Colley A, Halpern J, Paul S, et al. Factors associated with oncology patients' involvement in shared decision-making during chemotherapy. Psychooncology 2016. http://dx.doi.org/10.1002/pon.4284.

60. Brom L, Hopmans W, Pasman HR, et al. Congruence between patients' preferred and perceived participation in medical decision-making: a review of the literature. BMC Med Inform Decis Mak 2014;14:25.

61. Sim JA, Shin JS, Park SM, et al. Association between information provision and decisional conflict in cancer patients. Ann Oncol 2015;26(9):1974–80.

62. Cooper Z, Hevelone N, Sarhan M, et al. Identifying patient characteristics associated with deficits in surgical decision making. J Patient Saf 2016. [Epub ahead of print].

63. Kim SP, Knight SJ, Tomori C, et al. Health literacy and shared decision making for prostate cancer patients with low socioeconomic status. Cancer Invest 2001; 19(7):684–91.

64. Polite BN, Cipriano-Steffens T, Hlubocky F, et al. An evaluation of psychosocial and religious belief differences in a diverse racial and socioeconomic urban cancer population. J Racial Ethn Health Disparities 2017;4(2):140–8.

65. Palmer NRA, Kent EE, Forsythe LP, et al. Racial and ethnic disparities in patient-provider communication, quality-of-care ratings, and patient activation among long-term cancer survivors. J Clin Oncol 2014;32:4087–94.

66. Tariman JD, Berry DL, Cochrane B, et al. Preferred and actual participation roles during health care decision making in persons with cancer: a systematic review. Ann Oncol 2010;21(6):1145–51.

67. Kehl KL, Landrum MB, Arora NK, et al. Association of actual and preferred decision roles with patient-reported quality of care: shared decision making in cancer care. JAMA Oncol 2015;1(1):50–8.

68. Rood JA, Van Zuuren FJ, Stam F, et al. Cognitive coping style (monitoring and blunting) and the need for information, information satisfaction and shared decision making among patients with haematological malignancies. Psychooncology 2015;24(5):564–71.

69. Cherlin E, Fried T, Prigerson HG, et al. Communication between physicians and family caregivers about care at the end of life: when do discussions occur and what is said? J Palliat Med 2005;8(6):1176–85.

70. Keating NL, Landrum MB, Rogers SO Jr, et al. Physician factors associated with discussions about end-of-life care. Cancer 2010;116(4):998–1006.

71. Buss MK, Lessen DS, Sullivan AM, et al. Hematology/oncology fellows' training in palliative care: results of a national survey. Cancer 2011;117(18):4304–11.

72. Fallowfield LJ, Jenkins VA, Beveridge HA. Truth may hurt but deceit hurts more: communication in palliative care. Palliat Med 2002;16(4):297–303.

73. Weissman DE. Decision making at a time of crisis near the end of life. JAMA 2004;292(14):1738–43.

74. Christakis NA, Lamont EB. Extent and determinants of error in doctors' prognoses in terminally ill patients: prospective cohort study. BMJ 2000;320(7233):469–72.

75. Wolf JH, Wolf KS. The Lake Wobegon effect: are all cancer patients above average? Milbank Q 2013;91(4):690–728.

76. Chen CH, Kuo SC, Tang ST. Current status of accurate prognostic awareness in advanced/terminally ill cancer patients: systematic review and meta-regression analysis. Palliat Med 2017;31(5):406–18.

77. Innes S, Payne S. Advanced cancer patients' prognostic information preferences: a review. Palliat Med 2009;23(1):29–39.

78. Shin DW, Cho J, Roter DL, et al. Attitudes toward family involvement in cancer treatment decision making: the perspectives of patients, family caregivers, and their oncologists. Psychooncology 2016. http://dx.doi.org/10.1002/pon.4226.

79. Goldstein NE, Back AL, Morrison RS. Titrating guidance: a model to guide physicians in assisting patients and family members who are facing complex decisions. Arch Intern Med 2008;168(16):1733–9.

80. Rodriguez KL, Barnato AE, Arnold RM. Perceptions and utilization of palliative care services in acute care hospitals. J Palliat Med 2007;10(1):99–110.

81. Gomes B, Calanzani N, Curiale V, et al. Effectiveness and cost-effectiveness of home palliative care services for adults with advanced illness and their caregivers. Cochrane Database Syst Rev 2013;(6):CD007760.

82. Davis MP, Temel JS, Balboni T, et al. A review of the trials which examine early integration of outpatient and home palliative care for patients with serious illnesses. Ann Palliat Med 2015;4(3):99–121.

83. Howie L, Peppercorn J. Early palliative care in cancer treatment: rationale, evidence and clinical implications. Ther Adv Med Oncol 2013;5(6):318–23.

84. Smith TJ, Temin S, Alesi ER, et al. American Society of Clinical Oncology provisional clinical opinion: the integration of palliative care into standard oncology care. J Clin Oncol 2012;30(8):880–7.

85. Higginson IJ, Evans CJ. What is the evidence that palliative care teams improve outcomes for cancer patients and their families? Cancer J 2010;16(5):423–35.

86. May P, Normand C, Morrison RS. Economic impact of hospital inpatient palliative care consultation: review of current evidence and directions for future research. Palliat Med 2014;17(9):1054–63.

87. Tangeman JC, Rudra CB, Kerr CW, et al. A hospice-hospital partnership: reducing hospitalization costs and 30-day readmissions among seriously ill adults. J Palliat Med 2014;17(9):1005–10.

88. Temel J, Greer J, Muzikansky A, et al. Early palliative care for patients with metastatic non-small-cell lung cancer. N Engl J Med 2010;363:733–42.

89. Bakitas MA, Tosteson TD, Li Z, et al. Early versus delayed initiation of concurrent palliative oncology care: patient outcomes in the ENABLE III randomized controlled trial. J Clin Oncol 2015;33(13):1438–45.

90. Liao K, Blumenthal-Barby J, Sikora AG. Factors influencing head and neck surgical oncologists' transition from curative to palliative treatment goals. Otolaryngol Head Neck Surg 2017;156(1):46–51.

91. Parhar S, Rogers SN, Lowe D. Perspectives of the multidisciplinary team on the quality of life of patients with cancer of the head and neck at 2 years. Br J Oral Maxillofac Surg 2015;53(9):858–63.

92. Timon C, Reilly K. Head and neck mucosal squamous cell carcinoma: results of palliative management. J Laryngol Otol 2006;120:389–92.

93. Lin YL, Lin IC, Liou JC. Symptom patterns of patients with head and neck cancer in a palliative care unit. J Palliat Med 2011;14(5):556–9.

94. Enomoto LM, Schaefer EW, Goldenberg D, et al. The cost of hospice services in terminally ill patients with head and neck cancer. JAMA Otolaryngol Head Neck Surg 2015;141(12):1066–74.

95. Shuman AG, Yang Y, Taylor JM, et al. End-of-life care among head and neck cancer patients. Otolaryngol Head Neck Surg 2011;144(5):733–9.

96. Copp G, Field D. Open awareness and dying: the use of denial and acceptance as coping strategies by hospice patients. NT Res 2002;7:188–227.

97. Foy AJ, Filippone EJ. The case for intervention bias in the practice of medicine. Yale J Biol Med 2013;86(2):271–80.

98. Payer L. Medicine & culture: varieties of treatment in the United States, England, West Germany, and France. New York: H. Holt; 1988.

99. Jin J, Sklar GE, Min Sen Oh V. Factors affecting therapeutic compliance: a review from the patient's perspective. Ther Clin Risk Mana 2008;4(1):269–86.

100. Eaddy MT, Cook CL, O'Day K, et al. How patient cost-sharing trends affect adherence and outcomes: a literature review. P T 2012;37(1):45–55.

101. Easterbrook PJ, Gopalan R, Berlin JA, et al. Publication bias in clinical research. Lancet 1991;337(8746):867–72.

102. Emerson GB, Warme WJ, Wolf FM, et al. Testing for the presence of positive-outcome bias in peer review: a randomized controlled trial. Arch Intern Med 2010;170(21):1934–9.

103. Sciubba JJ. End-of-life care in the head and neck cancer patient. Oral Dis 2016; 22(8):740–4.

104. Peluso Ede T, Blay SL. Public stigma in relation to individuals with depression. J Affect Disord 2009;115(1–2):201–6.

105. Barber B, Dergousoff J, Nesbitt M, et al. Depression as a predictor of postoperative functional performance status (PFPS) and treatment adherence in head and neck cancer patients: a prospective study. J Otolaryngol Head Neck Surg 2015;44:38.

106. Lin BM, Starmer HM, Gourin CG. The relationship between depressive symptoms, quality of life, and swallowing function in head and neck cancer patients 1 year after definitive therapy. Laryngoscope 2012;122(7):1518–25.
107. Laurence B, Mould-Millman NK, Nero KE Jr, et al. Depression and hospital admission in older patients with head and neck cancer: analysis of a national healthcare database. Gerodontology 2016;22(8):740–4.
108. Barber B, Dergousoff J, Slater L, et al. Depression and survival in patients with head and neck cancer: a systematic review. JAMA Otolaryngol Head Neck Surg 2016;142(3):284–8.
109. Kim SA, Roh JL, Lee SA, et al. Pretreatment depression as a prognostic indicator of survival and nutritional status in patients with head and neck cancer. Cancer 2016;122(1):131–40.
110. Oberaigner W, Sperner-Unterweger B, Fiegl M, et al. Increased suicide risk in cancer patients in Tyrol/Austria. Gen Hosp Psychiatry 2014;36(5):483–7.
111. Kam D, Salib A, Gorgy G, et al. Incidence of suicide in patients with head and neck cancer. JAMA Otolaryngol Head Neck Surg 2015;141(12):1075–81.
112. Singer S, Danker H, Dietz A, et al. Screening for mental disorders in laryngeal cancer patients: a comparison of 6 methods. Psychooncology 2008;17(3):280–6.
113. Lloyd-Williams M, Spiller J. Which depression screening tools should be used in palliative care? Palliat Med 2003;17(1):40–3.
114. Ruetters D, Keinki C, Schroth S, et al. Is there evidence for a better health care for cancer patients after a second opinion? A systematic review. J Cancer Res Clin Oncol 2016;142(7):1521–8.
115. Chiou SJ, Wang SI, Liu CH, et al. Outpatient-shopping behavior and survival rates in newly diagnosed cancer patients. Am J Manag Care 2012;18(9):488–96.
116. Tam KF, Cheng DK, Ng TY, et al. The behaviors of seeking a second opinion from other health-care professionals and the utilization of complementary and alternative medicine in gynecologic cancer patients. Support Care Cancer 2005;13(9):679–84.
117. Mellink WA, Henzen-Logmans SC, Bongaerts AH, et al. Discrepancy between second and first opinion in surgical oncological patients. Eur J Surg Oncol 2006;32(1):108–12.
118. Bergamini C, Locati L, Bossi P, et al. Does a multidisciplinary team approach in a tertiary referral centre impact on the initial management of head and neck cancer? Oral Oncol 2016;54:54–7.
119. Morrow M, Jagsi R, Alderman AK, et al. Surgeon recommendations and receipt of mastectomy for treatment of breast cancer. JAMA 2009;302:1551–6.
120. Barton PL, Newhouse JP, Rand Corporation. Second surgical opinion programs: a review of the literature. Santa Monica (CA): Rand; 1989.
121. Whyte WH. 1950 September, Fortune, "is anybody listening?" New York: Time, Inc; p. 77, Quote Page 174. *often misattributed to George Bernard Shaw*.
122. Aslakson RA, Wyskiel R, Shaeffer D, et al. Surgical intensive care unit clinician estimates of the adequacy of communication regarding patient prognosis. Crit Care 2010;14:R218.
123. Tongue JR, Epps HR, Forese LL. Communication skills for patient-centered care: research-based, easily learned techniques for medical interviews that benefit orthopaedic surgeons and their patients. J Bone Joint Surg Am 2005;87:652–8.
124. Almack K, Cox K, Moghaddam N, et al. After you: conversations between patients and healthcare professionals in planning for end of life care. BMC Palliat Care 2012;11:15.

125. Available at: http://www.vitaltalk.org/clinicians/establish-rapport?vtitle=ask-tell-ask. Accesed September 21, 2016.
126. The AM, Hak T, Gerard Koëter G, et al. Collusion in doctor-patient communication about imminent death: an ethnographic study. BMJ 2000;321(7273):1376–81.
127. Friedrichsen M, Milberg A. Concerns about losing control when breaking bad news to terminally ill patients with cancer: physicians' perspective. J Palliat Med 2006;9(3):673–82.
128. Bousquet G, Orri M, Winterman S, et al. Breaking bad news in oncology: a meta-synthesis. J Clin Oncol 2015;33(22):2437–43.
129. Geltner P. Emotional communication: countertransference analysis and the use of feeling in psychoanalytic technique. Routledge; 2013.
130. Whalen PJ, Rauch SL, Etcoff NL, et al. Masked presentations of emotional facial expressions modulate amygdala activity without explicit knowledge. J Neurosci 1998;18(1):411–8.
131. Ruddick W. Hope and deception. Bioethics 1999;13(3–4):343–57.
132. Winner M, Wilson A, Ronnekleiv-Kelly S, et al. A singular hope: how the discussion around cancer surgery sometimes fails. Ann Surg Oncol 2016;24(1):31–7.
133. Portnoy DB, Paul K, Han J, et al. Physicians' attitudes about communicating and managing scientific uncertainty differ by perceived ambiguity aversion of their patients. Health Expect 2013;16(4):362–72.
134. Perlstein WM, Elbert T, Stenger VA. Dissociation in human prefrontal cortex of affective influences on working memory-related activity. Proc Natl Acad Sci U S A 2002;99(3):1736–41.
135. Available at: http://www.vitaltalk.org/sites/default/files/quick-guides/NURSEfor VitaltalkV1.0.pdf.
136. Hillen MA, de Haes HC, van Tienhoven G, et al. Oncologists' non-verbal behavior and analog patients' recall of information. Acta Oncol 2016;55(6):671–9.
137. Marschner L, Pannasch S, Schulz J, et al. Social communication with virtual agents: the effects of body and gaze direction on attention and emotional responding in human observers. Int J Psychophysiol 2015;97(2):85–92.
138. Epstein RM, Duberstein PR, Fenton JJ, et al. Effect of a patient-centered communication intervention on oncologist-patient communication, quality of life, and health care utilization in advanced cancer: the VOICE randomized clinical trial. JAMA Oncol 2017;3(1):92–100.
139. Dwamena F, Holmes-Rovner M, Gaulden CM, et al. Interventions for providers to promote a patient-centred approach in clinical consultations. Cochrane Database Syst Rev 2012;(12):CD003267.
140. Arnold RM, Back AL, Barnato AE, et al. The Critical Care Communication project: improving fellows' communication skills. J Crit Care 2015;30(2):250–4.
141. Tulsky JA, Arnold RM, Alexander SC, et al. Enhancing communication between oncologists and patients with a computer-based training program: a randomized trial. Ann Intern Med 2011;155(9):593–601.
142. Raper SE, Gupta M, Okusanya O. Improving communication skills: a course for academic medical center surgery residents and faculty. J Surg Educ 2015;72(6):e202–11.
143. Barry MJ, Edgman-Levitan S. Shared decision making–pinnacle of patient-centered care. N Engl J Med 2012;366(9):780–1.

A Story in Black and White

Radiologic Evaluation in the Multidisciplinary Setting

Ali R. Sepahdari, MD*, Banafsheh Salehi, MD

KEYWORDS

- Multidisciplinary • Head and neck radiology • Neuroradiology

KEY POINTS

- Radiologist engagement is essential to the success of a multidisciplinary conference.
- Logistical considerations of conference time and conference room setup are critical in ensuring optimal imaging review.
- By emphasizing unique clinical and academic benefits that are related to the conference, multidisciplinary team leaders can help ensure that active participation in the conference is a high priority for the radiologist.

RADIOLOGY, CRITICAL TO MULTIDISCIPLINARY CARE MODEL

Multidisciplinary clinical conferences (eg, tumor boards) that bring numerous specialists to the table, including radiologists, are critical to cancer care to reach the goal of providing a personalized treatment plan to any and every patient with cancer.

The continuing demand for the review of radiology findings at meetings is a testament to the perceived value and success of such reviews. One of the experienced benefits of a tumor board is the opportunity for medical, surgical and radiation oncologists, radiologists, and pathologists to meet together to build a stronger connection and a common ground with respect to terminology and expression in formal reports. Communication has improved between radiologists and clinicians, both in the provision of pertinent information to radiology at the time of request and the provision of formal reports from radiology whose meaning is clear to clinicians. Furthermore, technological developments in radiology make the choice of investigation and the

Disclosure Statement: The authors have nothing to disclose.
Department of Radiology, Scripps Clinic Medical Group, University of California, Los Angeles, 757 Westwood Plaza, Suite 1621D, Los Angeles, CA 90095, USA
* Corresponding author.
E-mail address: alisepahdari@gmail.com

Otolaryngol Clin N Am 50 (2017) 709–716
http://dx.doi.org/10.1016/j.otc.2017.03.007
0030-6665/17/© 2017 Elsevier Inc. All rights reserved.

oto.theclinics.com

interpretation of results more complex than in the past, so the meetings serve as an important opportunity for updating professional knowledge and continuing professional development.[1] Prior studies have recognized the impact of head and neck multidisciplinary team meetings in changing the clinical management in almost a third of the cases.[2] In academic centers, there also seems to be a connection between multidisciplinary meeting involvement and opportunities to collaborate in research projects.

ROLE OF THE RADIOLOGISTS IN MULTIDISCIPLINARY TEAM MEETINGS

As multidisciplinary care continues to evolve, radiologists are encouraged to provide image interpretation in tumor boards. In the current world of dynamic and advanced cancer care and subsequently more complex and advanced cancer imaging, a high level of expertise and ongoing engagement with the multidisciplinary group is necessary to optimize the radiologist's contribution.

Several different models exist for radiologist participation in multidisciplinary conferences, each of which is considered next.

Radiologist Presents Cases on the Production Picture Archiving and Communication System

For approximately a century after Roentgen discovered the X ray, medical images were interpreted from hardcopy films. The emergence of cross-sectional imaging, beginning with computed tomography (CT) in the 1970s and MRI in the 1980s, led to larger and more complicated image data sets, consisting of hundreds or thousands of individual images. This change, along with the increase in computer technology, spurred the development of filmless image interpretation in the 1990s. Filmless systems are referred to as picture archiving and communications systems (PACS). Over the past decade, most medical centers in the United States have adopted PACS, to the extent that many recently trained physicians have never interpreted images from film.

PACS runs on custom software purchased from a vendor. This software allows viewing and manipulation of digital images that are in a standardized format called digital imaging and communications in medicine (DICOM). PACS workstations are optimized for viewing of large image sets, including simultaneous display of multiple comparison studies. PACS workstations also allow the radiologist to create saved custom presentation states, or bookmarks. Initially, the use of PACS required expensive, high-power computer workstations that were typically only installed in radiology departments. Continued improvement in computer hardware, with dramatic reduction in costs, have now allowed for almost any modern computer to run a production PACS client.

Use of a production-quality PACS system for image presentation at multidisciplinary conference is the most popular choice among radiologists and also among most multidisciplinary team members, specifically in centers with a high volume of cases presented in each session. Rapid navigation through images from multiple studies, including current and comparison scans, allows for interactive image review to address specific questions. Use of a production PACS client also allows the radiologist to make efficient use of conference preparation time, by creating saved presentation states that streamline image presentation in conference. Furthermore, many PACS viewers allow the radiologist to create a conference folder for all of the week's cases, making the transitions between cases smooth.

Radiologist Presents Cases Using a Picture Archiving and Communication System Thin Client (eg, Web Picture Archiving and Communication System)

As described earlier, radiologists typically conduct their daily work with the use of a high-quality production PACS software package. On the other hand, nonradiologist physicians typically access medical images through a modified version of PACS, that is, a thin client. Thin client PACS viewers have less intensive hardware requirements and are often accessed as a Web application, removing the need to install the software on a specific computer. Essentially, any computer that can connect to the hospital network is a mini-PACS workstation.

Thin client PACS is an attractive option for image presentation at multidisciplinary conference because of its convenience. If all that is required is a Web-connected computer and a screen, then the task of finding a suitable conference room is considerably easier. Despite this convenience, there are drawbacks to this approach. First, thin client PACS viewers typically load and navigate images much less efficiently than a production (ie, thick client) PACS. Second, they often do not allow for creation of conference lists and saved presentation states to streamline conference flow. Finally, thin client PACS viewers often have different user interfaces from production PACS; as a result, the radiologist may not present the images as effectively.

Radiologist Presents Cases From Compact Discs

Many multidisciplinary conferences include cases that received initial imaging workup at an outside facility. Because of considerations of patient comfort, speed of workup, cost, and insurance coverage, it is often impossible to repeat the imaging workup at the site of the tumor board. As a result, the radiologist must interpret outside imaging that is usually submitted in DICOM format on a compact disc (CD).

Outside CDs typically come loaded with an image viewer program that must be launched from the CD. Although it is convenient for the clinician to bring these CDs to the conference and ask for a review, the authors strongly advise against this. First, it is the authors' experience that the image viewer programs included on these CDs often fail to load on the conference computer because of software incompatibility issues. Second, scrolling and navigation through images that are loading from a CD is often slow and stilted, with skips and lags. Third, a viewer application running from a CD can strain the resources of the presentation computer and cause computer freezes and crashes with associated delays. Fourth, the radiologist will often be unfamiliar with the image navigation software and, therefore, less effective in image review. Fifth, the images will not be saved on a local server for later review after the conference. Finally, this technique does not allow the radiologist adequate opportunity to preview the images and prepare for conference.

When outside images must be reviewed, the authors strongly recommend that they be loaded into the native PACS system that the radiologist uses for in-house work, to capture all of the advantages noted earlier. There may be some resistance from the local radiology department to this, as some may think that housing the images on a local PACS implies some responsibility for interpretation of the images. In addition, there are often costs associated with the upload and storage of images. Nevertheless, it is worthwhile to work closely with the radiology department to overcome these obstacles. There is a growing trend among radiology departments to import outside images and provide second readings, driven in part by the desire to avoid repeated medical radiation exposure.[3] It may help to emphasize that additional follow-up scans are expected to be performed through the local department for these patients.

As a worst-case scenario, if outside images cannot be loaded into the hospital PACS, the authors recommend copying all images onto the hard drive of the presentation computer and viewing them with a single DICOM viewer. A variety of third-party DICOM viewer software packages are available for Windows and Mac, containing much of the same functionality as a production PACS system. Many of the advantages of in-house PACS use can be captured with the use of this method.

Radiologist Prepares Electronic Slides of Key Images

It is customary for the pathologist at a tumor board to only show a few representative images, and the radiologist can adopt the same method. There are some advantages to this approach, most notably the high efficiency of image review during the conference session.

There are many disadvantages to this approach. First, it eliminates the opportunity to review additional findings and address specific questions that are not included in the key images. Furthermore, creation of electronic slide presentations with key images is time consuming for the radiologist and impractical when many cases are presented.

Surgeon or Oncologist Presents the Images, and the Radiologist Who Attends the Tumor Board Offers Input as Requested

This style is not favored in most of the centers, as image presentation and review is a key part in the final interpretation; it is more consistent, efficient, and accurate when provided by radiologists. Nevertheless, this may be the only choice available if the radiologist is not able to make a significant commitment to the conference.

WHICH RADIOLOGIST SHOULD STAFF THE TUMOR BOARDS?

Head and neck cancer is a challenging topic, given the wide variety of treatment options available, the complexity of the anatomy, and the dependence of the treatment plan on imaging information. Diagnostic radiology is a 5-year residency program that includes a preliminary year in medicine, surgery, or transitional year training. During the 4 years of training in radiology, residents are trained to interpret studies of every modality, involving every body part. Training in interpretation of head and neck cancer imaging is a small fraction of the residency program, and most graduates have difficulty with interpreting these scans at the end of the training program.

A subset of radiologists, approximately 10% to 20%, pursue 1 or 2 years of fellowship training in diagnostic neuroradiology, which includes head and neck imaging in addition to brain and spine imaging. Radiologists with this fellowship training should be sought for staffing of tumor boards and for interpretation of imaging studies in patients with known or suspected head and neck cancer. The authors recommend identifying at least 2 radiologists to share the tumor board staffing responsibilities, so that gaps in coverage can be minimized.

In many academic centers, there is often a subset of the group of diagnostic neuroradiologists that has additional training, interest, or experience in head and neck imaging. Ideally, these individuals should be identified and specifically recruited to participate in head and neck tumor boards. Radiologists with this added level of subspecialization are able to contribute greater degrees of nuance and better identify subtle findings that can dramatically alter treatment plans. These radiologists are more likely to be abreast of the current literature in the field and make contributions toward improving and evolving the clinical practice.

OVERCOMING OBSTACLES TO RADIOLOGIST INVOLVEMENT

Obtaining buy-in and involvement from the radiologist is a critical step in ensuring a consistent and highly functional interdisciplinary conference. By understanding the obstacles to radiologist involvement, the team leader can better overcome them.

The job of the radiologist has changed dramatically over the last generation. Small increases in the number of radiologists trained each year have not kept pace with the proliferation of imaging studies related to increasingly efficient utilization of scanners and increasing numbers of CT and magnetic resonance scanners. An increasing number of imaging studies are being ordered through the emergency department.[4] These STAT examinations must be interpreted rapidly whenever they are performed, and there is an increasing demand for subspecialist-level interpretation. As a result, radiologists are moving more toward shift work to cover longer hours and must spend more time physically at a workstation in order to satisfy the need for rapid turnaround time. Large hospital systems are increasingly investing in outpatient imaging centers, many of which are geographically remote from the main hospital, in order to serve a growing patient base. These outpatient centers typically require an on-site radiologist. New radiologist responsibilities, in addition to continued responsibility for image-guided interventions, administrative duties, and teaching duties in academic centers, create limits on radiologist availability for multidisciplinary conferences. Radiologists are forced to triage and prioritize competing demands, including multidisciplinary conference coverage.

It is helpful to communicate with the radiologist early in the process of setting up a new multidisciplinary team, so that the meetings can be arranged at a time when he or she is available. Ideally, a standing meeting can be set for a time when all essential parties regularly expect to be available. In the early stages, ad hoc meetings based on times when all essential parties are available can be helpful in testing out the suitability of various potential meeting times.

It is also helpful to create and emphasize downstream benefits for radiologists that staff multidisciplinary conferences. In an academic center, this may mean creating opportunities for radiologists to contribute to publications that are led by the surgeon or oncologist. Occasional unsolicited letters of thanks for contributions to a multidisciplinary team, copied to radiology department leadership, can provide internal and external rewards for the radiologist that fuel further contributions. Feedback on cases presented at the interdisciplinary conference, with particular attention to cases whereby the image interpretation influenced patient management, is an invaluable source of continuing education for the radiologist and will reinforce the clinical importance of the conference.

The use of the conference as a teaching tool for radiology residents and fellows can also help the radiologist kill 2 birds with one stone, increasing the attractiveness of the task. Finally, in academic and private practice settings alike, it is helpful to emphasize the role of the multidisciplinary conference as a driver of future imaging studies and related revenue.

WHICH IMAGING STUDIES SHOULD BE REVIEWED?

The radiologist needs time to review the images before the tumor board. This point cannot be stated firmly enough, and treating physicians should resist the urge to make last-minute add-ons if an accurate and thorough image review is desired. The most recent imaging must obviously be available as well as all relevant prior studies. If the most recent imaging was more than 1 to 2 months ago, serious consideration should be given to repeating the imaging before the conference. Significant changes can occur within a short time.

It is optimal to have all the images available at least 2 working days before the tumor board to give adequate time to the presenting radiologist to review all the images and preferably create saved presentation states on the PACS system. At the very least, the radiologist should have the images 1 day before the conference. If patients will receive a new relevant radiology examination on the day of or day before the tumor board, it is important to inform the radiologist about the pending scan.

HOW TO MAKE THE TUMOR BOARD SCHEDULE AND PATIENT LIST

Based on the volume of the cases and complexity of the cases, the tumor board schedule may vary in each institution to be weekly, biweekly, or monthly. It is important to have a consistent schedule for the tumor boards, including the date, time, approximate number of presented cases, location of the meeting, and the computer and PACS system that is used for image presentation. This schedule will allow the team to plan in advance and avoid any technical difficulty at the time of the presentation related to a new and unfamiliar location and equipment.

It is recommended to keep the list of the patients at 8 or fewer for each 1-hour session, ideally fewer than 6, to have enough time to focus on complex cases that will benefit the most from a multidisciplinary approach. It is helpful to have an experienced and organized scheduler to coordinate between the multidisciplinary team, make the list in a timely manner, and e-mail the list to all group members, including the radiologists. The scheduler should have the list of the attendees that are expecting to receive the list on a regular basis and also update it frequently to include the new faculty, fellows, and residents based on the policies and expectations of each department and section. It is important to keep in mind that tumor board lists have protected health information (PHI) and have to be compliant with the Health Insurance Portability and Accountability Act (HIPAA). Avoid e-mailing PHI to personal e-mail addresses or to those who are no longer considered a part of the team, such as graduated residents and fellows.

The conference list should include a brief 1- to 2-sentence statement of the clinical history and the reason for presentation at the conference. This statement will ensure an efficient, high-impact discussion that is focused on the most salient issues of each case.

HOW TO OPTIMIZE THE RADIOLOGY CONTRIBUTION TO MULTIDISCIPLINARY TEAM MEETINGS

Multidisciplinary conference participation is a challenging but worthwhile demand on the modern radiologist's time. Solutions to promote radiologist engagement include demonstration of the benefits of multidisciplinary conference to hospital administrators to justify additional resources required, improving conference workflow efficiency, and ensuring this increased workload is accurately represented and remunerated in individual job plans.[5]

Tumor boards require a lengthy preparation for radiologists to provide a concise, accurate, and efficient image presentation that answers the questions that the team might have. Studies have shown that an average radiologist's curriculum consists of conferences and tutorials making 14% and informal case discussions making 10% of the workload.[6] Having protected time on the radiologist's schedule to prepare for multidisciplinary meetings is essential to sustain the contribution over the long-term. Strong communication with radiology department leadership can help smooth this path.

Providing the essential data for the radiologist's review in a timely fashion is critical for optimal radiology input at the meeting. This timely provision will include early release of the list of the patients for each week, uploading the relevant outside facility images at least 2 working days in advance, and providing clinical history in advance, preferably included in the patient list. In academic centers, it may be helpful to assign a resident to preview the cases with the radiologist in order to give critical clinical information and identify the key clinical questions in each case.

HOW THE AUTHORS ACHIEVED SUCCESSFUL RADIOLOGIST INVOLVEMENT IN MULTIDISCIPLINARY CARE AT UNIVERSITY OF CALIFORNIA, LOS ANGELES

The head and neck cancer tumor board occurs weekly at the University of California, Los Angeles (UCLA), presenting 4 to 8 cases each week based on the number and complexity of new cases. Cases are submitted for presentation by the surgeon, medical oncologist, or radiation oncologist; an assigned coordinator updates the list and e-mails it to all the members.

The tumor board takes place in a conference room that is equipped with a production PACS system and large monitors for better image review. The quality of the image display and availability of this conference room was a top consideration in selecting the site for the meeting, even taking priority over physician schedule preference. The date and time of the tumor board is the same each week. The case review with the radiologist occurs from 2 PM to 3 PM, and multiple clinicians see the patients in rapid succession from 3 PM to 5 PM (the radiologist is not present for this component). The early afternoon time allows the staffing radiologist to attend regardless of whether he is scheduled for a morning or evening clinical shift. The head and neck tumor board is always staffed by one of the 2 head and neck imagers at UCLA, both of whom are fellowship trained in diagnostic neuroradiology, with additional training in head and neck imaging beyond the standard 1-year fellowship. These two radiologists report nearly all of the head and neck cancer cases and are, therefore, often familiar with the tumor board cases in advance, which helps with accuracy and consistency of the reports as well as the image review at the meeting.

The cases are reviewed in detail by the staffing radiologist before the meeting. As the meeting time is limited, the initial imaging presentation for each case is limited to less than 3 minutes to allow time for further discussion and questions that clinicians might have about the imaging. This type of summarized and precise image presentation requires detailed preparation by the radiologist, including saving a presentation state for each scan that allows the relevant studies and images to be rapidly displayed. Neuroradiology fellows and radiology residents attend the meeting during their head and neck rotations but do not present the cases.

The authors have found this to be an efficient and effective model for multidisciplinary collaboration in the treatment of patients with head and neck cancer. The authors' head and neck tumor board has served as a gateway toward research collaboration and cross-departmental teaching initiatives and continuous quality improvement. Active participation in the head and neck tumor board is a focal point in the ongoing quest to fulfill the clinical and academic mission at UCLA.

REFERENCES

1. Kane B, Luz S, O'Briain DS, et al. Multidisciplinary team meetings and their impact on workflow in radiology and pathology departments. BMC Med 2007;5:15.
2. Brunner M, Gore SM, Read RL, et al. Head and neck multidisciplinary team meetings: effect on patient management. Head Neck 2015;37:1046–50.

3. West OC. Second opinion readings on outside studies: should we bother? Appl Radiol 2012;41:6–9.
4. Levin DC, Rao VM, Parker L, et al. Analysis of radiologists' imaging workload trends by place of service. J Am Coll Radiol 2013;10:760–3.
5. Balasubramaniam R, Subesinghe M, Smith JT. The proliferation of multidisciplinary team meetings (MDTMs): how can radiology departments continue to support them all? Eur Radiol 2015;25:3679–84.
6. MacDonald SLS, Cowan IA, Floyd RA, et al. Measuring and managing radiologist workload: a method for quantifying radiologist activities and calculating the full-time equivalents required to operate a service. J Med Imaging Radiat Oncol 2013;57:551–7.

Through the Glass Brightly

Pathology Review in the Multidisciplinary Setting

Margaret Brandwein-Weber, MD

KEYWORDS

- Intraoperative assessment • AJCC Staging • Frozen sections

KEY POINTS

- Hospital-centered academic surgical pathologists are essential members of multidisciplinary head and neck tumor boards with respect to final diagnosis, tumor classification, staging, and collaborating on treatment decisions.
- The upcoming eighth American Joint Cancer Committee contains important shifts in staging paradigms.
- A working, multidisciplinary head and neck tumor board is composed of many dedicated professionals (surgeons, radiologists, pathologists, oncologists, radiation therapists, dentists, oral surgeons, nurses, speech therapists, trainees, tumor registrars, and so forth) who contribute their individual pieces of patient data.
- This weekly congregation of head and neck specialists results in a special, concerted, and dynamic process of data integration into a holistic matrix view of the patients.
- Despite all the technological advances in communication, the fundamentals of human interactions still apply: there is no better substitute for a regular, working, multidisciplinary head and neck tumor board.

MULTIDISCIPLINARY PATHOLOGY

Hospital-centered academic surgical pathologists can clearly prove their worth in this value-based medical economy and could be described as the doctors' doctor. Pathologists are essential in the context of multidisciplinary head and neck tumor boards with respect to final diagnosis, tumor classification, staging, and contributing to treatment decisions. The higher role of the doctor's doctor can be further appreciated in the following analogy. The Rambam (Rabbi Moses ben Maimon), a renowned twelfth century Jewish philosopher, prolific author, and physician,

Disclosure: The author has nothing to disclose.
Mount Sinai West, 1000 Tenth Avenue, NY, NY 10019, USA
E-mail address: Margaret.Brandwein@MountSinai.org

Otolaryngol Clin N Am 50 (2017) 717–732
http://dx.doi.org/10.1016/j.otc.2017.03.008
0030-6665/17/© 2017 Elsevier Inc. All rights reserved.

oto.theclinics.com

wrote, "Teach a man to fish, and you feed him for a lifetime."[1] Teaching a trade that leads to financial self-sufficiency represents the eighth and highest rung of charity. What is the seventh rung of charity? "Giving to the poor without knowing to whom one gives, and without the recipient knowing from who he received."[1] This relationship perfectly mirrors that of the pathologist and patient. Medicine is plied with the utmost integrity and dedication to unknown recipients. The lack of secondary gain from direct patient acknowledgment elevates this relationship even higher than that between patient and clinician.

It is intuitive that the work-up for patients with head and neck cancer includes review of relevant pathology slides and reports from other institutions. The most dramatic rationale for this best practice would be a significant disagreement in diagnosis. All clinicians can bear witness to anecdotal disasters resulting from lack of second institutional review. One case that comes to mind is that of a woman with a lingual thyroid that became symptomatic during pregnancy. A biopsy from the ulcerated region revealed vascular proliferation; this was misdiagnosed as angiosarcoma at another institution. Second pathology review did not occur. The tongue base tumor was resected (**Fig. 1**) and a radical neck dissection was also performed. In the ensuing legal dispute, that pathologist's sterling reputation did not abrogate the breech of the hospital's policy for mandated second reviews.

Second institutional review of pathology slides may affect the work-up of resection specimens. For instance, **Fig. 2** shows an 88-year old woman with a history of basal cell carcinoma. In the context of basal cell carcinoma, the perineural inflammation was dismissed as being caused by prior surgeries. Had the prior biopsies been reviewed, the pathologist would have seen that the cancer was squamous carcinoma and the suspicion for malignancy in this specimen would have increased. However, it was persistent pain that lead to the pathology case being revisited. **Fig. 3** shows infiltrating squamous carcinoma as highlighted with Cam 5.2, and the diagnostic revision.

Even in the absence of diagnostic revision, second institutional review can assist pathologists during intraoperative diagnosis. Intraoperative margin assessment usually precedes examination of the malignancy. Knowing the face of the enemy can improve the accuracy of intraoperative diagnoses. For example, the distinction between spindle cell variant of squamous carcinoma and tissue reaction can be treacherous during frozen section assessment if the malignancy has not been reviewed (**Fig. 4**).

In addition, the enhanced communication inherent in second institutional review of pathology slides builds a so-called economy of trust between pathologist and surgeon. In contrast, lack of communication quickly erodes trust, could waste time and efforts, and might harm patients. Consider the following example. The clinical information provided for a salvage laryngectomy stated that, "The patient is a 61-year old man with squamous cell carcinoma of the larynx. Treated with chemo and radiation. Completed this treatment 9/2011."[1] The date of the current surgery was 5 months after treatment; this was within the expected time frame of treatment failure. The salvage laryngectomy revealed ulceration, fibrosis, and radiation atypia. No malignancy was found after sampling the entire mucosal surface. This type of exhaustive specimen sampling consumes valuable time for the trainee, the histology laboratory, and the attending pathologist. The pathologist was left with the following questions: was a biopsy from another institution incorrectly diagnosed as recurrent cancer? The prior biopsy was requested for review; it correctly represented the original cancer diagnosis. The laryngectomy was performed for a nonfunctional larynx. This history was never conveyed in the preoperative history or even during conversations with the sphinxlike

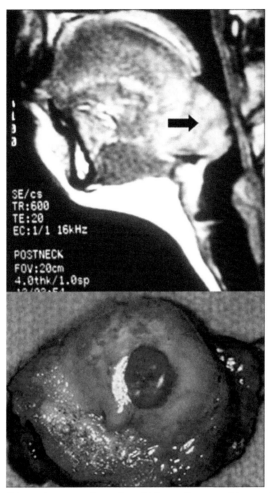

Fig. 1. (*Upper panel*) Ectopic tongue base thyroid (*arrow*) encroaching on the epiglottis; this woman's symptoms worsened with pregnancy. (*Bottom panel*) The lingual thyroid is predominantly submucosal and focally ulcerated.

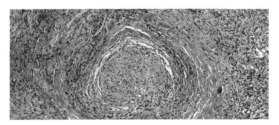

Fig. 2. The clinical information stated that this patient was undergoing reexcision for a basal cell carcinoma. The histology reveals prominent perineural inflammation and fibrosis. Because the pathologist was searching for residual basal cell carcinoma, the nature of some subtle epithelial strands was not investigated (H&E, low power magnification).

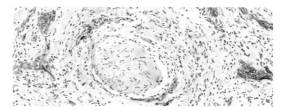

Fig. 3. Deeper sections and immunohistochemistry for keratin (Cam 5.2, shown here) confirmed the presence of squamous carcinoma and led to a belated diagnostic revision (Hemotoxylin counterstain, low power magnification).

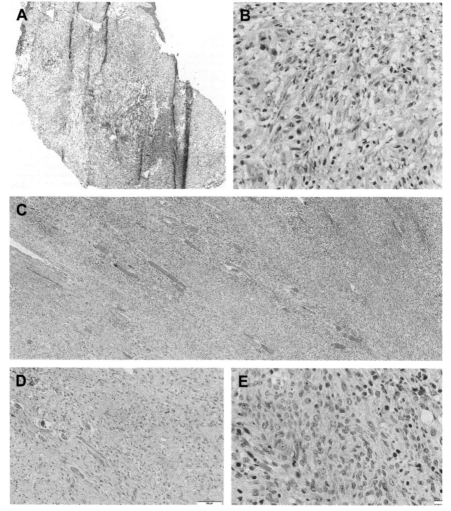

Fig. 4. (*A*, *B*) Frozen section histology of reactive tissue at laryngectomy stoma. Distinguishing this spindle cell reaction during intraoperative consultation from the recurrent spindle cell variant of squamous carcinoma (*C–E*) is simple if the sarcoma has been previously reviewed (H&E, [*A*, *C*, *D*] low power; [*B*, *E*] high power magnification).

surgeon, thus resulting in unacceptable waste of time and effort. Trust was severely eroded.

CHANGES IN AMERICAN JOINT CANCER COMMITTEE STAGING

The upcoming eighth American Joint Cancer Committee (AJCC) contains important shifts in staging paradigms, which are now discussed. The wealth of reported outcome data highlight the need for a new staging schema for human papillomavirus (HPV)–mediated oropharyngeal cancers. Oral cavity squamous carcinomas are now to be staged according to tumor depth of invasion. In addition, the rationale for introducing some new variables is data collection and validation; extranodal extension (ENE) in non-HPV–mediated cancers is in this category.

Since the 1990s the incidence of tonsil and tongue base high-risk (HR) HPV–mediated cancers has continued to increase.[2–4] Demographically, HR-HPV–mediated oropharyngeal cancers represent a novel disease occurring more often in young, healthy individuals with little or no tobacco exposure. This cancer is highly responsive to treatment and ongoing clinical trials are investigating whether deescalation of multimodality therapy can decrease treatment-related toxicities without sacrificing cure.[5–8] The data support that patients with HPV-mediated oropharyngeal cancers present with lower T stage and higher N stage compared with non-HPV–mediated cancers, and that the current AJCC staging schema is a poor outcome discriminator for these cancers.[8] Therefore, a new staging system was needed.

The eighth AJCC will separate pharyngeal malignancies into 3 separate chapters: (1) nasopharyngeal carcinoma, (2) HPV-mediated (p16-overexpressing) oropharyngeal cancers, and (3) p16-negative oropharyngeal and hypopharyngeal cancers. The rationale for selecting p16 overexpression by immunohistochemistry as a stage classifier is that (1) it is an established, robust surrogate biomarker for HPV-mediated carcinogenesis, limited to the context of oropharyngeal cancer; (2) p16 immunohistochemistry is inexpensive, has near-universal availability, and is fairly straightforward to read (**Fig. 5**); (3) it is also an independent positive prognosticator in the context of oropharyngeal carcinoma and HPV/p16 discordance. The outcome for patients with oropharyngeal cancers harboring transcriptionally active HR-HPV, but p16 silenced, is similar to that of patients with HPV-negative/p16-negative oropharyngeal cancers.[9] In contrast with p16 immunohistochemistry, direct HR-HPV detection by in situ hybridization (ISH) is expensive and not universally available, rendering it suboptimal for worldwide adoption. HPV-ISH is a send-out test in many institutions, which increases turnaround time. Probe sensitivity and specificity can be variable. HPV-ISH is recommended in addition to p16, and Epstein Barr Virus encoded small RNAs, for the workup of metastatic cervical carcinoma of unknown primary. **Figs. 6** and **7** highlight some

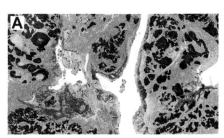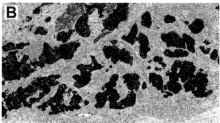

Fig. 5. (*A, B*) Diffuse, robust p16 overexpression is typical of an HR-HPV–mediated tonsillar carcinoma (hemotoxylin counterstain, [*A*] low power magnification; [*B*] high power magnification).

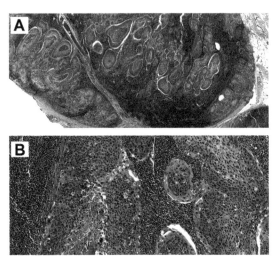

Fig. 6. (*A*, *B*) Inside-out maturation is a distinctive finding of HR-HPV–mediated tonsillar carcinoma. The peripheral rim of tumor islands is composed of flattened keratinizing tumor cells. This finding is distinct from the usual non-HPV–mediated keratinizing squamous carcinoma, which reveals central keratinization (H&E, [*A*] low power magnification; [*B*] high power magnification).

unique histologic features of HPV-mediated oropharyngeal cancer. The rationale for the new stage grouping comes from a study of 704 patients with surgically managed p16+ oropharyngeal cancers, (plus or minus adjuvant therapy) from the United States and United Kingdom.[9] The performance of the seventh AJCC staging criteria was compared with a new proposed staging system derived by the conjunctive consolidation method, which showed the best predictive performance with a cut point of 4 positive cervical lymph nodes (**Fig. 8**). The new stage groupings are presented in **Table 1**.

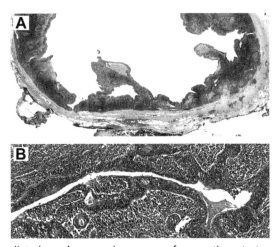

Fig. 7. HR-HPV–mediated oropharyngeal cancer can form cystic metastases in cervical lymph nodes, whereas the primary carcinoma is usually solid. It is unnecessary to document ENE for p16+ oropharyngeal cancers. (*A*) Uniloculated cystic metastases. (*B*) The metastatic carcinoma forms a ribbonlike (transitional) pattern with variable tumor maturation appearing as flattened keratinizing cells (H&E, [*A*] low power magnification; [*B*] high power magnification).

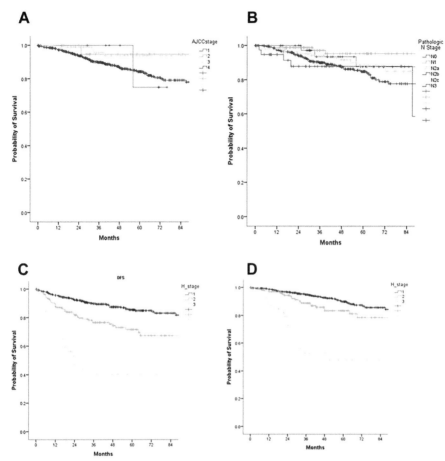

Fig. 8. (*A*) Overall survival for 704 patients with p16+ oropharyngeal cancer treated by primary surgery, plus or minus adjuvant therapy, by the seventh AJCC staging criteria. The overlapping curves represent poor outcome discrimination. (*B*) Overall survival for the same patient group by current pathologic N staging: overlapping curves show poor predictive performance. (*C, D*) Disease-free and overall survival, respectively, using eighth AJCC staging criteria (see **Table 1**).

The retrospective multicenter study of more than 3000 patients published by Ebrahimi and colleagues[10] serves as the rationale for important changes in the staging of oral cavity cancer. Tumor depth of invasion is measured from the level of intact basement membrane in adjacent normal mucosa (**Fig. 9**). A word of caution is warranted here. Tumor thickness is often incorrectly interchanged with depth of invasion (DOI). DOI is a marker of biological aggression with respect to invasion. **Fig. 9** shows an exophytic tumor, DOI (blue) is less than tumor thickness (white). In contrast, **Fig. 10** shows a thin, ulcerated carcinoma; correct assessment of DOI (blue) upstages this to T2. Ebrahimi and colleagues[10] examined DOI as a continuous variable. They showed that DOI cut points of 5 and 10 mm yield the best fit of data for T stage and disease-specific survival. They also show improved correlation of this revised T schema compared with the current seventh AJCC definitions. **Table 2** presents the new T-stage groups for oral cavity cancers.

Table 1
Eighth American Joint Cancer Committee staging schema for p16 overexpressing oropharyngeal cancers

T Category	T Criteria
T1	Tumor ≤2 cm
T2	Tumor >2 cm, ≤4 cm
T3	Tumor >4 cm extension to lingual surface of epiglottis
T4	Moderately advanced local disease (invades larynx, extrinsic muscle of tongue, medial pterygoid, hard palate, mandible, or beyond)

N Category	N Criteria (Pathologic)
NX	Regional lymph nodes cannot be assessed
pN0	No regional lymph node metastasis
pN1	Metastasis in ≤4 lymph nodes
pN2	Metastasis in >4 lymph nodes

When T Is:	And N Is:	And M Is:	Then Stage Group Is:
T0/T1/T2	N0/N1	M0	I
T0/T1/T2	N2	M0	II
T3/T4	N0/N1	M0	II
T3/T4	N2	M0	III
Any T	Any N	M1	IV

It is important to emphasize that p16 overexpression is only a validated and clinically relevant biomarker in the context of oropharyngeal carcinoma. At present, p16 status is clinically irrelevant as an HPV surrogate biomarker for oral squamous carcinomas.[11] Extranodal cancer extension is also added to the eighth AJCC staging schema for oral, hypopharyngeal, laryngeal, and p16-negative oropharyngeal cancers; it is irrelevant for p16+ oropharyngeal cancers.[7] The best clinicopathologic data to support this come from 2 studies on 350 patients with oral and laryngeal cancer[12] and 245 patients with oral cancer.[13] Both studies confirm significantly decreased disease-specific survival (DSS) on multivariate analysis, dependent on the degree of ENE. Prabhu and colleagues[12] showed that grade 4 ENE (obliteration of residual lymph node) was

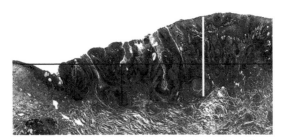

Fig. 9. The terms depth of invasion (DOI) and tumor thickness have been used interchangeably, which is incorrect. The white bar represents maximum tumor thickness. The blue bar is DOI. The horizon is established at the level of the basement membrane relative to the closest intact squamous mucosa. The greatest DOI is measured by dropping a "plumb line"[1] from the horizon (H&E, low power magnification).

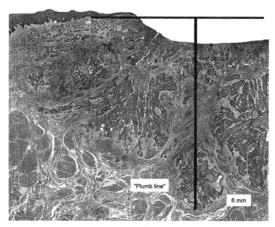

Fig. 10. DOI in an ulcerated carcinoma. Noe how tumor thickness would be deceptively thinner than DOI (H&E, low power magnification).

independently associated with decreased DSS (P = .01; hazard ratio, 2.44). Wreesman and colleagues[13] showed that major ENE (cut point 1.7 mm by receiver operating curve analysis) independently predicts decreased DSS on multivariate analysis (P = .001; hazard ratio, 3.37). **Table 3** presents the new N stage categories. Data will be collected as ENE_n (ENE none), ENE_m (ENE microscopic; $\leq$2 mm) and ENE_g (Gross ENE; ENE > 2 mm). However, any ENE upstages N status. Of note, metastatic carcinoma showing smooth bulging of the lymph node capsule is not considered ENE (**Figs. 11** and **12**).

THE RISK MODEL

The risk model is a validated prognostic schema for patients with oral cavity squamous carcinoma.[14–16] In a study of 299 patients with low-stage oral cavity cancer, the author showed that both the high-risk classification, and worst pattern of invasion (WPOI) 5 alone are significantly predictive of disease-free survival and DSS, adjusted

Table 2	
Eighth American Joint Cancer Committee T staging schema for oral cavity cancers	
T1	DOI ≤2 cm, ≤5 mm
T2	≤2 cm DOI >5 mm and ≤10 mm Or >2 cm but ≤4 cm and DOI ≤10 mm
T3	Tumor >4 cm or any tumor DOI >10 mm
T4a	Moderately advanced local disease, invading through cortical bone, or involving the inferior alveolar nerve, floor of mouth, or skin of face. Tumor invades adjacent structures only (eg, through cortical bone of the mandible or maxilla, or involves the maxillary sinus or skin of the face) Note: superficial erosion of bone/tooth socket (alone) by a gingival primary is not sufficient to classify a tumor as T4
T4b	Very advanced local disease, invading masticator space, pterygoid plates, or skull base, and/or encases the internal carotid artery

Table 3
N staging for oral, hypopharyngeal, laryngeal, and p16-negative oropharyngeal cancers

N Category	
NX	Regional lymph nodes cannot be assessed
N0	No regional lymph node metastasis
N1	One ipsilateral lymph node ≤3 cm no ENE
N2	One ipsilateral lymph node ≤3 cm and ENE+ One ipsilateral LN >3 cm but <6 cm, or multiple ipsilateral, bilateral, or contralateral lymph nodes ≤6 cm no ENE
N2a	One ipsilateral or contralateral node ≤3 cm and ENE+ or 1 ipsilateral node >3 cm but <6 cm no ENE
N2b	Multiple ipsilateral nodes ≤6 cm, no ENE
N2c	Metastasis in bilateral or contralateral lymph nodes, none >6 cm in greatest dimension and ENE−
N3	Metastasis in a lymph node >6 cm in greatest dimension and ENE− Or in a single ipsilateral node >3 cm in greatest dimension and ENE+ Or multiple ipsilateral, contralateral, or bilateral nodes any with ENE+
N3a	One LN >6 cm, no ENE
N3b	Metastasis in a single ipsilateral node >3 cm in greatest dimension and ENE+ Or multiple ipsilateral, contralateral, or bilateral nodes any with ENE+

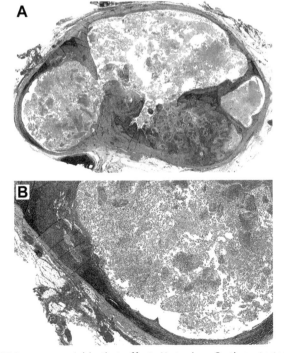

Fig. 11. (*A, B*) ENE is now a variable that affects N staging. Cystic metastasis that stretches, but does not breach, the lymph node capsule should be classified as ENE negative (H&E, [*A*] low power magnification; [*B*] high power magnification).

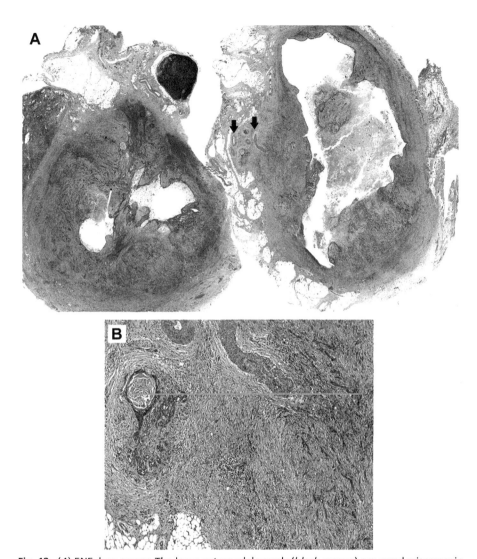

Fig. 12. (*A*) ENE, low power. The large extranodal vessels (*black arrows*) are good microscopic landmarks. Microscopic ENE (ENE$_{mi}$) is defined as ENE less than or equal to 2 mm. Macroscopic (gross) ENE (ENE$_{ma}$) is defined as either ENE apparent to the naked eye at the time of dissection, or extension greater than 2 mm beyond the lymph node capsule microscopically. ENE$_{ma}$ includes obliterated lymph node architecture with carcinoma in soft tissues. Either ENE$_{mi}$ or ENE$_{ma}$ is considered ENE+ for pN staging. (*B*) If the lymph node capsule is obliterated by desmoplasia, where is the reference point for measurement? Flip down the microscope condenser and look for the refraction of residual capsular collagen to estimate its position. Here, the green line is more than 2 mm from the estimated lymph node boundary and should be classified as ENE$_g$ (H&E, [*A*] low power magnification; [*B*] high power magnification).

for stage, age, margins, medical center, and treatment, in regression analysis, considering competing risks (**Table 4**). WPOI-5 described a dispersed tumor pattern of invasion (**Figs. 13–15**). WPOI-5 alone constitutes high-risk classification; however, patients may be classified as high risk for a combination of other histologic features.

Table 4
Phase II validation study: 299 patients with low-stage oral cavity cancer

Locoregional Recurrence	DF	Standard Error	P	Hazard Ratio	95% CI
WPOI-4, WPOI-5 vs WPOI-3	1	0.432	.0029	3.63	1.56, 8.47
WPOI-5	1	0.475	.0001	6.34	2.50, 16.09
Risk category	1	0.633	.0050	9.16	2.65, 31.66
DSS	**DF**	**Standard Error**	**P**	**Hazard Ratio**	**95% CI**
WPOI-5	1	0.475	.0001	6.34	2.50, 16.09
Risk category	1	0.633	.0005	9.55	2.65, 31.66

	Sensitivity (%)	Specificity (%)	NPV (%)	PPV (%)
WPOI-3	100.0	0	—	18.7
WPOI-4	89.3	38.3	93.9	25.0
WPOI-5	35.7	88.5	85.7	41.7
Low Risk	100.0	0	—	18.7
Intermediate Risk	98.2	14.8	97.3	21.0
High Risk	58.9	70.8	88.2	31.7

Abbreviations: CI, confidence interval; DF, degrees of freedom; NPV, negative predictive value; PPV, positive predictive value.

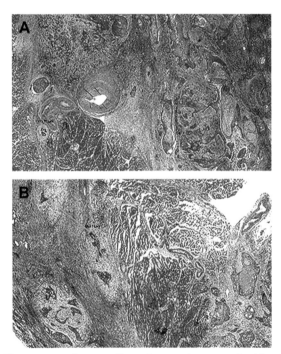

Fig. 13. WPOI-5. The context of tumor dispersion can be recognized by the abundance of skeletal muscle between tumor islands. (*A, B*) Both green lines measure a distance of more than 0.1 mm between satellites (H&E, [*A*] low power magnification; [*B*] high power magnification).

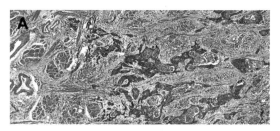

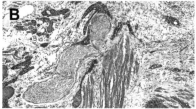

Fig. 14. (*A*) WPOI-5. Strandy pattern of invasion is often classifiable as WPOI-5. (*B*) This strandy pattern is also often associated with perineural invasion (H&E, [*A*] low power magnification; [*B*] high power magnification).

The positive predictive value (PPV) of WPOI-5 alone is greater than the PPV for high-risk classification (41.7% vs 31.7%, respectively, for locoregional recurrence), and this is the justification for migrating from the full risk model, which assesses 3 variables, to the single cut point of WPOI-5/not WPOI-5, as a strategy to increase transportability of this predictor.

The author has shown that WPOI-5 can predict occult cervical metastasis, studying 152 patients with T1/T2 oral cancers, with clinicoradiographic negative necks, undergoing elective neck dissection (END). This finding is relevant given the lack of a standardized approach for these patients, and that technetium 99m lymphoscintigraphy (sentinel node biopsy) is not commonly performed in the United States by head and neck surgeons. The overall rate of occult metastatic disease in this cohort was 31 out of 152 (20%), as expected (Velosa C, Shi Q, Stevens TM, et al, unpublished data, 2017). When stratified for WPOI, the rates of occult positive lymph nodes were 45% and 10% for patients with WPOI-5 and WPOI-3/WPOI-4, respectively, allowing the conclusion that WPOI-5 is significantly predictive of occult positive cervical nodes ($P<.0001$). The author suggests that WPOI assessment can be incorporated into the decision tree for selecting patients for END.

In addition, the risk model has the potential to change the standard of care for low-stage oral cancers classified as high risk/WPOI-5; retrospective observational data are necessary to support a clinical trial. Sample size estimates predict that at least 400 patients will be necessary to detect a 1.5-fold difference in mean time to disease progression ($\alpha = 0.5$, 80% power). Despite being underpowered, **Fig. 16** shows a Kaplan-Meier analyses showing good separation of curves for patients receiving adjuvant radiotherapy for DSS just justifying further data accrual.

BRINGING IT ALL TOGETHER AT TUMOR BOARD

A working, multidisciplinary head and neck tumor board is composed of many dedicated professionals (surgeons, radiologists, pathologists, oncologists, radiation therapists, dentists, oral surgeons, nurses, speech therapists, trainees, tumor registrars, and so forth) who contribute their individual pieces of patient data. This weekly

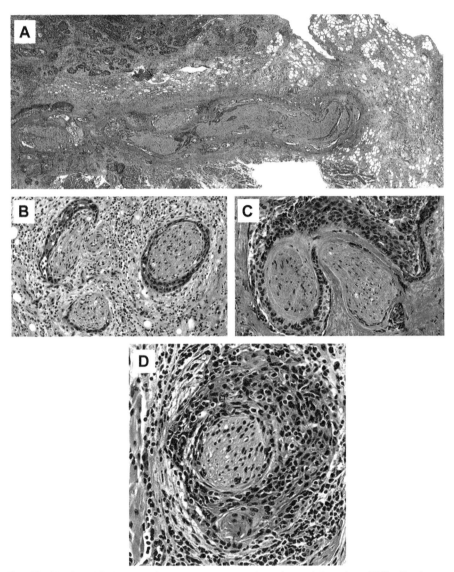

Fig. 15. (A–D) WPOI-5 secondary to extratumoral perineural invasion (PNI). Carcinoma should show a specific architectural relationship with nerve, such as wrapping around nerves, in order to be classified as PNI (H&E, [A] low power magnification; [B,C,D] high power magnification).

congregation of head and neck specialists results in a special, concerted, and dynamic process of data integration into a holistic matrix view of the patients. The board creates a impression of each particular patient, with the patient's particular comorbidities, personal proclivities, and specific diagnosis with the relevant histologic and molecular features. What then is the rationale for the treatment choices? What are the unknown factors? A certain synergy occurs in this process; the interactions result in a product greater than the sum of the parts. Despite all the technological advances in communication, the fundamentals of human interactions still

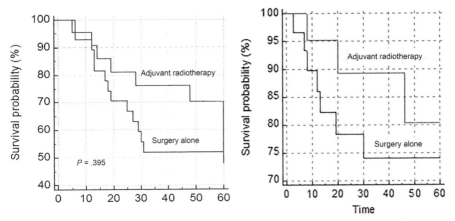

Fig. 16. Disease-free survival for 100 high-risk patients (*left*) and 55 patients with WPOI-5 low-stage oral cavity cancer (*right*) when stratified for surgery alone, versus surgery plus adjuvant radiotherapy. Although statistical significance is not achieved because of small sample size, the good separation of both curves justifies continuing patient accrual.

apply: there is no better substitute for a regular, working, multidisciplinary head and neck tumor board.

REFERENCES

1. Maimonides M. Mishneh Torah. Laws of Gifts to the poor. 10:7–14.
2. Gillison ML, D'Souza G, Westra W, et al. Distinct risk factor profiles for human papillomavirus type 16 positive and human papillomavirus type 16 negative head and neck cancers. J Natl Cancer Inst 2008;100:407–20.
3. Kreimer A, Clifford G, Boyle P, et al. Human papillomavirus types in head and neck squamous cell carcinomas worldwide: a systematic review. Cancer Epidemiol Biomarkers Prev 2005;14:467–75.
4. Ang KK, Harris J, Wheeler R, et al. Human papillomavirus and survival of patients with oropharyngeal cancer. N Engl J Med 2010;363:24–35.
5. Chera BS, Amdur RJ, Tepper J, et al. Phase 2 trial of de-intensified chemoradiation therapy for favorable-risk human papillomavirus–associated oropharyngeal squamous cell carcinoma. Int J Radiat Oncol Biol Phys 2015;93(5):976–85.
6. Masterson L, Moualed D, Liu ZW, et al. De-escalation treatment protocols for human papillomavirus-associated oropharyngeal squamous cell carcinoma: a systematic review and meta-analysis of current clinical trials. Eur J Cancer 2014;50: 2636–48.
7. Amini A, Jasem J, Jones BL, et al. Predictors of overall survival in human papillomavirus-associated oropharyngeal cancer using the National Cancer Data Base. Oral Oncol 2016;56:1–7.
8. Isayeva T, Xu J, Dai Q, et al. African Americans with oropharyngeal carcinoma have significantly poorer outcomes despite similar rates of human papillomavirus-mediated carcinogenesis. Hum Pathol 2014;45:310–9.
9. Haughey BH, Kallogjeri D, Goldberg R, et al. Pathologic staging for HPV-related squamous carcinoma of the oropharynx. J Clin Oncol, in press.
10. Ebrahimi A, Gil Z, Amit M, et al. International Consortium for Outcome Research (ICOR) in Head and Neck Cancer, primary tumor staging for oral cancer and a

proposed modification incorporating depth of invasion: an international multi-center retrospective study. JAMA Otolaryngol Head Neck Surg 2014;140:1138–48.

11. Isayeva T, Xu J, Ragin C, et al. The protective effect of p16(INK4a) in oral cavity carcinomas: p16(Ink4A) dampens tumor invasion-integrated analysis of expression and kinomics pathways. Mod Pathol 2015;28:631–53.

12. Prabhu RS, Hanasoge S, Magliocca KR, et al. Extent of pathologic extracapsular extension and outcomes in patients with nonoropharyngeal head and neck cancer treated with initial surgical resection. Cancer 2014;120:1499–506.

13. Wreesmann VB, Katabi N, Palmer FL, et al. Influence of extracapsular nodal spread extent on prognosis of oral squamous cell carcinoma. Head Neck 2016;38(Suppl 1):E1192–9.

14. Brandwein-Gensler M, Teixeira M, Lewis C, et al. Oral squamous cell carcinoma: histological risk assessment, but not margin status, is strongly predictive of local disease-free and overall survival. Am J Surg Pathol 2005;29:167–78.

15. Brandwein-Gensler M, Smith RV, Wang B, et al. Validation of the histological risk model in a new patient cohort with primary head and neck squamous cell carcinoma. Am J Surg Pathol 2010;34:676–88.

16. Li Y, Bai S, Carroll W, et al. Validation of the risk model: high-risk classification and tumor pattern of invasion predict outcome for patients with low-stage oral squamous cell carcinoma. Head Neck Pathol 2013;7:211–23.

New Frontiers in Surgical Innovation

Ryan S. Jackson, MD[a], Cecelia E. Schmalbach, MD, MSc[b],*

KEYWORDS

- Stereolithic modeling • Sentinel node biopsy • Transoral robotic surgery
- Intraoperative imaging

KEY POINTS

- Sentinel node biopsy is considered standard of care and now incorporated into the staging algorithm for intermediate-thickness head and neck cutaneous melanoma and head and neck Merkel cell carcinoma.
- Stereolithic modeling has the potential to improve anatomic restoration and to decrease intraoperative time for complex craniomaxillofacial trauma reconstruction.
- Transoral robotic surgery (TORS) was first approved by the Food and Drug Administration for T1/2 malignancies and its use has grown to include advanced disease including skull base and parapharyngeal space. The potential benefit is decreased rates of tracheostomy and gastrostomy tubes.
- The American Academy of Otolaryngology–Head and Neck Surgery/Foundation has published a position statement on intraoperative use of computer-aided surgery to endorse its use in appropriately selected cases for surgical assistance. Most endoscopic sinonasal surgeons agree that image-guided surgery is not routinely required; it is an important adjunct in performing safe endoscopic sinonasal surgery.

INTRODUCTION

It is an exciting time for head and neck (HN) surgical innovation with numerous advances in the perioperative planning and intraoperative management of patients with cancer, trauma patients, and individuals with congenital defects. The broad and rapidly changing realm of HN surgical innovation precludes a comprehensive summary. This article highlights some of the most important innovations from

Disclosure Statement: R.S. Jackson has nothing to disclose. C.E. Schmalbach has received teaching honorarium for AO North America Craniomaxillofacial Trauma Consortium (nonprofit).
[a] Head and Neck Oncology and Microvascular Reconstructive Surgery, Department of Otolaryngology–Head and Neck Surgery, Washington University School of Medicine, 660 South Euclid Avenue, Campus Box 8115, St Louis, MO 63110, USA; [b] Clinical Affairs, Department of Otolaryngology–Head & Neck Surgery, Indiana University School of Medicine, Fesler Hall, 1130 West Michigan Street, Suite 400, Indianapolis, IN 46202, USA
* Corresponding author.
E-mail address: cschmalb@iu.edu

Otolaryngol Clin N Am 50 (2017) 733–746
http://dx.doi.org/10.1016/j.otc.2017.03.009
0030-6665/17/© 2017 Elsevier Inc. All rights reserved.

oto.theclinics.com

preoperative planning with sentinel node biopsy (SNB) and three-dimensional (3D), stereolithic (SL) modeling to intraoperative innovations, such as transoral robotic surgery (TORS) and intraoperative navigation. Future surgical innovations, such as intraoperative optical imaging of surgical margins, is also highlighted.

STAGING: SENTINEL NODE BIOPSY

Regional metastasis remains the most important prognostic factor for mucosal and cutaneous HN cancers,[1] thus underscoring the importance of accurate staging to ensure that patients receive adequate treatment. Traditionally, selective/elective neck dissections (SND) are performed to identify occult, micrometatastic stage III regional disease.[2] In doing so, the first three draining echelons are dissected, yielding up to 40 lymph nodes for histopathologic evaluation. Given time and cost constraints, pathologists bivalve the node and apply hematoxylin and eosin (H&E) staining. However, occult nodal disease is often small volume and often consists of individual metastatic cells.[3] Furthermore, many cancers to include melanoma[4] and Merkel cell carcinoma[5] (MCC) require specific immunohistochemical staining (IHCS) because the cancer goes undetected on traditional H&E staining alone. SNB now provides a minimally invasive means of harvesting the first individual draining nodes (as opposed to entire nodal basins) for histopathologic review. In doing so, the pathologist has the ability to perform thorough evaluation to include microsectioning of each individual sentinel lymph node (SLN) and IHCS when indicated.

On the day of surgery, patients are brought to the nuclear medicine suite to undergo intradermal injection of a radioactive sulfur colloid. Delayed imaging, usually in the form of lymphoscintigraphy, is performed and serves as the surgeon's road map as to the number and laterality of sentinel nodes. This imaging is exceedingly helpful for midline lesions, which have the ability to drain bilaterally. More recently, many institutional have transitioned to the use to fused single-photon emission computed tomography (SPECT)/computed tomography (CT) imaging, which provides increased anatomic information through the use of gamma rays. Stoffels and colleagues[6] performed a prospective melanoma study comparing SNB using traditional lymphoscintigraphy (n = 254) with SPECT/CT (n = 149). A total of 38 (9.4%) had melanomas of the HN region. SPECT/CT altered surgical planning in 22% of the cases. Specifically, the anticipated location of the SLN was changed in 73% of the cases and a smaller incision was achieved in 27% of the SPECT/CT cases. More importantly, the yield of SLNs in the setting of SPECT/CT was statistically higher at 2.4 versus 1.87 nodes in the lymphoscintigraphy group ($P<.001$). Not only did SPECT/CT afford a higher yield in the number of harvested nodes, the identified metastatic rate was also higher at 34% compared with 21% ($P = .04$). With a mean follow-up of 28.8 months, disease-free survival was improved with the use of SPECT/CT (94% vs 79%; $P = .02$). Lastly, multivariate analysis identified the use of SPECT/CT as a statistically significant variable impacting disease-free survival ($P = .02$).

Following the radioactive injection, SNB patients are brought to the operating room where they undergo general anesthesia followed by a second intradermal injection of blue dye (**Fig. 1**). Given the close proximity of the primary HN tumor and associated draining lymphatics, the primary tumor is usually excised first to prevent radioactive "shine through." Once excised, SLNs are identified using the gamma probe. A 2-to-3-cm incision is made over the area of radioactivity. Using blunt dissection, auditory queues from the radioactivity, and visual cues from the blue dye, the SLN is harvested and sent to pathology. The one exception is the parotid nodal basin where a traditional modified Blair incision is recommend for cosmetic purposes (**Fig. 2**).[7] Studies have

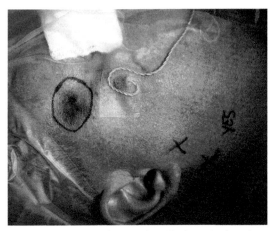

Fig. 1. Right temple T2b melanoma with two identified sentinel nodes marked X. Both the radioactive colloid injection and intraoperative blue dye have been injected.

demonstrated that in experienced hands, SNB is performed safely in the HN region to include the parotid gland.[8–10] Patients with a positive SNB ideally return to the operating room for completion neck dissection and, if indicated, parotidectomy. The remaining patients with a negative SND are observed closely, thus sparing any additional morbidity, mortality, and cost associated with traditional neck dissections.

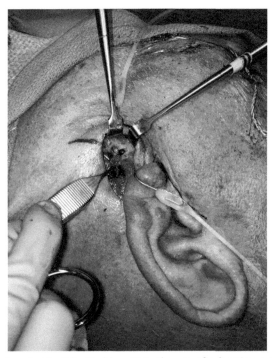

Fig. 2. Left sentinel node identified in blue. Note the use of a facial nerve monitor to safely harvest nodes in the parotid basin.

The largest single institutional study investigating the role of SNB in HN melanoma was conducted at the University of Michigan.[9] A total of 353 patients were staged using the technique and prospectively followed for a mean of 48 months (12-month minimum requirement). Safety was demonstrated with no major complications to include cranial nerve injury. A total of 283 patients were observed following a negative SNB. A total of 4.2% of patients with local control went on to fail regionally in a previously mapped nodal basin (false omission rate). The 95.8% negative predictive value of a negative SNB was considered accurate, and the authors concluded that a patient with a negative SNB could be observed closely for recurrent disease. In addition, the authors found that the status of the SLN (negative vs positive) was prognostic for disease-free recurrence and overall survival.

Currently, SNB remains the most accurate staging modality for melanoma, more so than PET or MRI.[11] SNB is considered standard of care for intermediate-thickness HN melanoma as indicated by its incorporation into the current American Joint Committee on Cancer staging system and National Comprehensive Cancer Network practice guidelines.[12]

In addition to cutaneous melanoma, SNB is also considered standard of care for MCC.[13] This rare neuroendocrine cancer unfortunately couples the high regional recurrence rate of melanoma with the high local recurrence rate of cutaneous squamous cell carcinoma (cSCC) and basal cell carcinoma.[14] MCC has a propensity for neurotropic spread, with patients often dying of local recurrence at the skull base. MCC is a diagnostic challenge for the dermatopathologist given the spindle-celled appearance and need for MCC-specific IHCS to differentiate it from other small round blue cell tumors. The original study investigating the role of SNB for HN MCC identified an occult rate of nodal metastasis in 20%.[5] However, all patients harboring occult metastasis were negative on traditional H&E staining and it was only after IHCS for CK-20 that the metastatic disease was identified and the patients were accurately staged. Such diagnostic challenges again underscore the importance of providing the pathologist with the highest risk, first echelon individual SLNs for thorough histologic evaluation.

The role of SNB in cSCC remains promising but investigational. Systematic review of the literature investigating the role of SNB specific to HN cSCC identified five articles from 11 countries for a total of 73 patients meeting inclusion criteria. Three of the 73 patients (4.6%) failed in a previously mapped nodal basin.[15] This finding is promising given the close approximation to the previously reported 4.2% false rate of omission in melanoma where the SNB technique is considered standard of care. Future investigation is required, likely in the setting of a multi-institutional trial, to determine which patients with cSCC will truly benefit from this staging modality. One likely group is the immunosuppressed transplant population, which carries a significant risk of developing skin cancer compared with the general patient population.[16]

Although most HN SNB research has focused on cutaneous cancers, the technique has been successfully applied to mucosal tumors as well, especially within the oral cavity. Broglie and colleagues[17] conducted a prospective trial of 79 patients with oral cavity and oropharynx cancer. The 5-year regional control rate for patients with a negative SNB was 96% compared with only 74% for patients with a positive SNB. The study concluded that the SNB technique is safe and accurate for small T1/T2 tumors.

Civantos and colleagues[18] performed a systematic review of the literature, which included more than 60 clinical trials investigating the application of SNB in the setting of mucosal HN cancer. The overall predictive value of a negative SNB was between 90% and 100%, and safety was demonstrated. One of the added bonuses to the use of SNB was the identification of aberrant nodal drainage patterns, not uncommon for HN lymphatics, which are often deemed watershed in nature. SNB allowed for the identification of at-risk nodes, which would have been missed in a traditional SND. In 2015 the National Comprehensive Cancer Network formally incorporated SNB into the treatment algorithm for patients with T1/2 oral cavity cancer involving the buccal mucosa, floor of mouth, oral tongue, hard palate, and retromolar trigone.[2] If patients are clinically N0, primary section with or without SNB can is advocated.

PREOPERATIVE PLANNING: STEREOLITHIC MODELING

The primary goal in HN reconstruction is restoration of function to include mastication, occlusion, deglutition, articulation, and airway patency.[19] Long-term tracheostomy tubes and gastrostomy tubes are avoided, thus improving patient quality of life. The secondary goal in HN reconstruction is bony and soft tissue restoration to minimize aesthetic deformity.

One area of surgical innovation is preoperative 3D virtual planning with SL modeling. Using state-of-the-art digital imaging and communications in medicine (DICOM) software (**Fig. 3**), a new virtual model of the mandible (**Fig. 4**), midface, or cranium (**Fig. 5**) is reproduced, often using the uninjured side as a mirror image. In brief, DICOM images are translated into an SL model via a 3D printer, which layers an ultrathin photopolymer material. The accuracy of SL models is reported to be within 0.016 mm.[20] This innovation proves invaluable for delayed, secondary bone reconstruction where significant bony lost has led to fibrosis and soft tissue contracture. SL modeling has numerous preoperative planning applications to include the construction of preformed titanium plates, custom arch bars, preformed cranioplasty plates, custom orbital plates, and tracheal splints/scaffolds.[21] Additionally it is used to construct templates for osteotomy design and spatial repositioning, which can aid in bony free tissue transfer.[22]

D'Urso and colleagues[23] conducted the first prospective trial investigating the application of SL for craniomaxillofacial (CMF) surgery. Forty-five patients enrolled in the study and underwent 3D imaging (CT or MRI) with SL construction in the preoperative setting. Experienced CMF surgeons were given a questionnaire after viewing traditional preoperative imaging, after viewing traditional imaging with the associated SL model, and then postoperatively. Surgeons noted that SL modeling was superior to traditional imaging alone in the following areas: operative planning ($P<.01$), diagnosis ($P<.01$), measurement accuracy ($P<.05$), and operative time reduction (18%). These

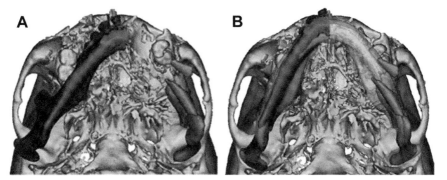

Fig. 3. Left mandibular defect following a self-inflicted gunshot wound (*A*) and DICOM planning with virtual reconstruction of defect illustrated in *aqua* (*B*).

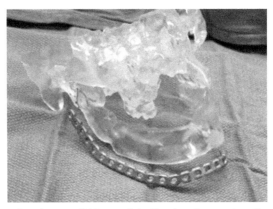

Fig. 4. Three-dimensional stereolithic model allowing for prebending of the titanium mandibular reconstruction plate before surgery.

improvements led to an estimated cost effectiveness of $1031 (AUS). In addition, patients were given the opportunity to examine and review the model before surgical consent. Patients noted improvement in understanding of the surgical procedure and consent when given the SL model (*P*<.0001).

Dzieglelewski and colleagues[24] investigated the application of 3D SL modeling for reconstruction of a hemimandibular defect using a crossover study. Ten experienced surgeons bent a mandibular reconstruction plate free hand and using an SL model of the same defect. A standardized completed model was used as the control. The free-handed plates consistently led to increase in intercondylar distance and intra-angular splay, both of which can cause undo tension and torsional forces on the temporomandibular joint. In addition it took an average of 11 minutes longer to free hand the titanium plate.

Precision in the CMF region is imperative given the potential impact on sight for midface reconstruction and occlusion/mastication for mandibular reconstruction. In essence, advances in DICOM, 3D printing, and associated SL modeling provide an innovative means for "laboratory surgery," thereby minimizing traditional operative

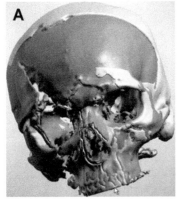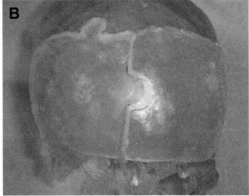

Fig. 5. DICOM imaging of (*A*) craniotomy defect (*gray*) following high-speed motor vehicle accident and (*B*) associated stereolithic model.

time and length of anesthesia. Many cite improved accuracy (and therefore function/quality of life) and time as the justification to offset any additional cost incurred with SL modeling, which ranges from $800 to $3500 (US) compared with $400 to 800 for conventional CT scanning.

INTRAOPERATIVE NAVIGATION

Intraoperative navigation during endoscopic sinonasal surgery has become increasingly popular over the past two decades with a recent survey demonstrating increased use.[25] Advantages include improved anatomic localization and safety in revision sinus surgery, patients with significant mucosal disease, and sinonasal tumors. Its use has been advocated when the risk of surgical complications is highest.[26] Like any other technology, there is associated cost related to the use of intraoperative image guidance, which has been estimated at a 6.7% increase with its use for endoscopic sinus surgery.[27] Therefore, its use as an intraoperative tool must improve patient outcomes, decrease morbidity, and be cost effective.

Ramakrishnan and colleagues[28] performed a review of the literature to determine if image guidance decreases surgical complications and improves surgical outcomes in endoscopic sinus surgery. They determined that the use of intraoperative image guidance has not clearly been shown to decrease surgical complications or improve outcomes. Their investigation was limited by the currently available grade C evidence. However, Dalgorf and colleagues[29] found a lower risk of operative complications in selected populations in a systematic review and meta-analysis on the use of intraoperative image guidance in endoscopic sinus surgery. They found in their meta-analysis of 14 included studies that major complications and total complications were less in patients undergoing endoscopic sinus surgery with image-guided assistance.

Based on expert opinion and consensus, the use of intraoperative image guidance has been recommended as an option based on clinical judgment. The American Academy of Otolaryngology–Head and Neck Surgery has published a position statement on intraoperative use of computer-aided surgery to endorse its use in appropriately selected cases for surgical assistance.[30] Most endoscopic sinonasal surgeons agree that image-guided surgery, although not necessary for routine sinus surgeries, is an important adjunct and has significant advantages in performing safe endoscopic sinonasal surgery. Future investigations need to define clear uses of intraoperative image-guided surgery that improve patient outcomes, reduce surgical morbidity, and are cost effective.

SURGICAL MANAGEMENT: TRANSORAL ROBOTIC SURGERY

Robotic surgery in the HN region has become increasingly popular over the past decade and it has renewed interest in primary surgery for upper aerodigestive tract malignancies. A surgical-based approach with or without adjuvant therapy for oropharyngeal cancer has been one of the recommended treatments for oropharyngeal malignancies. Unfortunately, this anatomic location is difficult to expose with direct transoral surgery. Therefore, splitting of the lower lip with mandibulotomy, mandibulectomy, or pharyngotomy has frequently been necessary to gain access, resulting in the necessity of a tracheotomy and gastrostomy tube. Complications have been reported at 60% with such approaches, and include fistula, dysarthria, dysphagia, malocclusion, hardware failure, and cosmetic deformity.[31–35] Therefore, until recently, the treatment paradigm for many HN upper aerodigestive tract malignancies has shifted from an open surgical approach to a nonsurgical radiation-based approach.

Recent advances in technology, mainly transoral laser microsurgery and TORS collectively termed transoral surgery, have been developed to allow improved transoral access to the oropharynx and larynx, avoiding the morbidity associated with an open approach in many cases. This shift has revitalized the interest in a primary surgical approach for selected upper aerodigestive tract malignancies. TORS offers several advantages over transoral laser microsurgery: improved visualization with the addition of 30° endoscopes, articulating instrumentation, tremor damping, and a shorter learning curve. Unfortunately, TORS currently does not offer haptic feedback and has limited access to certain hypopharyngeal and laryngeal lesions given the current size limitations of the robotic system.

TORS for HN lesions was first reported by Hockstein and colleagues[36] by demonstrating the ability of using the da Vinci surgical system (Intuitive Surgical Inc, Sunnyvale, CA) in the oropharynx and larynx of a mannequin. Multiple investigations were then performed in the laboratory setting to determine the feasibility and safety of such a system in humans.[37–39] TORS was first reported for oropharyngeal squamous cell carcinoma by O'Malley and colleagues[40] in 2006 and by Weinstein and colleagues[38] and Solares and Strome[41] in 2007 for supraglottic laryngeal cancers. The da Vinci surgical system was first approved by the Food and Drug Administration for abdominal surgery in 2000 and was later approved for TORS in 2009 for T1 and T2 malignancies and benign lesions. With growing experience, robotics in otolaryngology has been used to successfully treat even more advanced disease and has been adapted for use in thyroidectomy, neck dissection, skull base surgery, and access to parapharyngeal space masses.[42–46]

The current system most widely in use, the da Vinci surgical system, consists of three main components: (1) the surgeon console, (2) the patient cart, and (3) the vision cart. The surgeon console is a remote-operating console that allows 3D high-definition visualization of the operative field provided by the endoscope mounted on the patient cart (**Fig. 6**). The surgeon console is also the master control for the robotic arms. The patient cart consists of three or four robotic arms controlled at the surgeon console. One of the arms controls the endoscope and two or three additional arms control the wristed articulating instruments (**Fig. 7**). The vision cart is connected to the endoscope and its image processing software provides the visualization of the surgical field. This system is not a true robot, because it makes no autonomous actions.

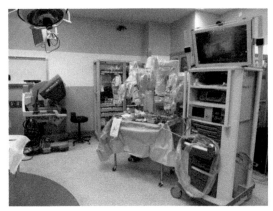

Fig. 6. Da Vinci surgical system consisting of, from left to right, the surgeon console, the patient cart, and the vision cart. (*Courtesy of* Intuitive Surgical, Sunnyvale, CA.)

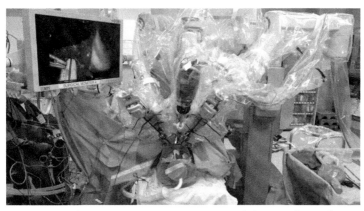

Fig. 7. Da Vinci surgical system patient cart consisting of three or four robotic arms that are controlled by the surgeon at the surgeon console. (*Courtesy of* Intuitive Surgical, Sunnyvale, CA.)

Instead, it is a master-slave system that requires surgeon control for every movement. In addition to the robot, the surgical assistant seated at the head of the bed is supplied with several instruments, including suction, suction cautery, endoscopic bipolar, and endoscopic clip appliers. This allows for potentially four instruments working in the oropharynx simultaneously.

A common criticism of robotic surgery in general is the lack of haptic feedback. Although a reported limitation, this does not seem to have limited the ability to safely and effectively resect lesions transorally under robotic assistance. A recent investigation has demonstrated visual feedback may adequately substitute for haptic feedback in expert users.[47]

A major limitation of robotic-assisted surgery is that it has been pioneered by nonotolaryngologists to gain access for urologic and pelvic procedures. The most commonly used robotic system (da Vinci) was not developed for use in otolaryngology and the limitations of fitting three endoscopic arms into the mouth are evident. As a result, there are several factors defined by Rich and colleagues[48] as the eight "Ts" that limit transoral resectability (teeth, trismus, tori, transverse dimensions of the mandible, tongue, tilt, prior treatment, and tumor factors). Improvements in the da Vinci platform with single site robotics[49] and new robotics systems, such as the Medrobotics Flex Robotic System (Medrobotics Corp, Raynham, MA)[50] to overcome some of these access limitations are a testament to the utility of robotics in the future of otolaryngology–HN surgery.

The role of robotic surgery in benign and malignant disorders of the HN has yet to be established. At the current time, robotics offers a new way of thinking to allow access to the oropharynx with less morbidity than traditional open approaches. Increasing competition will improve existing robotic platforms and allow for development of new platforms to address the limitations of existing robotic systems.

Short- and long-term investigations have demonstrated favorable functional outcomes after robotic surgery for oropharyngeal lesions while maintaining oncologic outcomes.[51–55] Despite the feasibility of using robotics in the HN, one must be critical of the data on robotic surgery. The added benefit of this technology must be found to outweigh the cost, and functional and oncologic outcomes should be investigated in clinical trials, such as ECOG 3311.

Lastly, there is currently no standardization for education and credentialing for the use of robotic surgery in otolaryngology. Recently, committees within the American Head and Neck Society and the American Academy of Otolaryngology–Head and Neck Surgery have proposed recommendations for training and credentialing robotic surgeons.[56] These recommendations will continue to evolve as new robotic platforms, techniques, and surgical indications arise.

FUTURE INNOVATIONS: INTRAOPERATIVE IMAGING OF TUMOR MARGINS

One promising area for future HN surgical innovation is the identification and associated management of intraoperative margins. The need for clear surgical margins to achieve local tumor control is well recognized. However, surgeons are faced intraoperatively with the challenge of poor tumor margin visualization and subdermal/submucosal extension not visible to the human eye. Although preoperative imaging techniques, such as CT, PET, and MRI, are imperative to staging and surgical planning, these modalities are not sensitive in detecting intraoperative tumor localization and margin planning. Real-time, intraoperative optical imaging has the potential to improve surgery success in achieving negative margins, thereby decreasing the need for additional surgeries.[57] Although a comprehensive review of all imaging modalities is beyond the scope of this article, this exciting area of innovation warrants brief review.

Several innovative optical imaging techniques to include raman spectroscopy, confocal microscopy, and fluorescence imaging have been developed for intraoperative tumor margin guidance.[58–61] Ideally these innovations improve localization at the gross and microscopic level. Most recently, dynamic optical contrast imaging has been developed at University of California Los Angeles as a novel modality for intraoperative tumor margin delineation.[62] Dynamic optical contrast imaging can rapidly distinguish HN SCC from normal tissue, yielding wide-field visual contrast consistent with histology. Dynamic optical contrast imaging can now be used as an intraoperative instrument for directed frozen section analysis, and ultimately for real-time intraoperative tumor margin demarcation. An intraoperative instrument to image cancer tissue would provide the potential to significantly improve the sensitivity and accuracy of determining true margins thus enabling the surgeon to save healthy tissue and improve patient outcomes. Significant advances have been achieved in real-time optical imaging strategies for intraoperative tumor identification and margin assessment. Optical imaging holds great promise in achieving the highest percentage of negative surgical margins.

REFERENCES

1. Rowe DE, Carroll RJ, Day CL Jr. Prognostic factors for local recurrence, metastasis, and survival rates in squamous cell carcinoma of the skin, ear, and lip. Implications for treatment modality selection. J Am Acad Dermatol 1992;26(6):976–90.
2. Head & neck cancers. National Comprehensive Cancer Network. v.2.2016. Available at: http://www.nccn.org. Accessed October 22, 2016.
3. Wagner JD, Davidson D, Coleman JJ 3rd, et al. Lymph node tumor volumes in patients undergoing sentinel lymph node biopsy for cutaneous melanoma. Ann Surg Oncol 1999;6(4):398–404.
4. Joseph E, Brobeil A, Glass F, et al. Results of complete lymph node dissection in 83 melanoma patients with positive sentinel nodes. Ann Surg Oncol 1998;5(2):119–25.

5. Schmalbach CE, Lowe L, Teknos TN, et al. Reliability of sentinel lymph node biopsy for regional staging of head and neck Merkel cell carcinoma. Arch Otolaryngol Head Neck Surg 2005;131(7):610–4.

6. Stoffels I, Boy C, Poppel T, et al. Association between sentinel lymph node excision with or without preoperative SPECT/CT and metastatic node detection and disease-free survival in melanoma. JAMA 2012;308(10):1007–14.

7. Lohuis PJ, Tan ML, Bonte K, et al. Superficial parotidectomy via facelift incision. Ann Otol Rhinol Laryngol 2009;118(4):276–80.

8. Schmalbach CE, Nussenbaum B, Rees RS, et al. Reliability of sentinel lymph node mapping with biopsy for head and neck cutaneous melanoma. Arch Otolaryngol Head Neck Surg 2003;129(1):61–5.

9. Erman AB, Collar RM, Griffith KA, et al. Sentinel lymph node biopsy is accurate and prognostic in head and neck melanoma. Cancer 2012;118(4):1040–7.

10. Loree TR, Tomljanovich PI, Cheney RT, et al. Intraparotid sentinel lymph node biopsy for head and neck melanoma. Laryngoscope 2006;116(8):1461–4.

11. Melanoma. National Comprehensive Cancer Network. v.3.2016. Available at: http://www.nccn.org. Accessed October 22, 2016.

12. Schmalbach CE, Bradford CR. Is sentinel lymph node biopsy the standard of care for cutaneous head and neck melanoma? Laryngoscope 2015;125(1):153–60.

13. Merkel cell carcinoma. National Comprehensive Cancer Network. v.1. 2017. Available at: http://www.nccn.org. Accessed October 22, 2016.

14. Schmalbach CE. Merkel cell carcinoma. In: Weber R, Moore B, editors. Cutaneous malignancy of the head and neck: a multidisciplinary approach. San Diego (CA): Plural Publishing Inc; 2011.

15. Ahmed MM, Moore BA, Schmalbach CE. Utility of head and neck cutaneous squamous cell carcinoma sentinel node biopsy: a systematic review. Otolaryngol Head Neck Surg 2014;150(2):180–7.

16. Garrett GL, Lowenstein SE, Singer JP, et al. Trends of skin cancer mortality after transplantation in the United States: 1987 to 2013. J Am Acad Dermatol 2016;75(1):106–12.

17. Broglie MA, Haile SR, Stoeckli SJ. Long-term experience in sentinel node biopsy for early oral and oropharyngeal squamous cell carcinoma. Ann Surg Oncol 2011;18(10):2732–8.

18. Civantos FJ, Stoeckli SJ, Takes RP, et al. What is the role of sentinel lymph node biopsy in the management of oral cancer in 2010? Eur Arch Otorhinolaryngol 2010;267(6):839–44.

19. Chang EI, Hanasono MM. State-of-the-art reconstruction of midface and facial deformities. J Surg Oncol 2016;113(8):962–70.

20. Barrera JE, Schmalbach CE. Preoperative planning for delayed head and neck surgery. In: Brennan JA, Holt GR, Thomas RW, editors. Otolaryngology–head and neck surgery combat casualty care in Operation Iraqi Freedom and Operation Enduring Freedom. Fort Sam Houston (TX): Borden Institute; 2015. p. 441–51.

21. Kaye R, Goldstein T, Zeltsman D, et al. Three dimensional printing: a review on the utility within medicine and otolaryngology. Int J Pediatr Otorhinolaryngol 2016;89:145–8.

22. Matros E, Santamaria E, Cordeiro PG. Standardized templates for shaping the fibula free flap in mandible reconstruction. J Reconstr Microsurg 2013;29(9):619–22.

23. D'Urso PS, Barker TM, Earwaker WJ, et al. Stereolithographic biomodelling in cranio-maxillofacial surgery: a prospective trial. J Craniomaxillofac Surg 1999; 27(1):30–7.
24. Dziegielewski PT, Zhu J, King B, et al. Three-dimensional biomodeling in complex mandibular reconstruction and surgical simulation: prospective trial. J Otolaryngol Head Neck Surg 2011;40(Suppl 1):S70–81.
25. Justice JM, Orlandi RR. An update on attitudes and use of image-guided surgery. Int Forum Allergy Rhinol 2012;2(2):155–9.
26. Stankiewicz JA, Lal D, Connor M, et al. Complications in endoscopic sinus surgery for chronic rhinosinusitis: a 25-year experience. Laryngoscope 2011; 121(12):2684–701.
27. Gibbons MD, Gunn CG, Niwas S, et al. Cost analysis of computer-aided endoscopic sinus surgery. Am J Rhinol 2001;15(2):71–5.
28. Ramakrishnan VR, Orlandi RR, Citardi MJ, et al. The use of image-guided surgery in endoscopic sinus surgery: an evidence-based review with recommendations. Int Forum Allergy Rhinol 2013;3(3):236–41.
29. Dalgorf DM, Sacks R, Wormald PJ, et al. Image-guided surgery influences perioperative morbidity from endoscopic sinus surgery: a systematic review and meta-analysis. Otolaryngol Head Neck Surg 2013;149(1):17–29.
30. American Academy of Otolaryngology–Head and Neck Surgery. Intra-operative use of computer aided surgery. Available at: http://www.entnet.org/content/intra-operative-use-computer-aided-surgery. Accessed October 25, 2016.
31. Sessions DG. Surgical resection and reconstruction for cancer of the base of the tongue. Otolaryngol Clin North Am 1983;16(2):309–29.
32. Babin R, Calcaterra TC. The lip-splitting approach to resection of oropharyngeal cancer. J Surg Oncol 1976;8(5):433–6.
33. Moore DM, Calcaterra TC. Cancer of the tongue base treated by a transpharyngeal approach. Ann Otol Rhinol Laryngol 1990;99(4 Pt 1):300–3.
34. Zeitels SM, Vaughan CW, Ruh S. Suprahyoid pharyngotomy for oropharynx cancer including the tongue base. Arch Otolaryngol Head Neck Surg 1991;117(7): 757–60.
35. Gopalan KN, Primuharsa Putra SH, Kenali MS. Suprahyoid pharyngotomy for base of tongue carcinoma. Med J Malaysia 2003;58(4):617–20.
36. Hockstein NG, Nolan JP, O'Malley BW, et al. Robotic microlaryngeal surgery: a technical feasibility study using the daVinci surgical robot and an airway mannequin. Laryngoscope 2005;115(5):780–5.
37. Hockstein NG, Nolan JP, O'Malley BW Jr, et al. Robot-assisted pharyngeal and laryngeal microsurgery: results of robotic cadaver dissections. Laryngoscope 2005;115(6):1003–8.
38. Weinstein GS, O'Malley BW Jr, Snyder W, et al. Transoral robotic surgery: supraglottic partial laryngectomy. Ann Otol Rhinol Laryngol 2007;116(1):19–23.
39. Hockstein NG, O'Malley BW Jr, Weinstein GS. Assessment of intraoperative safety in transoral robotic surgery. Laryngoscope 2006;116(2):165–8.
40. O'Malley BW, Weinstein GS, Snyder W, et al. Transoral robotic surgery (TORS) for base of tongue neoplasms. Laryngoscope 2006;116(8):1465–72.
41. Solares CA, Strome M. Transoral robot-assisted CO_2 laser supraglottic laryngectomy: experimental and clinical data. Laryngoscope 2007;117(5):817–20.
42. Kang SW, Jeong JJ, Nam KH, et al. Robot-assisted endoscopic thyroidectomy for thyroid malignancies using a gasless transaxillary approach. J Am Coll Surg 2009;209(2):e1–7.

43. Shin YS, Hong HJ, Koh YW, et al. Gasless transaxillary robot-assisted neck dissection: a preclinical feasibility study in four cadavers. Yonsei Med J 2012; 53(1):193–7.

44. Kim WS, Lee HS, Kang SM, et al. Feasibility of robot-assisted neck dissections via a transaxillary and retroauricular ("TARA") approach in head and neck cancer: preliminary results. Ann Surg Oncol 2012;19(3):1009–17.

45. Hanna EY, Holsinger C, DeMonte F, et al. Robotic endoscopic surgery of the skull base: a novel surgical approach. Arch Otolaryngol Head Neck Surg 2007; 133(12):1209–14.

46. Arshad H, Durmus K, Ozer E. Transoral robotic resection of selected parapharyngeal space tumors. Eur Arch Otorhinolaryngol 2013;270(5):1737–40.

47. Meccariello G, Faedi F, AlGhamdi S, et al. An experimental study about haptic feedback in robotic surgery: may visual feedback substitute tactile feedback? J Robot Surg 2016;10(1):57–61.

48. Rich JT, Milov S, Lewis JS, et al. Transoral laser microsurgery (TLM) +/- adjuvant therapy for advanced stage oropharyngeal cancer: outcomes and prognostic factors. Laryngoscope 2009;119(9):1709–19.

49. Holsinger FC. A flexible, single-arm robotic surgical system for transoral resection of the tonsil and lateral pharyngeal wall: next-generation robotic head and neck surgery. Laryngoscope 2016;126(4):864–9.

50. Remacle M, M N Prasad V, Lawson G, et al. Transoral robotic surgery (TORS) with the Medrobotics Flex System: first surgical application on humans. Eur Arch Otorhinolaryngol 2015;272(6):1451–5.

51. de Almeida JR, Byrd JK, Wu R, et al. A systematic review of transoral robotic surgery and radiotherapy for early oropharynx cancer: a systematic review. Laryngoscope 2014;124(9):2096–102.

52. Moore EJ, Olsen KD, Kasperbauer JL. Transoral robotic surgery for oropharyngeal squamous cell carcinoma: a prospective study of feasibility and functional outcomes. Laryngoscope 2009;119(11):2156–64.

53. Dziegielewski PT, Teknos TN, Durmus K, et al. Transoral robotic surgery for oropharyngeal cancer: long-term quality of life and functional outcomes. JAMA Otolaryngol Head Neck Surg 2013;139(11):1099–108.

54. Cohen MA, Weinstein GS, O'Malley BW Jr, et al. Transoral robotic surgery and human papillomavirus status: oncologic results. Head Neck 2011;33(4):573–80.

55. de Almeida JR, Li R, Magnuson JS, et al. Oncologic outcomes after transoral robotic surgery: a multi-institutional study. JAMA Otolaryngol Head Neck Surg 2015;141(12):1043–51.

56. Gross ND, Holsinger FC, Magnuson JS, et al. Robotics in otolaryngology and head and neck surgery: recommendations for training and credentialing: a report of the 2015 AHNS education committee, AAO-HNS robotic task force and AAO-HNS sleep disorders committee. Head Neck 2016;38(Suppl 1):E151–8.

57. Frangioni JV. New technologies for human cancer imaging. J Clin Oncol 2008; 26(24):4012–21.

58. de Boer E, Moore LS, Warram JM, et al. On the horizon: optical imaging for cutaneous squamous cell carcinoma. Head Neck 2016;38(Suppl 1):E2204–13.

59. Chen Y, Dai J, Zhou X, et al. Raman spectroscopy analysis of the biochemical characteristics of molecules associated with the malignant transformation of gastric mucosa. PLoS One 2014;9(4):e93906.

60. Braga JC, Macedo MP, Pinto C, et al. Learning reflectance confocal microscopy of melanocytic skin lesions through histopathologic transversal sections. PLoS One 2013;8(12):e81205.

61. Hwang JY, Park J, Kang BJ, et al. Multimodality imaging in vivo for preclinical assessment of tumor-targeted doxorubicin nanoparticles. PLoS One 2012;7(4): e34463.
62. Tajudeen B, Taylor Z, Sherman A, et al. Dynamic optical contrast imaging as a novel modality to rapidly distinguish head and neck squamous cell carcinoma (HNSCC) from surrounding normal tissue. Cancer 2017;123(5):879–86.

It Takes Two: One Resects, One Reconstructs

Shabnam Ghazizadeh, MD[a], Edward C. Kuan, MD, MBA[a], Jon Mallen-St. Clair, MD[b], Elliot Abemayor, MD, PhD[c], Quang Luu, MD[d], Vishad Nabili, MD[d], Maie A. St. John, MD, PhD[e],*

KEYWORDS

- Head and neck oncology • Reconstruction • Microvascular • Surgical technique
- Two-team approach

KEY POINTS

- In planning for resection of head and neck defects, a thorough understanding of the preoperative anatomy, expected surgical defect, and options for reconstruction should be communicated between the teams.
- Each case of head and neck surgery is unique and so requires an individualized approach for management.
- A 2-team approach to simultaneous ablation and reconstruction of head and neck tumors should be highly considered and can contribute to obtaining optimal outcomes and decreased operative time.

TISSUE IS THE ISSUE

Through all phases of care, the care of patients with advanced head and neck cancer is a multidisciplinary effort. Demonstrably, optimal control of disease requires oncologic resection of tumors with adequate margins, which can require extensive resection involving soft tissue, bone, cartilage, and/or neurovascular structures. The resulting defects can often result in devastating physical and functional deficits associated with a significant decrease in quality of life.[1,2] This consideration is especially

Disclosure Statement: The authors have nothing to disclose.
[a] Department of Head and Neck Surgery, University of California, Los Angeles Medical Center, 10833 Le Conte Avenue, CHS 62-132, Los Angeles, CA 90095, USA; [b] UCSF, 10833 Le Conte Avenue, San Francisco, CA 90095, USA; [c] UCLA Head and Neck Cancer Program, Department of Head and Neck Surgery, University of California, Los Angeles Medical Center, 10833 Le Conte Avenue, CHS 62-132, Los Angeles, CA 90095, USA; [d] Division of Facial Plastic and Reconstructive Surgery, Department of Head and Neck Surgery, University of California, Los Angeles Medical Center, 10833 Le Conte Avenue, CHS 62-132, Los Angeles, CA 90095, USA; [e] UCLA Head and Neck Cancer Program, Jonsson Comprehensive Cancer Center, David Geffen School of Medicine at UCLA, Los Angeles, CA, USA
* Corresponding author.
E-mail address: mstjohn@mednet.ucla.edu

Otolaryngol Clin N Am 50 (2017) 747–753
http://dx.doi.org/10.1016/j.otc.2017.03.010
0030-6665/17/© 2017 Elsevier Inc. All rights reserved.
oto.theclinics.com

significant within the boundaries of the head and neck, where tumors surround and involve structurally complex and functionally critical anatomy. Given the advances in free tissue reconstruction, the vast majority of defects can be reconstructed using free flaps. Although previous work has suggested that secondary free flap reconstruction is feasible and associated with high success,[3] immediate reconstruction of tissue defects is preferred, because recipient vessels are more easily accessible near the surgical field, and fibrosis and scarring associated with secondary reconstructions can be avoided.

One of the most significant advances in the ability to care for head and neck cancer patients effectively is having a 2-team operative collaboration. Multiple institutions have advocated a 2-team surgical approach, which includes an oncologic team, responsible for effective and complete tumor ablation, as well as a team that reconstructs the resulting defect with optimal form and function. Additional surgical subspecialists should be involved when needed; for example, neurosurgery and vascular surgery may be required in the event of intracranial extent or involvement of critical vascular structures. A significant advantage of the 2-team approach is that it allows the oncologic team to ensure adequate resection with wider tumor free margins, thereby potentially facilitating increased local control of the tumor and optimal patient survival. In this dynamic, the oncologic team is free to resect to tumor-free margins without undue concern about conserving local tissue for reconstructive efforts. By shifting the responsibility of reconstructive planning to the reconstructive team, a 2-team approach allows the ablative surgeon to remove as much tissue as required to accomplish a 3-dimensional, tumor-free margin. The reconstructive team is then called on to reconstruct the defect and to maximize speech and swallow outcomes while preserving form when possible. Through this approach, operations can be combined into a single major effort to facilitate single-stage functional and aesthetic restoration.

THE STATE OF CURRENT OPINION

In 1980, Freiberg and Bartlett[4] described a 10-year experience with a 2-team reconstructive and ablative approach for complex head and neck cancers at Toronto East General and Orthopedic Hospital. At this time, immediate reconstructive techniques were limited to skin grafts and locoregional tissue transfers, and more definitive reconstruction usually involved multistaged flap transfers. Definitive, immediate reconstruction is now the preferred modality for head and neck cancers, because recipient vessels are typically easily accessible near the surgical field, and the fibrosis and scarring associated with secondary reconstructions are avoided. Advances in techniques and free tissue transfers allow for reliable single-stage reconstruction after radical surgical resections.[5] As the complexity of microvascular techniques advances, oncologic surgeons are increasingly reliant on the teamwork and expertise of reconstructive surgeons. A 2-team approach can provide great benefit for patients throughout the comprehensive treatment of head and neck cancers.

There are differing opinions regarding the timing of the reconstructive operation for immediate, single-stage reconstructions. Simultaneously raising tissue flaps for reconstruction, as the oncologic resection is underway, enables decreased operative times. Thus, minimizing fluid shifts and blood loss, decreasing risk of pressure sores and ulcers, and lessening the chance for neuropathic injuries, such as brachial plexus palsy from prolonged incorrect patient positioning. It can also facilitate communication between the surgical teams regarding boundaries and size of the defect intraoperatively. However, some institutions feel that the reconstruction should only start when the resection has been completed. Reconstruction performed sequentially with the oncologic surgeon delays raising the tissue flap until the exact 3-dimensional nature of the defect can be appreciated. This can enable the reconstructive surgeon to tailor the free tissue to match more closely the defect, and avoids the possibility of inadequate tissue coverage by the free tissue transfer. This maneuver can also allow the ablative surgeon to have freedom to complete the resection with less concern for timing or reconstructive consequences of tissue loss. The timing of the reconstruction is institution dependent, with advocates for both approaches. At the University of California at Los Angeles (UCLA), we feel that a thorough review of the clinical examination and preoperative imaging allows accurate prediction of the anticipated defect; thus, simultaneous free flap harvest is our preferred method. Future clinical research will likely define if there are advantages to delaying the reconstruction using objective outcomes measures. A list of commonly used free tissue flaps as well as the feasibility for simultaneous operations are shown in **Table 1**.

As reconstructive techniques have become more advanced, they have also come to occupy a significant portion of preoperative planning and operative time. Compared with locoregional reconstruction, reconstruction with free tissue transfer results in a significantly longer operative time (9 hours 35 minutes vs 4 hours 58 minutes).[6] Several studies have shown that increased operative time is associated significantly with an increased risk of free flap failure as well as other postoperative complications.[7,8] In a National Surgical Quality Improvement Program analysis of single-stage, fibular, free tissue reconstruction, operations lasting longer than 11 hours were associated significantly with increased duration of hospital stay (>10 days), which is further correlated with increased cost and risk for complications.[7] Although there are little to no data regarding the amount of time saved by 2-team simultaneous ablation and donor harvest compared with a single surgeon or sequential approach, given the complexity of many free flap transfers it is likely to be tremendous.

There are few studies evaluating outcomes of 2-team surgical management for ablation and immediate reconstruction. One study looked at the effectiveness of a 2-team surgical approach for immediate implant-based reconstruction after breast cancer surgery and found that surgeons who worked together on fewer than 150 procedures had higher rates of infection.[9] Another study evaluating the impact of surgeon–surgeon familiarity on patient outcomes after mastectomy with immediate reconstruction reported that, among high-volume surgeons, complication rates were not affected by the team's experience with each other, but more so patient characteristics and risk factors.[10] There were no similar studies performed regarding

Table 1
Intraoperative burden of free tissue transfer used for head and neck reconstruction

Free Tissue Transfer Donor Site	Tissue Types	Compatible With 2-Team Simultaneous Surgery?
Forearm	Soft tissue $\pm$ bone	Yes
Anterolateral Thigh Free Flap	Soft tissue	Yes
Fibula	Soft tissue, bone	Yes
Rib	Soft tissue	Yes
Scapula	Soft tissue, bone	No
Iliac crest	Soft tissue, bone	Yes
Latissimus dorsi	Soft tissue	Yes (UCLA yes others no)

Abbreviation: UCLA, University of California at Los Angeles.

outcomes of 2-team operations in the head and neck region in particular. However, it remains obvious that careful preoperative and intraoperative planning and communication between the ablative and reconstructive teams is critical in ensuring the highest quality of patient care.

THE UNIVERSITY OF CALIFORNIA AT LOS ANGELES EXPERIENCE

At UCLA, the Head and Neck Surgery Department uses a 2-team ablation and reconstruction approach for the majority of cases, and all cases involving free tissue transfer. Tumor resection is performed by the ablative team. The reconstruction is performed primarily by a microvascular fellowship–trained otolaryngologist and a facial plastic and reconstructive fellow and occasionally by a plastic surgeon trained in microvascular surgery. Each team has a distinct surgical setup with dedicated technicians who are kept separate to prevent cross-contamination of the donor and recipient sites. Both the ablative and reconstructive donor fields are prepped separately and draped in the usual sterile fashion.

Single-stage reconstruction using simultaneous teams allows for efficient use of operating room time, and is the approach used by our institution. At the onset of marking the facial and/or neck skin, there is open communication between the 2 teams to ensure that when possible, aesthetic principles of surgical subunits are preserved, extended, or modified when possible. During the resection there is communication between the head and neck surgeon and the reconstructive team with regard to reconstructive planning including vessel isolation (eg, choice of recipient vessels, vessel length), extent of resection, final defect size, and tumor margins. Intraoperatively, the ablative team is responsible for oncologic control through complete resection of the tumor with adequate negative margins as well as preliminary isolation of recipient vessels for anastomosis and sequential closure of the surgical site after the reconstruction has been performed. The 2-team approach allows the ablative surgeon to remove as much tissue as required without undue concern for the reconstructive consequences, with constant communication with the reconstructive team regarding the margins of tissue loss.

The reconstructive team is responsible for harvesting the donor tissue with adequate dimensions for full coverage, closure of the donor site, insetting of the donor tissue, and microvascular anastomosis of vessels. The reconstruction team also plans for flap surveillance, whether it be with an implantable Doppler, percutaneous needle prick, or, in the majority of our cases, transcutaneous Doppler monitoring of the arterial pedicle marked by a nonabsorbable suture. The reconstructive team is responsible for communicating the flap monitoring protocol to nursing staff and house staff who follow the patient after surgery. Ultimately, there is fluidity between the 2 teams, which allows for comprehensive care of the patient with the goal of achieving the best possible surgical outcome.

Free tissue transfer patients require a period of postoperative recovery in the hospital, during which both operative teams monitor patients. At UCLA, flap checks are primarily performed by nursing staff, as well as by the head and neck surgery inpatient service twice daily, or more frequently as needed. Patient recovery is generally structured along 2 main flap protocols based on whether a tracheostomy was done intraoperatively, as seen in **Table 2**. A similar 10-day postoperative clinical care pathway was evaluated by Dautremont and colleagues,[11] which showed improved clinical outcomes and reduced cost compared with prepathway control cohort.

Although the operative planning is discussed conjointly between the 2 surgeons, a major advantage of a 2-team approach is the division of preoperative and

Flap Protocol	5-Day Protocol (No Tracheostomy)	7-Day Protocol (Patients Requiring Tracheostomy)
Table 2		
UCLA head and neck department in-patient flap protocol		
POD 0	Nil per os Baseline laboratory studies PCA	Nil per os Baseline laboratory studies Chest radiography PCA
POD 1	Begin diet or tube feeds Physical therapy	Deflate tracheostomy cuff Begin tube feeds Physical therapy Begin teaching family regarding tracheostomy and gastrostomy care
POD 2	Remove bladder Foley catheter Continue advancing diet Discontinue IV fluids Discontinue PCA, initiate oral pain regimen	Remove bladder Foley catheter Bolus tube feeds Discontinue IV fluids Discontinue PCA, initiate oral pain regimen
POD 3	No changes	No changes
POD 4	No changes	Downsize tracheostomy
POD 5	Remove donor site cast and splint Remove drains, sutures, staples Discharge	Tracheostomy capping trial
POD 6	N/A	Decannulate Possible oral feeding trial
POD 7	N/A	Remove donor site cast and splint Remove drains, sutures, staples Discharge

Abbreviations: IV, intravenous; N/A, not applicable; PCA, Patient-controlled analgesia; POD, postoperative day; UCLA, University of California at Los Angeles.

postoperative responsibilities. When executed appropriately, this can allow each surgeon to provide expert management and facilitate a comprehensive multidisciplinary approach to treatment. Most often, patients with oncologic tumors present to head and neck surgery clinic. The primary surgeon is tasked with oncologic workup and coordinating care in a multidisciplinary setting. This includes preoperative imaging, tumor staging, presentation of the case at tumor board or other multidisciplinary conferences, planning for adjunctive chemotherapy and/or radiation therapy, and directing preoperative referrals to services like dentistry and reconstructive surgery. The ablative surgeon will also prepare the patient for preoperative medical clearance and order any necessary laboratory and imaging studies. After surgery, the head and neck ablative surgeon manages the follow-up of pathology, adjuvant treatments, symptom management, and referral to rehabilitation consults, and directs oncologic surveillance.

Simultaneously, the reconstructive surgeon provides both preoperative and postoperative input regarding reconstructive planning and follow-up. Preoperatively, the reconstructive surgeon is responsible for evaluation of patients' history and comorbidities and candidacy for free tissue transfer surgery. The surgeon performs a thorough clinical examination to determine the appropriate technique and flap selection based on the requirements and goals of reconstruction. The assessment also includes appraisal of recipient vessels with regard to length and caliber, evaluation of the donor site, and vascular imaging for evaluation of donor vessels (eg, MRI of the lower extremities for fibular flaps). During the postoperative period, the reconstructive team monitors flap tissue perfusion and viability as well as manages wound care issues. Long-term follow-up to evaluate for additional reconstructive needs such as tissue debulking or wound complications are also performed by the reconstructive team.

The success of a head and neck operation is based on numerous factors, one of the most important being preoperative planning. Before coordinating a date, the 2 teams should have a preconceived plan in place. Careful consideration of surgical approach, extent of resection, and possible complications, as well as reconstructive options, makes these operations among the most complex and challenging, but also rewarding, in our field. Early involvement and intraoperative cooperation between ablative and reconstructive surgeons can facilitate optimal care for patients.

RECOMMENDATIONS

Many patients undergoing surgery for head and neck cancer have defects that cannot be repaired by primary closure, skin grafting, or pedicled rotational flaps, and require free tissue transfers. The 2-team approach to ablation and reconstruction is critical to the comprehensive care of head and neck cancer patients. There are limited data regarding the outcomes of simultaneous versus sequential approach to immediate, single-stage reconstruction. The experience at our institution with simultaneous reconstruction is as described, and facilitates efficiency intraoperatively as well as collaboration for a comprehensive surgical treatment. A multidisciplinary, carefully planned and carefully executed approach to head and neck surgery should be highly considered.

REFERENCES

1. Terrell JE, Ronis DL, Fowler KE, et al. Clinical predictors of quality of life in patients with head and neck cancer. Arch Otolaryngol Head Neck Surg 2004; 130(4):401–8.
2. Verdonck-de Leeuw IM, Buffart LM, Heymans MW, et al. The course of health-related quality of life in head and neck cancer patients treated with chemoradiation: a prospective cohort study. Radiother Oncol 2014;110(3):422–8.
3. Iseli TA, Yelverton JC, Iseli CE, et al. Functional outcomes following secondary free flap reconstruction of the head and neck. Laryngoscope 2009;119(5): 850–60.
4. Freiberg A, Bartlett GS. Two-team approach to surgery for head and neck cancer. Can J Surg 1980;23(1):35–8.
5. Blackwell KE. Unsurpassed reliability of free flaps for head and neck reconstruction. Arch Otolaryngol Head Neck Surg 1999;125(3):295–9.
6. McCrory AL, Magnuson JS. Free tissue transfer versus pedicled flap in head and neck reconstruction. Laryngoscope 2002;112(12):2161–5.
7. Offodile AC 2nd, Aherrera A, Wenger J, et al. Impact of increasing operative time on the incidence of early failure and complications following free tissue transfer? A risk factor analysis of 2,008 patients from the ACS-NSQIP database. Microsurgery 2017;37(1):12–20.
8. Wong AK, Joanna Nguyen T, Peric M, et al. Analysis of risk factors associated with microvascular free flap failure using a multi-institutional database. Microsurgery 2015;35(1):6–12.

9. Gfrerer L, Mattos D, Mastroianni M, et al. Assessment of patient factors, surgeons, and surgeon teams in immediate implant-based breast reconstruction outcomes. Plast Reconstr Surg 2015;135(2):245e–52e.

10. Seth AK, Hirsch EM, Kim JY, et al. Two surgeons, one patient: the impact of surgeon-surgeon familiarity on patient outcomes following mastectomy with immediate reconstruction. Breast 2013;22(5):914–8.

11. Dautremont JF, Rudmik LR, Yeung J, et al. Cost-effectiveness analysis of a postoperative clinical care pathway in head and neck surgery with microvascular reconstruction. J Otolaryngol Head Neck Surg 2013;42:59.

Advances in Radiation Oncology: What to Consider

John V. Hegde, MD, Allen M. Chen, MD, Robert K. Chin, MD, PhD*

KEYWORDS

- Radiation • Chemoradiation • Head and neck cancer • Proton therapy • HPV
- TORS • IMRT • IMPT

KEY POINTS

- Further refinement to intensity-modulated radiotherapy (IMRT) planning continues to improve long-term swallowing and xerostomia outcomes.
- Deintensified therapy with dose de-escalated radiotherapy and transoral robotic surgery (TORS) are both potentially practice changing in head and neck cancer treatment.
- The optimal adjuvant therapies after TORS are still being defined.
- Modern proton therapy seems to reduce short-term and long-term toxicity for head and neck cancer treatment compared with contemporary IMRT, and it may further improve as intensity-modulated proton therapy (IMPT) continues to develop.

INTRODUCTION

Changing patient demographics and advances in radiation therapy techniques have significantly altered the head and neck cancer landscape. This review discusses active areas of investigation and technological improvements that are changing the practice of radiation oncology. IMRT continues to be refined to maximize quality of life (QOL) while maintaining excellent locoregional control outcomes. For example, additional exploration into radiation dose constraints to normal structures for treatment planning has yielded further QOL improvements. Deintensified regimens in the human papilloma virus (HPV)-related setting have emerged using different strategies, including reduced radiation dose regimens and the incorporation of TORS.

Technology is also playing a significant role. Functional imaging with novel PET promises to refine tumor targeting and treatment delivery as well as stratification of risk according to treatment response. Modern proton therapy has illustrated favorable

Disclosure Statement: None.
Department of Radiation Oncology, University of California, Los Angeles, David Geffen School of Medicine, 200 UCLA Medical Plaza, Suite B265, Los Angeles, CA 90095, USA
* Corresponding author.
E-mail address: rkchin@mednet.ucla.edu

Otolaryngol Clin N Am 50 (2017) 755–764
http://dx.doi.org/10.1016/j.otc.2017.03.011
0030-6665/17/© 2017 Elsevier Inc. All rights reserved.

QOL outcome gains in head and neck cancer and will likely continue to improve with the optimization and more widespread use of IMPT.

IMPROVEMENTS IN INTENSITY-MODULATED RADIOTHERAPY TO IMPROVE SWALLOWING AND XEROSTOMIA OUTCOMES

With the implementation of IMRT for head and neck cancer in the 2000s, various dosimetric parameters to the pharyngeal constrictors and larynx have been correlated with aspiration risk, stricture risk, and patient-reported and observer-reported swallowing scores.[1–3] These have been applied successfully to reduce dysphagia in patients undergoing chemoradiation for head and neck cancer.[4] More recently, the mean dose to the floor of mouth (encompassing 3 suprahyoid and 2 extrinsic tongue muscles) was associated with an increased risk of aspiration.[5] In addition, a recent study from the MD Anderson Cancer Center (MDACC) noted that in addition to the pharyngeal constrictors, the mylo/geniohyoid complex, genioglossus, and anterior digastric muscle doses were associated with chronic radiation-associated dysphagia.[6]

Previously, parotid-sparing IMRT showed reduce xerostomia rates in multiple randomized studies.[7,8] More recently, submandibular-sparing techniques have been used to improve xerostomia outcomes.[9] In a series of 125 patients who underwent definitive chemoradiation with and without bilateral submandibular sparing for node-positive oropharyngeal carcinoma, no locoregional failures occurred outside the treatment field and 2-year locoregional control rates were similar regardless of whether bilateral submandibular sparing was used. Patient-reported and observer-reported xerostomia scores were both significantly improved with submandibular sparing. Mean dose to the oral cavity, which contains minor salivary glands, also seems to be a significant predictor of patient-reported and observer-reported xerostomia, even after adjusting for parotid gland and submandibular gland doses.[10]

The emphasis on swallowing- and salivary gland–sparing IMRT seems to have yielded long-term, durable improvements in QOL. A series from the University of Michigan reporting on swallowing- and salivary organ–sparing chemoradiation for locally advanced, HPV-related oropharyngeal carcinoma showed long-term stable or improved QOL at 6 years compared with QOL prior to treatment and at 2 years of follow-up.[11]

DEINTENSIFICATION OF RADIATION DOSE IN HUMAN PAPILLOMA VIRUS–RELATED OROPHARYNGEAL CARCINOMA

Conventional chemoradiation to 70 Gy with concurrent cisplatin[12] was established for locally advanced squamous cell carcinoma (SCC) of the head and neck in an era when much of the disease was related to alcohol and tobacco.[13] With the rapid rise in HPV-related oropharyngeal carcinoma, however, which is known to have a more favorable outcome,[14,15] there is a new focus on treatment deintensification. For example, multiple studies have indicated that a lower radiation dose may be sufficient for successful treatment given the compromised DNA repair capacity of HPV-related SCC tumor cells,[16] thus resulting in enhanced radiosensitivity. The pressing issue has been to identify means of de-escalating therapy without compromising disease control. **Table 1** lists several ongoing clinical trials assessing various deintensification regimens.

Differing approaches have emerged to identify suitable low-risk patients. One approach is to stratify patients according to response to initial treatment. Given the more robust response of HPV-related tumors to induction chemotherapy,[17] induction chemotherapy followed by lower-intensity chemoradiation to good responders is being explored to reduce the radiated volume and radiation dose to potentially reduce long-term toxicity. Multiple deintensification clinical trials have adopted this approach.[18,19]

Although induction chemotherapy provides a means of clearly identifying responders, there is often worry that decreased local toxicity from reduced radiotherapy dose may be negated by increased systemic toxicity from induction chemotherapy. As such, there is interest in identifying disease response in the setting of definitive concurrent chemoradiotherapy. For example, a phase 2 trial of deintensified chemoradiation for favorable-risk, HPV-related oropharyngeal SCC was recently completed in which pathologic complete response (pCR) was assessed after concurrent chemoradiation with weekly cisplatin and IMRT to a dose of 60 Gy.[20] The pCR rate was 86%, which is similar to the goal 2-year progression-free survival (PFS) rate used in several multi-institutional de-escalation trials (see **Table 1**). In this study, 39% of patients required a feeding tube for a median of 15 weeks. Major clinician-reported grade 3 or grade 4 acute toxicity rates were 39% for dysphagia, 34% for mucositis, 20% for appetite, and 18% for nausea. This regimen is being compared against radiotherapy alone to 60 Gy, delivered in accelerated fashion over 5 weeks, in the ongoing randomized phase 2 study, NRG-HN002 (see **Table 1**).

A third strategy has been to use functional imaging of tumor response to initial doses of radiotherapy to define risk groups. For example, in a recent prospective dose de-escalation trial for HPV-related oropharyngeal carcinoma, patients were imaged for hypoxia using F-18 and dynamic F-18 PET.[21] Tumor hypoxia was detected in all tumors pretreatment but resolved in 48% of patients within 1 week at either the primary site or regional lymph nodes. Patients who demonstrated resolution of hypoxia within the regional lymph nodes (30%) qualified for a 10-Gy dose reduction to the lymph nodes. Although long-term follow-up data continue to mature, the 2-year locoregional control rate was 100%, demonstrating the promise of safe dose reduction tailored to individual tumor response to radiotherapy.

EMERGING EVIDENCE FOR ADJUVANT THERAPY RECOMMENDATIONS AFTER TRANSORAL ROBOTIC SURGERY

In part due to interest in de-escalating treatment intensity and its related morbidity, primary surgical treatment of early-stage head and neck cancer, in particular oropharyngeal SCC, has been increasing.[22] The early experience of TORS has been encouraging, with outcomes of a large, multi-institutional retrospective analysis of a cohort with predominantly oropharyngeal cancer revealing 2-year rates for locoregional control and overall survival of 91.8% and 91%, respectively[23]; 31.3% had adjuvant radiotherapy and 21.3% had adjuvant chemoradiation.

The National Comprehensive Cancer Network guidelines for SCC of the head and neck for postoperative adjuvant therapy generally recommend adjuvant treatment for the following features: T3-T4 tumors, N2-N3 nodal disease, perineural invasion (PNI), lymphovascular invasion (LVSI), extracapsular extension (ECE), or positive margins.[24] Adjuvant therapy after TORS, however, is an evolving area of research for adjuvant therapy guidelines, especially given the increase in HPV-related disease rates. In a recent National Cancer Database study of T1-T2 oropharyngeal SCC treated with primary surgical resection, positive surgical margins were present in 24% and ECE in 25%. For patients eligible for single-modality therapy (T1-T2 and N0-N1 disease), 33% had positive surgical margins and/or ECE, and 47% had at least 1 adverse pathologic feature, including T3-T4 disease, N2-N3 disease, positive surgical margins, and/or ECE.[22] These findings indicate that approximately half of patients with clinically

Table 1
Select human papilloma virus–related, oropharyngeal carcinoma treatment deintensification studies using a reduced radiation dose or primary transoral robotic surgery

Study	Phase	No. Patients	Inclusion Criteria	Study Arms	Primary Endpoint	Major Reported Outcomes
University of North Carolina[20]	2	43	T0-T3, N0-N2c, M0 Minimal/remote smoking history	Single-arm 60 Gy IMRT with weekly concurrent cisplatin (30 mg/m^2)	pCR by biopsy of primary site and by dissection of pretreatment-positive lymph node regions	pCR rate of 86% Common Terminology Criteria for Adverse Events (CTCAE) grade 3–4 toxicity and Patient-Reported CTCAE severe–very severe symptoms: mucositis 34%/45%, general pain 5%/48%, nausea 18%/52%, vomiting 5%/34%, dysphagia 39%/55%, and xerostomia 2%/75% 39% required a feeding tube.
NRG-HN002	2	296 (target accrual)	T1-T2, N1-N2b or T3, N0-N2b, M0 ≤10 pack-year smoking history.	Arm 1: 60 Gy in 6 wk with concurrent weekly cisplatin Arm 2: 60 Gy in 5 wk using 6 fractions per week	2-y PFS rate of ≥85%	N/A
ECOG 1308[35]	2	90	Stage III-IV resectable	Induction chemotherapy: paclitaxel, cisplatin, and cetuximab for 3 cycles. After induction: Arm 1: patients with a complete response at the primary site receive 54 Gy in 27 fractions with cetuximab. Arm 2: standard dose (69.96 Gy in 33 fractions) with cetuximab is given to all other patients.	PFS at 2 y	Median follow-up time 35.4 months. 70% had complete clinical response. For 54 Gy arm: 2-year PFS was 80%, and 2-y OS was 94%. 1 late-grade 3 toxicity occurred in 1 reduced-dose patient (hypomagnesemia at 30 mo). For entire cohort: 2-year PFS of 78% and OS of 91%

	Phase	Enrollment	Eligibility	Treatment arms	Primary endpoint	
ORATOR[27]	2	68 (target accrual)	T1-T2, N0-N2, ≤3 cm in size, no imaging evidence of ECE. Likely negative margins at surgery and unlikely to require chemotherapy	Arm 1: RT ± chemotherapy: RT alone with N0 disease, and concurrent chemotherapy with N1-N2 disease Arm 2: TORS with selective neck dissection ± adjuvant (chemo)radiation High-risk features determine adjuvant therapy.	QOL using MD Anderson Dysphagia Inventory	N/A
ECOG 3311	2	377 (estimated enrollment)	Stage III, IVa, or IVb No primary tumor or nodal metastases fixed to the carotid artery, skull base, or cervical spine	Patients classified by risk status, then assigned to the appropriate treatment group, with intermediate-risk patients randomized to 1–2 treatment arms. Arm 1 (low risk): TORS Arm 2 (intermediate risk): TORS with low-dose IMRT for 5 wk (5 d/wk) Arm 3 (intermediate risk): TORS with standard-dose IMRT for 6 wk (5 d/wk) Arm 4 (high risk): TORS with standard-dose chemoradiation (IMRT for 6–7 wk, 5 d/wk, with cisplatin or carboplatin weekly during radiation)	PFS at 2 y, accrual rate, risk distribution, and incidence of grade 3–4 bleeding events	N/A

early-stage disease may need some type of adjuvant treatment after TORS for oropharyngeal SCC.

Several retrospective series illustrate different adjuvant treatment trends with TORS and report on early outcomes. A series of 114 patients with p16-positive, oropharyngeal SCC treated with primary TORS at the University of Pennsylvania had a favorable 2-year locoregional failure rate of 3.3% and distant failure rate of 8.4%; 9% had T3-T4 tumors, 63% had N2b-N3 disease, 33% had ECE, 35% had LVSI, and 14% had PNI.[25] In this cohort, 78% had adjuvant radiation, and 43% had concurrent chemoradiation. The only significant factor for recurrence was the use of radiation for adjuvant treatment (hazard ratio 0.20; $P = .02$). Chemotherapy use was not significant for recurrence. These studies suggest the need for careful selection of patients undergoing TORS to minimize the risk of needing adjuvant radiotherapy, and thus paradoxically escalating treatment intensity.

The utility of adjuvant radiotherapy based on standard indications, even in patients with HPV-related disease, was demonstrated in a small series from the Mayo Clinic that evaluated relapse after TORS alone in patients with HPV-positive oropharyngeal SCC with intermediate-risk (T3-T4 disease, N2 disease, PNI, or LVSI) or high-risk (positive margins or ECE) features for which adjuvant radiation or chemoradiation traditionally is offered.[26] A 20% risk of locoregional relapse was seen, with relapses seen at a median of 4.8 months. ECE was associated with a 43% risk of locoregional relapse. Despite the large proportion of locoregional relapse in this cohort, all patients were successfully salvaged with re-resection and adjuvant radiotherapy with/without chemotherapy.

Ultimately, because the primary reason for the utilization of TORS is to deintensify treatment to improve QOL, randomized studies between TORS with or without adjuvant therapy versus definitive (chemo)radiotherapy like the ORATOR study, which evaluates both oncologic outcomes and QOL, will best determine the optimal strategy for treatment.[27]

EARLY EXPERIENCES WITH MODERN PROTON THERAPY

Proton therapy has been long admired for the unique physical properties of its beam: low-energy deposition on entrance, a rapid rise in deposition within the Bragg peak, followed by negligible dose on exiting the target.[28] This contrasts with photon therapy with conventional radiation, in which more dose is deposited on both entrance and exit. For much of its existence, however, the superior treatment algorithms with IMRT for photon beams have blunted the advantages of proton therapy in clinical use. This is rapidly changing, because these same advanced planning algorithms are now available for proton therapy, known as IMPT.

An early report of 15 patients from MDACC has supported the feasibility of IMPT for reducing head and neck cancer treatment morbidity through its improved normal tissue–sparing properties.[29] With a median follow-up time of 28 months, the overall clinical complete response rate was 93.3%. No grade 5 toxicities were seen, and only 1 grade 4 toxicity was seen (vomiting). Acute toxicities included grade 1 to grade 2 xerostomia in 93.3%, but only 1 patient had grade 3 xerostomia; 38% had grade 3 dysphagia, whereas 40% had grade 3 mucositis. At 2 years, 66.7% continued to have grade 1 xerostomia.

A study of 50 patients with oropharyngeal SCC (98% HPV related) from MDACC treated with IMPT also noted encouraging results.[30] At 2-years, actuarial PFS was 88.6% and overall survival was 94.5%. Although a variety of treatment strategies were used (induction chemotherapy, TORS, concurrent chemoradiation, and radiation alone), no grade 4 or grade 5 toxicities were seen. Major acute toxicities included grade 3 dermatitis in 46%, grade 3 mucositis in 58%, and grade 3 dysphagia in 24%. Major late toxicities included greater than or equal to grade 2 dysphagia in 38%, greater than or equal to grade 2 xerostomia in 52%, and grade 2 dysgeusia in 28%.

A recent retrospective study from the Memorial Sloan Kettering Cancer Center (MSKCC) of 41 consecutive patients with major salivary gland tumors or cutaneous SCC treated with unilateral radiotherapy (no neck radiation contralateral to the site of disease) compared IMRT to proton therapy from 2011 to 2014, during which time institutional preference shifted from IMRT to proton therapy.[31] IMRT treatment plans showed significantly higher maximal doses to the brainstem (29.7 Gy vs 0.62 Gy relative biological effectiveness [RBE]) and spinal cord (36.3 Gy vs 1.88 Gy RBE), higher mean doses to the oral cavity (20.6 Gy vs 0.94 Gy RBE), contralateral parotid gland (1.4 Gy vs 0 Gy RBE), and contralateral submandibular gland (4.1 Gy vs 0 Gy RBE) compared with proton therapy. This improved normal tissue dosimetry translated into significantly lower rates of greater than or equal to grade 2 acute dysgeusia (5.6% vs 65.2%), mucositis (16.7% vs 52.2%), and nausea (11.1% vs 56.5%) for proton therapy compared with IMRT.

Recent experience of reirradiation with proton therapy has been reported by MSKCC as well, with promising results.[32] In a series of 92 patients, the incidence of locoregional failure at 12 months was 25.1%, distant metastasis-free survival was 84.0%, and overall survival was 65.2%. Acute greater than or equal to grade 3 toxicities for mucositis, dysphagia, esophagitis, and dermatitis were all less than 10%. Grade 3 or greater late toxicities for skin and dysphagia were seen in 8.7% and 7.1% of patients, respectively. One death was seen due to disease progression, whereas 2 patients had grade 5 toxicity due to treatment-related bleeding. By comparison, a previous MSKCC report of reirradiation for SCC of the head and neck with IMRT or 3-D conformal radiotherapy noted 1-year locoregional control and overall survival rates of approximately 60% for each outcome.[33] The University of Michigan experience[34] with IMRT-based reirradiation for recurrent SCC of the head and neck from 2008 to 2015 noted 25% of patients having severe ($\geq$ grade 3) long-term toxicity, including 80% of those patients being feeding tube–dependent and 19% with soft tissue damage.

There is significantly increased cost associated with proton therapy, as well as less access, because the high cost of a proton center. Recent studies with proton therapy for head and neck cancer, however, show appealing potential gains in morbidity and efficacy compared with IMRT, especially in the setting of reirradiation.

SUMMARY

In conclusion, radiation treatment continues to become more tailored in SCC of the head and neck with the use of state-of-the-art imaging and delivery techniques. The emergence of these technologies in tandem with clinical refinements in primary surgical techniques has shown the potential to improve long-term QOL in patients with head and neck cancer. Together with new considerations for concurrent and adjuvant therapy management, there is great promise for providing patients with head and neck cancer increasingly efficacious therapies with reduced toxicity.

REFERENCES

1. Feng FY, Kim HM, Lyden TH, et al. Intensity-modulated radiotherapy of head and neck cancer aiming to reduce dysphagia: early dose-effect relationships for the swallowing structures. Int J Radiat Oncol Biol Phys 2007;68(5):1289–98.

2. Caglar HB, Tishler RB, Othus M, et al. Dose to larynx predicts for swallowing complications after intensity-modulated radiotherapy. Int J Radiat Oncol Biol Phys 2008;72(4):1110–8.

3. Caudell JJ, Schaner PE, Desmond RA, et al. Dosimetric factors associated with long-term dysphagia after definitive radiotherapy for squamous cell carcinoma of the head and neck. Int J Radiat Oncol Biol Phys 2010;76(2):403–9.

4. Feng FY, Kim HM, Lyden TH, et al. Intensity-modulated chemoradiotherapy aiming to reduce dysphagia in patients with oropharyngeal cancer: clinical and functional results. J Clin Oncol 2010;28(16):2732–8.

5. Kumar R, Madanikia S, Starmer H, et al. Radiation dose to the floor of mouth muscles predicts swallowing complications following chemoradiation in oropharyngeal squamous cell carcinoma. Oral Oncol 2014;50(1):65–70.

6. Min M, Lin P, Lee M, et al. Prognostic value of 2-[(18)F] Fluoro-2-deoxy-D-glucose positron emission tomography-computed tomography scan carried out during and after radiation therapy for head and neck cancer using visual therapy response interpretation criteria. Clin Oncol 2016;28(6):393–401.

7. Kam MK, Leung SF, Zee B, et al. Prospective randomized study of intensity-modulated radiotherapy on salivary gland function in early-stage nasopharyngeal carcinoma patients. J Clin Oncol 2007;25(31):4873–9.

8. Nutting CM, Morden JP, Harrington KJ, et al. Parotid-sparing intensity modulated versus conventional radiotherapy in head and neck cancer (PARSPORT): a phase 3 multicentre randomised controlled trial. Lancet Oncol 2011;12(2):127–36.

9. Tam M, Riaz N, Kannarunimit D, et al. Sparing bilateral neck level IB in oropharyngeal carcinoma and xerostomia outcomes. Am J Clin Oncol 2015;38(4):343–7.

10. Little M, Schipper M, Feng FY, et al. Reducing xerostomia after chemo-IMRT for head-and-neck cancer: beyond sparing the parotid glands. Int J Radiat Oncol Biol Phys 2012;83(3):1007–14.

11. Vainshtein JM, Moon DH, Feng FY, et al. Long-term quality of life after swallowing and salivary-sparing chemo-intensity modulated radiation therapy in survivors of human papillomavirus-related oropharyngeal cancer. Int J Radiat Oncol Biol Phys 2015;91(5):925–33.

12. Nguyen-Tan PF, Zhang Q, Ang KK, et al. Randomized phase III trial to test accelerated versus standard fractionation in combination with concurrent cisplatin for head and neck carcinomas in the Radiation Therapy Oncology Group 0129 trial: long-term report of efficacy and toxicity. J Clin Oncol 2014;32(34):3858–66.

13. Habbous S, Chu KP, Qiu X, et al. The changing incidence of human papillomavirus-associated oropharyngeal cancer using multiple imputation from 2000 to 2010 at a comprehensive cancer centre. Cancer Epidemiol 2013;37(6):820–9.

14. Ang KK, Harris J, Wheeler R, et al. Human papillomavirus and survival of patients with oropharyngeal cancer. N Engl J Med 2010;363(1):24–35.

15. Rischin D, Young RJ, Fisher R, et al. Prognostic significance of p16INK4A and human papillomavirus in patients with oropharyngeal cancer treated on TROG 02.02 phase III trial. J Clin Oncol 2010;28(27):4142–8.

16. Rieckmann T, Tribius S, Grob TJ, et al. HNSCC cell lines positive for HPV and p16 possess higher cellular radiosensitivity due to an impaired DSB repair capacity. Radiother Oncol 2013;107(2):242–6.

17. Fakhry C, Westra WH, Li S, et al. Improved survival of patients with human papillomavirus-positive head and neck squamous cell carcinoma in a prospective clinical trial. J Natl Cancer Inst 2008;100(4):261–9.

18. Masterson L, Moualed D, Masood A, et al. De-escalation treatment protocols for human papillomavirus-associated oropharyngeal squamous cell carcinoma. Cochrane Database Syst Rev 2014;(2):CD010271.
19. Yom SS, Gillison ML, Trotti AM. Dose de-escalation in human papillomavirus-associated oropharyngeal cancer: first tracks on powder. Int J Radiat Oncol Biol Phys 2015;93(5):986–8.
20. Chera BS, Amdur RJ, Tepper J, et al. Phase 2 trial of de-intensified chemoradiation therapy for favorable-risk human papillomavirus-associated oropharyngeal squamous cell carcinoma. Int J Radiat Oncol Biol Phys 2015;93(5):976–85.
21. Lee N, Schoder H, Beattie B, et al. Strategy of using intratreatment hypoxia imaging to selectively and safely guide radiation dose de-escalation concurrent with chemotherapy for locoregionally advanced human papillomavirus-related oropharyngeal carcinoma. Int J Radiat Oncol Biol Phys 2016;96(1):9–17.
22. Cracchiolo JR, Baxi SS, Morris LG, et al. Increase in primary surgical treatment of T1 and T2 oropharyngeal squamous cell carcinoma and rates of adverse pathologic features: national cancer data base. Cancer 2016;122(10):1523–32.
23. de Almeida JR, Li R, Magnuson JS, et al. Oncologic Outcomes After Transoral Robotic Surgery: A Multi-institutional Study. JAMA Otolaryngol Head Neck Surg 2015;141(12):1043–51.
24. Gooi Z, Fakhry C, Goldenberg D, et al. AHNS Series: Do you know your guidelines?Principles of radiation therapy for head and neck cancer: A review of the National Comprehensive Cancer Network guidelines. Head Neck 2016;38(7): 987–92.
25. Kaczmar JM, Tan KS, Heitjan DF, et al. HPV-related oropharyngeal cancer: Risk factors for treatment failure in patients managed with primary transoral robotic surgery. Head Neck 2016;38(1):59–65.
26. Funk RK, Moore EJ, Garcia JJ, et al. Risk factors for locoregional relapse after transoral robotic surgery for human papillomavirus-related oropharyngeal squamous cell carcinoma. Head Neck 2016;38(Suppl 1):E1674–9.
27. Nichols AC, Yoo J, Hammond JA, et al. Early-stage squamous cell carcinoma of the oropharynx: radiotherapy vs. trans-oral robotic surgery (ORATOR)–study protocol for a randomized phase II trial. BMC Cancer 2013;13:133.
28. Mendenhall NP, Malyapa RS, Su Z, et al. Proton therapy for head and neck cancer: rationale, potential indications, practical considerations, and current clinical evidence. Acta Oncol 2011;50(6):763–71.
29. Frank SJ, Cox JD, Gillin M, et al. Multifield optimization intensity modulated proton therapy for head and neck tumors: a translation to practice. Int J Radiat Oncol Biol Phys 2014;89(4):846–53.
30. Gunn GB, Blanchard P, Garden AS, et al. Clinical outcomes and patterns of disease recurrence after intensity modulated proton therapy for oropharyngeal squamous carcinoma. Int J Radiat Oncol Biol Phys 2016;95(1):360–7.
31. Romesser PB, Cahlon O, Scher E, et al. Proton beam radiation therapy results in significantly reduced toxicity compared with intensity-modulated radiation therapy for head and neck tumors that require ipsilateral radiation. Radiother Oncol 2016;118(2):286–92.
32. Romesser PB, Cahlon O, Scher ED, et al. Proton Beam Reirradiation for Recurrent Head and Neck Cancer: Multi-institutional Report on Feasibility and Early Outcomes. Int J Radiat Oncol Biol Phys 2016;95(1):386–95.
33. Riaz N, Hong JC, Sherman EJ, et al. A nomogram to predict loco-regional control after re-irradiation for head and neck cancer. Radiother Oncol 2014;111(3): 382–7.

34. Lee JY, Suresh K, Nguyen R, et al. Predictors of severe long-term toxicity after re-irradiation for head and neck cancer. Oral Oncol 2016;60:32–40.
35. Marur S, Li S, Cmelak A, et al. E1308: phase II trial of induction chemotherapy followed by reduced-dose radiation and weekly cetuximab in patients with HPV-associated resectable squamous cell carcinoma of the oropharynx- ECOG-ACRIN Cancer Research Group. J Clin Oncol 2016;35(5):490–7.

Precision Medicine
Genomic Profiles to Individualize Therapy

 CrossMark

Oscar E. Streeter Jr, MD[a],*, Phillip J. Beron, MD[b],
Prashant Natarajan Iyer, BE (Chem), MTPC, SCPM[c]

KEYWORDS

- Precision medicine • Big data • Genomic profiling • Immunotherapy
- Checkpoint inhibitors • Hyperthermia • Radiogenomics • Machine learning

KEY POINTS

- Precision medicine is generally understood to be the application of genotypic and Omics biomarkers to determine the most appropriate, outcome-driven treatment or therapy for individual patients.
- Information technology (IT)-enabled big data management and health care are becoming and will be required tools in the clinical kit to properly manage and leverage the complex data that result from genomic, clinic, financial, and behavioral data to benefit individualize patient care and outcomes by predicting for multiple stratified populations.
- Immunotherapy in 2017 has been most effective in checkpoint inhibitor medications.
- One of the novel immunomodulators is hyperthermia (HT) that is most effective in combination with radiation therapy (RT) or chemotherapy.

Precision medicine is an evolving term whose definition is changing as the influence of genomic and population big data biomarkers are becoming well understood.

WHAT IS PRECISION MEDICINE?

Precision medicine is generally understood as the application of genotypic and Omics biomarkers to determine the most appropriate, outcome-driven treatment of or therapy for individual patients. The authors agree with this definition but would like to extend it — in line with a more comprehensive and clinically relevant view, that is,

Disclosure Statement: O.E. Streeter and P.J. Beron have no disclosures. P.N. Iyer: Oracle Corporation, employer.
[a] The Center for Thermal Oncology, 2001 Santa Monica Boulevard, Suite 1190, Santa Monica, CA 90404, USA; [b] Department of Radiation Oncology, UCLA Health System, 200 UCLA Medical Plaza, Suite B265, Los Angeles, CA 90095, USA; [c] Healthcare Solutions, Oracle Corporation, 5805 Owens Drive, Pleasanton, CA 94588, USA
* Corresponding author.
E-mail address: ostreeter@thermaloncology.com

Otolaryngol Clin N Am 50 (2017) 765–773
http://dx.doi.org/10.1016/j.otc.2017.03.012
0030-6665/17/© 2017 Elsevier Inc. All rights reserved.

oto.theclinics.com

precision medicine is the determination and delivery of the "right therapy to the right patient at the right time."[1] The authors' view of precision medicine acknowledges a few realities that must be addressed via any multidisciplinary approach that combines people, behaviors, social determinants of health (a patients zip code has as much influence on their health as their genetic code), and their phenotypic data (**Fig. 1**). An integrated definition, such as the one used in this article, also addresses prevailing concerns about cost, access, and outcomes for individual patients and multidimensional stratified populations.

The authors posit that the definition of precision medicine that will enable oncology, chronic/acute care, and prevention/wellness must not only address the availability of genomics sequencing data and biomarkers but also do more on health variables that are constantly being defined. Although genomics at the point of care is fundamental to precision medicine, care at the bedside (in the facility or at home) also requires the acquisition, management, integration, clinician validation, and use of data from disparate sources, such as

1. Clinical care (imaging, electronic medical records [EMRs], computerised physician order entry [CPOE], clinical narratives, and sensor/device data)
2. Research (clinical research, trials, publications, results of data discovery, and secondary use)
3. Financial (cost, charges, affordability, income disparities, and credit scores)
4. External and patient-reported data that encompasses patient self-reported data on the Web and via smartphones; family and disease histories/lore that are not in the history and physical examination; environmental variables; behavior/sentiment data; and, increasingly, income/educational/cognitive disparities.

These data sources are varied, voluminous, and processed at high velocities (**Fig. 2**). There also is a corresponding need in the context of therapy and procedures to examine the veracity and value of data and information in enabling and supporting precision medicine. Supporting the natural evolution of precision medicine requires an

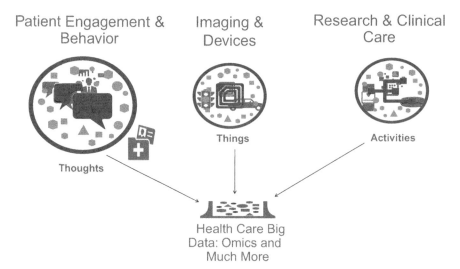

Fig. 1. Big data collection requires a central repository; processes need to be developed across institutions.

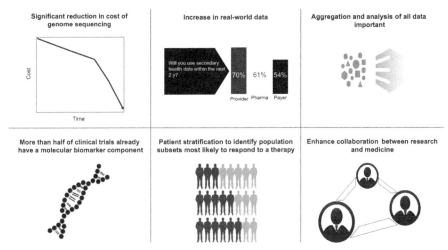

Fig. 2. The growth of big data.

understanding of the new world of big data technologies, analytics, and machine learning. It also needs recognition that a patient's data will no longer be created and used inside a facility's 4 walls or in its EMRs. In this new world of health care datafication, important patient (and other) information will be sourced from secondary use that involves integrated order-results workflows that are driven by

1. Incorporating molecular and clinical annotation by additional collaborators—molecular pathologists, consulting physicians, primary care providers, and other specialists
2. Machine learning–based, large-scale, affordable, and automated analysis of images, speech, video, and large text (clinical narratives, discharge summaries, and progress notes)
3. New data from smart devices, home monitors, telemedicine, medical images, and social networks (life and viral networks)
4. Separation of signal from noise—and incorporating actionable analytics, clinician feedback loops and approval, and annotation into clinical system workflows

IT-enabled big data management and health care should be a required tool in the clinical kit to properly manage and leverage the complex data that result from genomic, clinical, financial, and behavioral data that brings the biggest benefit to individual patients, their outcomes, and applying the new clinical guidelines and newly created knowledge by extrapolating or predicting for multiple stratified populations that can be expanded to cover new analytics dimensions beyond the diagnosis or disease, including

1. Demographics—gender, race, ethnicity, zip code, and so forth
2. Real-time, location-specific influences—suspended particulate (smog, forest fires, and disasters) or other carcinogens (eg, asbestos, human activities such as fracking)
3. Social determinants of health—examples are activities of daily living (ADL), physical activity, diet, education, and income
4. Patient outcomes, including the effect of a procedure or therapy on survival, recovery, and health management

Addressing key health determinants simultaneously at the population and individual levels and the integration of clinical/Omics/other relevant data are critical in delivering precision medicine. Relating individuals to both research cohorts and stratified populations by taking advantage of the latest software technologies—prescriptive analytics, big data integration, and machine learning—provide opportunities to create or use knowledge that has not existed before or is undiscovered.

Applying precision medicine into the clinical workflow generates preventative and diagnostic solutions to advance human care—bringing new targeted therapies, improved patient outcomes, and cost savings.[1]

GENOMIC PROFILING

To understand this evolving technology of genomic profiling,[2] a few terms need to be defined. Base pairs are 2 nucleotides on opposite complementary DNA or RNA strands that are connected by hydrogen bonds. Sequencing is a method of detecting single bases as they are incorporated into DNA template strands. Whole-exome sequencing is a technique for sequencing all the expressed genes in a genome.

Next-generation sequencing is the application of genome sequencers that with a single run of material can analyze more than 1.8 terabases (the amount of genetic sequence data equivalent to 10^{12} base pairs). The cost of sequencing has fallen approximately 10-fold over the last few years, with improved accuracy and speed, bringing the cost to less than $2000 with targeted, although limited at this point, improvement in care at the bedside. It is now available to most patients covered by insurance. Genomic data analysis is where newly identified sequences are aligned to a reference genome.

The first and best example of the success of precision medicine in oncology is imatinib mesylate (Gleevec, Novartis Pharma Services AG, Basel, Switzerland) used to treat chronic myeloid leukemia (CML) with the *BCR-ABL* translocation. CML is due to a clonal evolution, starting with the acquisition of the 9(9;22) (q34;q11) translocation (Philadelphia chromosome), which creates a fusion between the *BCR* and *ABL1* genes. Imatinib mesylate controls CML because it is an inhibitor of *ABL* family kinases, including the *BCR-ABL* fusion gene.[3]

Most squamous cell carcinomas of the head and neck respond to standard drug therapy. When the clonal composition of the pretreatment biopsy is compared over time, however, after drug treatment, there may be changes in clonal-mutation prevalence.[4] Sequencing reveals large changes in the abundance of specific clones that may give clues as to which genotypes may confer resistance and may be sensitive to intervention. Therefore, local recurrence or new metastatic sites should be biopsied and sequenced to determine which drug or other intervention may improve response. Therefore, surgeons play a key role in requesting the pathologist send both the primary tumor and recurrent/metastatic tumor for sequencing. An example of this process used in a multidisciplinary clinic is the Weill Cornell Medical College Institute for Precision Medicine. The process starts with clinical examination and consent, followed by metastatic tumor biopsy and whole-exome sequencing/biobanking of tissue for future reference. Results are discussed in a tumor board, with communication to the patient and referring physicians to guide treatment, and used to fuel translational research and development of new diagnostics and therapeutics.[5] A trial currently accruing patients that best demonstrates the application of precision medicine in oncology is the recently opened National Cancer Institute Molecular Analysis for Therapy Choice (NCI-MATCH) clinical trial. This precision medicine trial explores treating patients based on the molecular profile of tumors with the inclusion criteria of adult patients, solid tumors (including rare tumors and lymphomas), and tumors that no longer respond to standard treatment, with an accrual goal of approximately 3000 cancer patients screened with a tumor biopsy. Biopsied tumor tissue is submitted for gene sequencing to identify initially 143 gene mutations that may respond to a specific therapy (the list of gene mutations is expanding with new discoveries). If a patient's tumor has a genetic abnormality that matches one targeted by a drug used in the trial, the patient becomes eligible to join the treatment portion of NCI-MATCH. This is an important trial found at the Web site, clinicaltrials.gov, and includes a listing of the mutations examined and drugs useful for each mutation. It is an excellent resource for physicians in the clinics helping to individualize therapy and is constantly updated. As of the fall of 2016, more than 1000 clinical sites, across America, are participating in this trial. It is a federally sponsored trial and free to eligible patients with an estimated primary completion date of June 2022.[6]

Head and neck squamous cell carcinoma (HNSCC) is an immunosuppressive disease that when recurrent or metastatic responds to immunotherapy, such as checkpoint inhibitors that are available currently.[7] Ongoing trials are considering combining current immunotherapies with cancer vaccines. An open-access article by Robert Ferris provides a review of immunologic principles related to head and neck cancer, including the concept of cancer immunosurveillance and immune escape.[8] The authors recommend this article because it has figures describing immune escape and antigen presentation allowing recognition of tumor cells by immune system. Most importantly are tables listing the mechanisms of immune escape in HNSCC, monoclonal antibodies under investigation in HNSCC, and a detailed table of immunotherapy trials in HNSCC. Most clinicians will be working with checkpoint inhibitors and a brief discussion of this immunotherapy is warranted and illustrated in a free-access *JAMA Oncology* patient page.[9] Immune checkpoint inhibitor drugs can target either tumor cells or T cells. They block normal proteins on cancer cells or the proteins on T cells that respond to those "normal proteins."

The checkpoint inhibitors prevent tumor cells from attaching to T cells, allowing the T cells to stay activated. A response to immune checkpoint inhibitor treatment results in a brief increase in tumor size (pseudoprogression) due to the increase in the number of activated T cells that enter the tumor.

To evaluate genetic mutation changes in tumors when there may not be enough tissue for mutation analysis in a primary or metastatic biopsy or to monitor tumor response, there is an increasing use of analyzing cell-free DNA mutations (cfDNAs) in the plasma and circulating tumor cells (CTCs) in the buffy coat of a centrifuged peripheral blood draw (**Figs. 3** and **4**).[10,11] Every month there are more Clinical Laboratory Improvement (CLIA) certified tests for tumors in specific organs. Commercial companies have developed blood sampling techniques to profile and monitor for programmed death ligand-1 (PD-L1) expression, an important biomarker in immune-oncology treatment decision making and will play an increasing role in the treatment of head and neck cancers.

HYPERTHERMIA AS A NOVEL IMMUNE MODULATOR

HT is also a form of precision medicine. Because HT over the past 2 decades has been limited in the United States due to a lack of available equipment and trained practitioners who can deliver this modality between the temperature range of 41°C and 43°C, there is limited understanding of its role in stimulating a nontoxic immune response in practically all tumors. An important phase III trial reported long-term results comparing RT alone with RT plus HT to metastatic lymph nodes in stage IV head and neck patients.[12] This study was conducted in 1985 to 1986 to improve the outcome of fixed and inoperable (N3) metastatic lymph nodes in HNSCC in 41 patients with 46 metastatic lymph nodes. Because of the striking results of the

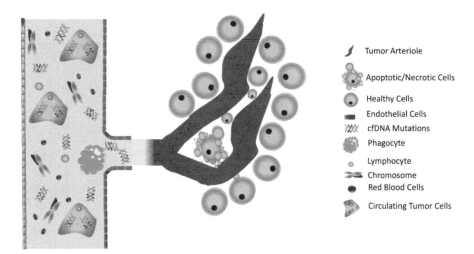

Fig. 3. Illustration of the origin of cfDNAs and CTCs from a milieu of apoptotic and necrotic fragments from tumors and other cellular fragments. (*Courtsey of* Oscar Streeter, MD, The Center for Thermal Oncology, Santa Monica, California.)

combined modality arm, the study was prematurely closed because of ethical reasons with a 5-year actuarial probability of nodal control of 24.2% for the radiation-only arm versus 68.6% in the RT plus HT arm. The actuarial survival of the 2 groups at 5 year favors the RT plus HT arm of 53.3% versus 0% ($P = .02$). Although metastatic disease developed in 19% of the patients, it was reduced in the RT plus HT arm to 12.5% vs 24% in the RT-alone arm. It is now known that HT not only has a direct cytotoxic effect but stimulates a natural immune response in the fever range of 39°C to 41°C by activation of heat shock proteins, generating important immune

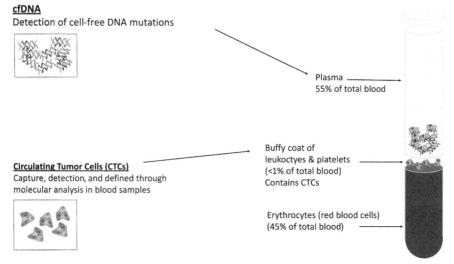

Fig. 4. Liquid biopsies. After centrifugation of a blood sample, cfDNA from shed tumors is detected from the plasma component of the supernatant, whereas CTCs are captured from the buffy coat component.

actions and increasing blood flow, effective in primary and metastatic disease.[13] The mechanisms of how HT can be used in metastatic disease as immunotherapy is because of the following effect on heated tumor cells: (1) an increase in the surface expression of MICA, a NKG2D ligand, and major histocompatibility class 1 (MHC 1), making the tumor cells more sensitive to lysis by natural killer (NK) cells and CD8[+] T cells, respectively, and (2) the release of heat shock proteins (HSPs), which activate NK cells and antigen-presenting cells (APCs). HSPs contain potential tumor antigens, and APCs take up the HSP-antigen complex and cross-present the antigen to CD8[+] T cells; (3) release of exosomes, which contain potential tumor antigens, and APCs take up the antigen and cross present the antigen to CD8[+] T cells; (4) immune cells, such as NK cells, CD8[+] T cells and dendritic cells, in the tumor also get heated and become activated; and (5) tumor vasculature becomes more permeable and may increase expression of the intercellular cell adhesion molecule (ICAM)-1, a protein expressed by the cancer cell with one function to facilitate signal transduction immune response. ICAM-1 also facilitates better immune trafficking between tumor cells and draining lymph nodes.

RADIOGENOMICS

Although the use of big data in health care research is still in its infancy, the potential of combining big data with information from comparative effectiveness research and EMR data with machine learning in the future will help with decision making on what type of therapy is best for individual patients, including informing individual patients of potential complications and risk of secondary cancers based on their genomic profile.[14] The challenges associated with implementing big data analytics in radiation oncology or in medical oncology are (1) validity of the training data set, (2) availability of public health and computer science experts, (3) silo ownership of the data, and (4) and the critical need to shift from deductive to inductive reasoning using new statistical and probabilistic tools from the field of machine learning (**Fig. 5**).

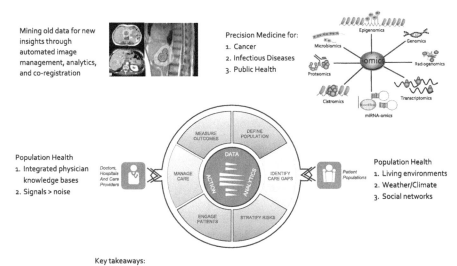

Key takeaways:
1. Precision medicine and population health are two sides of the same coin.
2. In healthcare, it is not always about searching for the needle in the haystack.
3. Big data analytics in precision medicine allows us to burn the hay to find the needle.

Fig. 5. Precision medicine applications.

WHAT IS MACHINE LEARNING?

Machine learning approaches problems as a doctor progressing through a residency would, starting with patient observation, using algorithms that sift through variables, and looking for combinations that reliably predict outcome. Ongoing research at Harvard Medical School and at the Perelman School of Medicine and Wharton School, University of Pennsylvania, have demonstrated that machine learning algorithms can predict death in metastatic cancer patients. This is accomplished by not only looking at known outcomes for a specific stage of cancer, but other variables such as infections during treatment, use of a wheelchair as well as other variables that are not ordinarily considered in determining prognosis. Obermeyer and Emanuel[15] predict prognostic algorithms will come into use in the next 5 years with several more years of prospective validation.

SUMMARY

Although there has been significant progress in the ability to sequence a person's genome in 1 sequencing process, the ability to aggregate all these data into a useful instrument to treat a single patient with cancer is a big data problem that will not be solved by any single institution. That type of computing power and transmitting that information across different platforms require a new type of thinking in medicine, the idea that the institution does not own the data, patients do, and must be part of a larger database tool that currently is in its infancy. For head and neck cancer patients, what can be used today is looking for a mutation that has a therapeutic target and understanding that the tumor will undergo clonal evolution and eventually become resistant. Also, a counterintuitive benefit for patients that is just as important is the ability to identify therapies of low value and avoiding adverse reactions.

REFERENCES

1. Oracle Health Sciences. Precision medicine: providing the right therapy to the right patient at the right time. 2016. Available at: http://www.oracle.com/us/industries/health-sciences/precision-medicine-info-2692756.pdf. Accessed October 1, 2016.
2. Green ED, Guyeer MS, National Human Genome Research Institute. Charting a course for genomic medicine from base pairs to bedside. Nature 2011; 470(7333):204–13.
3. Mohamed AN, Pemberton P, Zonder J, et al. The effect of imatinib mesylate on patients with Philadelphia chromosome-positive chronic myeloid leukemia with secondary chromosomal aberrations. Clin Cancer Res 2003;9(4):1333–7.
4. Aparicio S, Caldas C. The implications of clonal genome evolution for cancer medicine. N Engl J Med 2013;368(9):842–51.
5. Beltran H, Eng K, Mosquera JM, et al. Whole-exome sequencing of metastatic cancer and biomarkers of treatment response. JAMA Oncol 2015;1(4):466–74.
6. National Cancer Institute. NCI-MATCH: targeted therapy directed by genetic testing in treating patients with advanced refractory solid tumors or lymphomas (ClinicalTrials.gov Identifier: NCT02465060). 2015. Available at: https://clinicaltrials.gov/ct2/results?term=nct02465060. Accessed September 28, 2016.
7. Lalami Y, Awada A. Innovative perspectives of immunotherapy in head and neck cancer. From relevant scientific rationale to effective clinical practice. Cancer Treat Rev 2016;43:113–23.

8. Ferris RL. Immunology and immunotherapy of head and neck cancer. J Clin Oncol 2015;33(29):3293–304.
9. West H. Immune checkpoint inhibitors. JAMA Oncol 2015;1(1):115.
10. Diaz LA Jr, Bardelli A. Liquid biopsies: genotyping circulating tumor DNA. J Clin Oncol 2014;32(6):579–86.
11. Economopoulo P, Agelaki S, Perisanidis C, et al. The promise of immunotherapy in head and neck squamous cell carcinoma. Ann Oncol 2016;27(9):1675–85.
12. Valdagni R, Amichetti M. Report of long-term follow-up in a randomized trial comparing radiation therapy and radiation therapy plus hyperthermia to metastatic lymph nodes in Stage IV head and neck patients. Int J Radiat Oncol Biol Phys 1994;28(1):163–9.
13. Toraya-Brown S, Fiering S. Local tumor hyperthermia as immunotherapy for metastatic cancer. Int J Hyperthermia 2014;30(8):531–9.
14. Trifiletti DM, Showaalter TN. Big data and comparative effectiveness research in radiation oncology: synergy and accelerated discovery. Front Oncol 2015;5(274):1–5.
15. Obermeyer Z, Emanuel EJ. Predicting the future - big data, machine learning, and clinical medicine. N Engl J Med 2016;375(13):1216–9.

Systemic Treatment for Squamous Cell Carcinoma of the Head and Neck

Aditya V. Shetty, MD, Deborah J. Wong, MD, PhD*

KEYWORDS

- Chemoradiation • Cisplatin • Erbitux • PD-1 inhibition

KEY POINTS

- Head and neck cancers represent a diverse group of diseases with varied histopathologic features and outcomes.
- In patients with locally advanced squamous cell cancer of the head and neck, a multimodality treatment approach is recommended.
- The addition of platinum-based systemic therapy concurrently with radiation has been shown to be superior to radiation alone and is considered standard therapy for locally advanced disease.
- In the recurrent or metastatic setting, systemic treatment with chemotherapy is palliative.
- A subset of patients treated with PD-1 immunotherapy, however, may achieve durable responses.

INTRODUCTION

Head and neck cancer is a heterogeneous group of neoplasms arising in the oral cavity, nasopharynx, pharynx, larynx, or salivary glands. Although head and neck cancer can present with a variety of different histologic variants, squamous cell carcinomas of the head and neck (SCCHN) account for nearly 95% of the cases. A multidisciplinary treatment approach is recommended in all patients with head and neck cancer. The choice of treatment modality largely depends on the site and extent of the disease and the feasibility of organ preservation. Although stage I and II SCCHN is typically treated with radiotherapy or surgery, a multimodality treatment approach, including systemic therapy, is recommended for more advanced stages of the disease. The optimal sequencing of chemotherapy, radiotherapy, and surgery is still unclear. Although many chemotherapeutic agents have shown activity in SCCHN,

Division of Hematology-Oncology, UCLA Medical Center, 2825 Santa Monica Boulevard suite 200, Santa Monica, Los Angeles, CA 90404, USA
* Corresponding author.
E-mail address: DeWong@mednet.ucla.edu

Otolaryngol Clin N Am 50 (2017) 775–782
http://dx.doi.org/10.1016/j.otc.2017.03.013
0030-6665/17/Published by Elsevier Inc.

platinum-based therapy with either cisplatin or carboplatin is considered standard frontline therapy in inoperable or metastatic disease.

CONCURRENT CHEMORADIATION

The superiority of concurrent chemoradiation versus radiotherapy alone was first demonstrated in a study published in 1992. A total of 157 patients with previously untreated, unresectable advanced SCCHN were assigned to treatment with either alternating chemotherapy and radiotherapy or radiotherapy alone.[1] The median survival was noted to be 16.5 months in the combination arm and 11.7 months in the radiotherapy group. The 3-year survival was 41% in the combination arm and 23% in the radiotherapy arm. In a 5-year update to this study, overall survival (OS) was noted to be 24% in the combination group versus 10% in the radiotherapy group.[2] Five-year progression-free survival (PFS) was also noted to be significantly improved in the combination group at 21% and 9% in the radiotherapy group. In another trial, 295 unresectable patients were randomly to single daily radiation; to single daily radiation plus three cycles of concurrent cisplatin on Days 1, 22, and 43; or to a split course of single daily fractionated radiotherapy and three cycles of concurrent fluorouracil and cisplatin (CF) chemotherapy.[3] The 3-year OS rate was significantly improved with concurrent cisplatin and radiotherapy arms (37% vs 23%; $P = .014$) versus radiotherapy alone. No statistically significant differences in survival were observed with split course concurrent arm versus the radiotherapy arm (27% vs 23%).

Evidence also suggests that concurrent chemoradiotherapy leads to improved disease control versus radiotherapy not only in unresectable head and neck cancer but also in resectable cases of advanced head and neck cancer. A phase III study comparing the radiotherapy versus combination chemotherapy and radiotherapy in resectable stage III and IV head and neck cancer was undertaken.[4] A total of 100 resectable stages III and IV patients were randomized to either radiotherapy alone, 68 to 72 Gy at 1.8 to 2.0 Gy per day, or to radiotherapy with concurrent chemotherapy, consisting of 5-fluorouracil, 1000 mg/m^2/day and cisplatin 20 mg/m^2/day, both given as continuous intravenous infusions over 4 days beginning on Day 1 and Day 22 of the radiotherapy. Three-year relapse-free survival was noted to be higher in the combination arm at 67% versus 52% in the radiotherapy-alone arm. Successful primary site preservation was also noted to be improved in the combination arm at 57% versus 35% in the radiotherapy-alone arm. Development of metastases was also significantly lower in the combination arm compared with the radiotherapy arm alone (10% vs 2%). In a 5-year follow-up study, relapse-free survival (62% vs 51%) and development of metastasis (84% vs 75%) were noted to be improved in the combination arm.[5] No significant differences in OS were noted; however, 5-year OS was improved in patients who successfully achieved primary site preservation in the chemoradiotherapy arm.

The benefits of concurrent chemoradiation can also be seen in organ-preservation treatment of larynx and nasopharyngeal cancers. In the Intergroup RTOG 91-11 trial, 547 patients with locally advanced larynx cancer were randomly assigned to either induction cisplatin plus fluorouracil followed by radiotherapy, radiotherapy with concurrent administration of cisplatin, or radiotherapy alone.[6] At the 2-year mark larynx preservation was achieved in 88% in radiotherapy with concurrent cisplatin arm, 75% in the induction chemotherapy followed by radiotherapy arm, and 70% in radiotherapy arm alone. Locoregional control was also significantly better with concurrent chemoradiation (78% vs 61% in induction cisplatin plus fluorouracil followed by radiotherapy vs 56% in radiotherapy alone). With long-term follow-up, both arms treated with chemotherapy continued to have improved laryngectomy-free survival compared with the radiotherapy alone arm.[7] A randomized phase III trial was done to compare concurrent chemoradiotherapy with radiotherapy alone in 350 patients with locally advanced nasopharyngeal carcinoma.[8] Two-year PFS was significantly improved in the concurrent arm at 76% versus 69% in the radiotherapy alone arm. OS was also found to be significantly improved in concurrent chemoradiotherapy arm compared with radiotherapy arm alone (70.3% vs 58.6%).[9] Several meta-analyses have shown the benefit with the addition of chemotherapy to radiation in locally advanced nasopharyngeal cancer. In one meta-analysis consisting of 1528 patients from six randomized trials the addition of chemotherapy to radiotherapy improved PFS and OS by 34% and 20%, respectively, at 4 years.[10] In another meta-analysis consisting of 1753 from eight randomized trials a 6% absolute survival benefit was seen at 5 years with the addition of chemotherapy to radiotherapy.[11]

The improvement in outcomes with concurrent chemoradiation also results in increased toxicity. These include increased rates of grade 3 and 4 mucositis, increased rates of gastrostomy placement, and increased cytopenias.

INDUCTION THERAPY

Although concurrent chemoradiotherapy is considered the standard treatment of locally advanced head and neck cancer, multiple trials have been undertaken to assess the benefit of induction chemotherapy followed by radiotherapy or chemoradiotherapy. In a trial published in 2000, patients with oropharyngeal cancer for whom curative radiotherapy or surgery was considered feasible were randomly assigned to neoadjuvant chemotherapy followed by locoregional treatment.[12] Patients in the neoadjuvant arms were assigned to three cycles of cisplatin (100 mg/m^2) on Day 1 followed by a 24-hour infusion of fluorouracil (1000 mg/m^2/day) for 5 days every 21 days. Median survival was 5.1 years in neoadjuvant group, compared with median survival of 3.3 years in the locoregional arm.

Several trials have also compared with the addition of docetaxel to CF (TCF). In the TAX 323 trial, 358 patients with locoregionally advanced or unresectable disease were assigned to TCF or CF regimen for four cycles followed by radiation therapy.[13] The median PFS was significantly higher in the TCF arm (11.0 and 8.2 months in the TCF and CF induction arms). Response rates were also noted to be improved in the TCF induction arm compared with the CF arm (68% vs 54%). Median OS was also improved, 18.8 and 14.5 months with TCF and CF induction arms. In the TAX 324 trial, 501 patients with locoregionally advanced or unresectable disease were randomly assigned to either TCF or CF induction chemotherapy, followed by chemoradiotherapy with weekly carboplatin therapy plus radiotherapy.[14] The 3-year OS was 62% and 48% in TCF and CF induction arms. The median OS was substantially longer in the TCF arm, 71 months, compared with 30 months in the CF arm.

The GORTEC trial was a phase III designed to assess the feasibility of organ preservation in patients with pharyngeal and laryngeal cancer.[15] Patients were randomly assigned to receive three cycles of TCF or CF. Patients who had a response to therapy received radiotherapy with or without chemotherapy. Three-year larynx-preservation rate was improved in the TCF arm compared with the CF arm (70.3% vs 57.5%). Other trials have looked at induction chemotherapy with definitive radiotherapy regimens with the aim for organ preservation of the larynx and hypopharynx. In the phase III

VALCSG (the Department of Veterans Affairs Laryngeal Cancer Study Group) study 332 patients with stage III or IV laryngeal cancer were randomly assigned to receive either three cycles of CF chemotherapy and radiation therapy or to surgery and radiation therapy.[16] Two-year survival was 68% in both arms. Total laryngectomy was avoided in 64% of patients, and local failure was significantly higher and distant metastases significantly lower in the chemotherapy arm compared with the surgery arm. The EORTC (the European Organization for Research and Treatment Cancer) trial attempted to compare a larynx-preservation rate with induction chemotherapy plus definitive radiation therapy versus surgery with postoperative radiotherapy in patients previously untreated and operable hypopharyngeal cancer.[17] Complete response rates in the induction chemotherapy group were noted to be 54% in localized disease and 51% in locally advanced disease. The median survival was 44 and 25 months in induction arm and surgery arms. However, this was less than superiority margin and, therefore, the two treatment groups were considered equal. At the 3- and 5-year marks, organ preservation was 42% and 35%.

Several trials have also been done to assess the efficacy of induction chemotherapy followed chemoradiation versus chemoradiation alone. In the PARADIGM Trial, patients were randomly assigned to receive either induction chemotherapy with three cycles of TCF chemotherapy followed by concurrent chemoradiotherapy with either docetaxel or carboplatin or concurrent chemoradiotherapy alone with two cycles of bolus cisplatin.[18] No significant differences in OS were noted because 3-year OS was 73% in TCF arm compared with 78% in chemoradiotherapy arm alone ($P = .77$). In the DeCIDE trial patients with locally advanced N2 or N3 disease were assigned to two cycles of TCF induction chemotherapy followed with chemoradiotherapy or chemoradiotherapy alone.[19] At the 3-year mark, there were no significant changes in OS (75.0% and 73.0% in induction arm and chemoradiotherapy arms, respectively).

Overall, these trials demonstrate that the TCF regimen as induction chemotherapy significantly improved OS, PFS, and distant failure rates compared with CF for locally advanced head and neck cancer. However, the DeCIDE and PARADIGM trials failed to demonstrate a significant benefit with the addition of induction chemotherapy to chemoradiation. To date, there is no evidence to suggest that TCF induction chemotherapy followed by chemoradiotherapy is superior to chemoradiotherapy alone. Given this, chemoradiation alone is still considered the standard treatment of locally advanced head and neck cancer.

ADJUVANT THERAPY

Several trials have evaluated the benefit of chemoradiotherapy versus radiotherapy alone in the adjuvant setting. In the EORTC 22931 trial, 334 patients with locally advanced head and neck cancer were randomly assigned to adjuvant radiotherapy alone or concomitant chemoradiation with cisplatin at 100 mg/m^2 on Days 1, 22, and 43 of radiotherapy.[20] With a median follow-up of 5 years PFS and OS were both significantly improved. In the RTOG 9501 trial, 459 patients with resected high-risk head and neck cancer were randomly assigned to radiotherapy or to chemoradiation with concomitant cisplatin (100 mg/m^2, on Days 1, 22, and 43 of radiotherapy).[21] Although 2-year locoregional control and disease-free survival were improved in the chemoradiotherapy arm, no differences in OS were noted. In combined analysis of both the EORTC 22931 and RTOG 9501 trials only extracapsular nodal extension and positive surgical margins were found to be associated with the benefit from adjuvant chemoradiation.[22]

CYTOTOXIC CHEMOTHERAPY FOR METASTATIC AND RECURRENT HEAD AND NECK CANCER

Overall, the prognosis is poor for patients with metastatic head and neck cancer with median OS of less than 1 year.[23] Cisplatin, carboplatin, docetaxel, paclitaxel, fluoro-uracil, capecitabine, pemetrexed, and methotrexate have all been shown to have activity as single agents in recurrent or metastatic head and neck cancer, with response rates of 10% to 20%.[24] Although platinum doublet therapy has been shown to improve overall response rates over single-agent therapy, several phase III trials have failed to demonstrate an improvement in OS.[25,26]

THE ROLE OF EPIDERMAL GROWTH FACTOR RECEPTOR INHIBITION IN HEAD AND NECK CANCER

Overexpression of epidermal growth factor receptor is frequently observed in head and neck cancer and has been associated with a poor prognosis.[27] The benefit of cetuximab with concurrent radiotherapy was assessed in 424 patients with locally advanced head and neck cancer.[28] Following an initial loading dose at 400 mg/m^2, radiotherapy was administered with a weekly dose of 250 mg/m^2. In comparison with the radiotherapy group, locoregional control was significantly improved in patients treated with cetuximab plus radiotherapy (24.4 months vs 14.9 months). Median OS was also significantly improved in the cetuximab plus radiotherapy group because median OS was 49.0 months in the cetuximab plus radiotherapy group versus 29.3 months in the radiotherapy alone group. The side effects of cetuximab include infusion reactions, acneiform skin rash, hypomagnesemia, and hypokalemia. The group treated with cetuximab and radiotherapy compared with radiotherapy alone had increased incidence of infusion reactions (17% vs 1%, respectively) and acneiform skin rash (87% vs 10%, respectively). Other toxicities including mucositis were similar. The benefits of the addition of cetuximab in patients with recurrent or metastatic head and neck cancer were shown in the EXTREME trial.[29] In this phase III study, 442 patients with recurrent or metastatic head and neck cancer were assigned to receive platinum-based therapy alone (cisplatin or carboplatin and 5-fluorouracil) or platinum-based therapy plus cetuximab in the frontline setting. OS was improved with the addition of cetuximab to chemotherapy (10.1 vs 7.4 months). Although the EXTREME regimen improved OS, increased toxicity was noted, including increased rate of sepsis, skin rash, infusion reactions, and hypomagnesemia. Because crossover was not allowed on the study, it is unclear whether sequential treatment with cetuximab after progression on platinum-based chemotherapy would yield the same OS benefit compared with concurrent treatment. Nevertheless, based on these data, platinum/5-fluorouracil with cetuximab is a standard frontline treatment of recurrent/metastatic SCCHN.

IMMUNOTHERAPY FOR METASTATIC AND RECURRENT HEAD AND NECK CANCER

Immunotherapy using checkpoint inhibitors has been evaluated in the second-line setting. To date, several antibodies targeting the programmed cell death (PD-1) protein have been studied. In the Keynote-012 trial, pembrolizumab at 10 mg/kg every 2 weeks was assessed in 104 patients with recurrent or metastatic SCCHN.[30] Overall response was 18% in all patients, 25% in human papilloma virus–positive patients, and 14% in human papilloma virus–negative patients. A total of 65% of those who responded were continuing to respond at the time of final analysis. Median OS for all patients was noted to be 8 months. Nivolumab was assessed in the Checkmate-141 phase III trial.[31] A total of 361 patients with platinum-refractory, recurrent, or metastatic disease were randomly assigned to either nivolumab at 3 mg/kg every 2 weeks or to single-agent methotrexate, docetaxel, or cetuximab per the investigator's choice. Median OS was improved in the nivolumab arm (7.5 vs 5.1 months), with a 1-year survival rate of 36% in the nivolumab arm versus 16% in the chemotherapy. Objective response was also noted to be improved in the nivolumab group (13.3% vs 5.8%). In those with greater than 1% PD-L1 expression, OS was significantly increased with immunotherapy compared with chemotherapy (8.7 vs 4.6 months), whereas no significant differences in OS were noted in those with less than 1% PD-L1 expression. Based on these data, in 2016, the Food and Drug Administration granted accelerated approval to pembrolizumab and nivolumab for treatment of platinum refractory recurrent/metastatic SCCHN. Current studies are ongoing to delineate the role of immunotherapy in the frontline recurrent metastatic setting and in the definitive therapy and adjuvant settings.

SUMMARY

A multidisciplinary therapeutic approach is recommended for all patients with head and neck cancer. The use of platinum-based systemic therapy in combination with concurrent radiation has been shown to be superior to radiation alone in patients with locally advanced head and neck cancer and is considered the standard of care in these patients. Although induction therapy with TCF has been shown be to superior to induction therapy CF, no study to date has shown the benefit of induction chemotherapy to chemoradiation versus chemoradiation alone. Although several chemotherapeutic agents have shown to have activity in metastatic or recurrent head and neck cancer, prognosis is overall poor. Recently, several PD-1 inhibitors have shown benefit in recurrent or metastatic head and neck, with a subset of patients achieving durable responses.

REFERENCES

1. Merlano M, Vitale V, Rosso R, et al. Treatment of advanced squamous-cell carcinoma of the head and neck with alternating chemotherapy and radiotherapy. N Engl J Med 1992;327(16):1115–21.
2. Merlano M, Benasso M, Corvo R, et al. Five-year update of a randomized trial of alternating radiotherapy and chemotherapy compared with radiotherapy alone in treatment of unresectable squamous cell carcinoma of the head and neck. J Natl Cancer Inst 1996;88(9):583–9.
3. Adelstein DJ, Li Y, Adams GL, et al. An intergroup phase III comparison of standard radiation therapy and two schedules of concurrent chemoradiotherapy in patients with unresectable squamous cell head and neck cancer. J Clin Oncol 2003;21(1):92–8.
4. Adelstein DJ, Saxton JP, Lavertu P, et al. A phase III randomized trial comparing concurrent chemotherapy and radiotherapy with radiotherapy alone in resectable stage III and IV squamous cell head and neck cancer: preliminary results. Head Neck 1997;19(7):567–75.
5. Adelstein DJ, Lavertu P, Saxton JP, et al. Mature results of a phase III randomized trial comparing concurrent chemoradiotherapy with radiation therapy alone in patients with stage III and IV squamous cell carcinoma of the head and neck. Cancer 2000;88(4):876–83.
6. Forastiere AA, Goepfert H, Maor M, et al. Concurrent chemotherapy and radiotherapy for organ preservation in advanced laryngeal cancer. N Engl J Med 2003;349(22):2091–8.

7. Forastiere AA, Zhang Q, Weber RS, et al. Long-term results of RTOG 91-11: a comparison of three nonsurgical treatment strategies to preserve the larynx in patients with locally advanced larynx cancer. J Clin Oncol 2013;31(7):845–52.

8. Chan AT, Teo PM, Ngan RK, et al. Concurrent chemotherapy-radiotherapy compared with radiotherapy alone in locoregionally advanced nasopharyngeal carcinoma: progression-free survival analysis of a phase III randomized trial. J Clin Oncol 2002;20(8):2038–44.

9. Chan AT, Leung SF, Ngan RK, et al. Overall survival after concurrent cisplatin-radiotherapy compared with radiotherapy alone in locoregionally advanced nasopharyngeal carcinoma. J Natl Cancer Inst 2005;97(7):536–9.

10. Huncharek M, Kupelnick B. Combined chemoradiation versus radiation therapy alone in locally advanced nasopharyngeal carcinoma: results of a meta-analysis of 1,528 patients from six randomized trials. Am J Clin Oncol 2002; 25(3):219–23.

11. Baujat B, Audry H, Bourhis J, et al, MAC-NPC Collaborative Group. Chemotherapy in locally advanced nasopharyngeal carcinoma: an individual patient data meta-analysis of eight randomized trials and 1753 patients. Int J Radiat Oncol Biol Phys 2006;64(1):47–56.

12. Domenge C, Hill C, Lefebvre JL, et al, French Groupe d'Etude des Tumeurs de la Tete et du Cou(GETTEC). Randomized trial of neoadjuvant chemotherapy in oropharyngeal carcinoma. French Groupe d'Etude des Tumeurs de la Tete et du Cou (GETTEC). Br J Cancer 2000;83(12):1594–8.

13. Vermorken JB, Remenar E, van Herpen C, et al. Cisplatin, fluorouracil, and docetaxel in unresectable head and neck cancer. N Engl J Med 2007;357(17): 1695–704.

14. Posner MR, Hershock DM, Blajman CR, et al, TAX 324 Study Group. Cisplatin and fluorouracil alone or with docetaxel in head and neck cancer. N Engl J Med 2007; 357(17):1705–15.

15. Pointreau Y, Garaud P, Chapet S, et al. Randomized trial of induction chemotherapy with cisplatin and 5-fluorouracil with or without docetaxel for larynx preservation. J Natl Cancer Inst 2009;101(7):498–506.

16. The Department of Veterans Affairs Laryngeal Cancer Study Group. Induction chemotherapy plus radiation compared with surgery plus radiation in patients with advanced laryngeal cancer. N Engl J Med 1991;324(24):1685–90.

17. Lefebvre JL, Chevalier D, Luboinski B, et al. Larynx preservation in pyriform sinus cancer: preliminary results of a European Organization for Research and Treatment of Cancer phase III trial. EORTC Head and Neck Cancer Cooperative Group. J Natl Cancer Inst 1996;88(13):890–9.

18. Haddad R, O'Neill A, Rabinowits G, et al. Induction chemotherapy followed by concurrent chemoradiotherapy (sequential chemoradiotherapy) versus concurrent chemoradiotherapy alone in locally advanced head and neck cancer (PARADIGM): a randomised phase 3 trial. Lancet Oncol 2013;14(3):257–64.

19. Cohen EE, Karrison T, Kocherginsky M, et al. Decide: a phase III randomized trial of docetaxel (D), cisplatin (P), 5-fluorouracil (F) (TPF) induction chemotherapy (IC) in patients with N2/N3 locally advanced squamous cell carcinoma of the head and neck (SCCHN). J Clin Oncol 2012;30(15 Suppl (20 Suppl)):5500.

20. Bernier J, Domenge C, Ozsahin M, et al, European Organization for Research and Treatment of Cancer Trial 22931. Postoperative irradiation with or without concomitant chemotherapy for locally advanced head and neck cancer. N Engl J Med 2004;350(19):1945–52.

21. Cooper JS, Pajak TF, Forastiere AA, et al, Radiation Therapy Oncology Group. Postoperative concurrent radiotherapy and chemotherapy for high-risk squamous-cell carcinoma of the head and neck. N Engl J Med 2004;350(19):1937–44.

22. Bernier J, Cooper JS, Pajak TF, et al. Defining risk levels in locally advanced head and neck cancers: a comparative analysis of concurrent postoperative radiation plus chemotherapy trials of the EORTC (#22931) and RTOG (# 9501). Head Neck 2005;27(10):843–50.

23. Price KA, Cohen EE. Current treatment options for metastatic head and neck cancer. Curr Treat Options Oncol 2012;13(1):35–46.

24. Pfister DG, Ang KK, Brizel DM, et al, National Comprehensive Cancer Network. Head and neck cancers, version 2.2013. Featured updates to the NCCN guidelines. J Natl Compr Canc Netw 2013;11(8):917–23.

25. Jacobs C, Lyman G, Velez-Garcia E, et al. A phase III randomized study comparing cisplatin and fluorouracil as single agents and in combination for advanced squamous cell carcinoma of the head and neck. J Clin Oncol 1992; 10(2):257–63.

26. Forastiere AA, Metch B, Schuller DE, et al. Randomized comparison of cisplatin plus fluorouracil and carboplatin plus fluorouracil versus methotrexate in advanced squamous-cell carcinoma of the head and neck: a Southwest oncology group study. J Clin Oncol 1992;10(8):1245–51.

27. Kalyankrishna S, Grandis JR. Epidermal growth factor receptor biology in head and neck cancer. J Clin Oncol 2006;24(17):2666–72.

28. Bonner JA, Harari PM, Giralt J, et al. Radiotherapy plus cetuximab for squamous-cell carcinoma of the head and neck. N Engl J Med 2006;354(6):567–78.

29. Vermorken JB, Mesia R, Rivera F, et al. Platinum-based chemotherapy plus cetuximab in head and neck cancer. N Engl J Med 2008;359(11):1116–27.

30. Seiwert TY, Burtness B, Mehra R, et al. Safety and clinical activity of pembrolizumab for treatment of recurrent or metastatic squamous cell carcinoma of the head and neck (KEYNOTE-012): an open-label, multicentre, phase 1b trial. Lancet Oncol 2016;17(7):956–65.

31. Ferris RL, Blumenschein G, Fayette J, et al. Nivolumab for recurrent squamous-cell carcinoma of the head and neck. N Engl J Med 2016;375(19):1856–67.

Decision Making for Diagnosis and Management: A Consensus Comes to Life

Rebecca C. Hoesli, MD, Andrew G. Shuman, MD,
Carol R. Bradford, MD*

KEYWORDS

- Diagnosis and management • Decision making • Head and neck cancer
- Multidisciplinary team

KEY POINTS

- The diagnosis and treatment of head and neck cancer is extremely complex due to the wide diversity of tumor types, the complex anatomy of the head and neck, the significant functional morbidity of tumors and treatment, the variability in patient preferences and quality-of-life outcomes, and the rapid development of new treatments and therapies.
- Multiple medical providers are involved in a patient's care, and the multidisciplinary tumor boards provide a forum whereby they can share and discuss the intricacies of each individual patient's case.
- Patient-centric decision making requires a careful balance between quality of life and survival outcomes, and tends to rely heavily on professional recommendations.
- The treating oncology team should have a deep understanding of each individual patient's goals for care, and patient preferences should be incorporated in the discussion at the multidisciplinary tumor board.
- When recommendations are presented to the patient and decisions are to be finalized, the patient should benefit from the collective wisdom of a team of providers to achieve and implement a patient-centric and clinically sound consensus.

INTRODUCTION: ASSESSING FACTORS IN DECISION MAKING

The diagnosis and treatment of head and neck cancer remains challenging due to the complex interaction among tumor characteristics, patient demographics and preferences, and institutional capabilities. Head and neck cancers represent a diverse collection of neoplasms that differ in their location, type, and stage, all of which

Disclosure Statement: The authors have nothing to disclose.
Department of Otolaryngology–Head and Neck Surgery, Comprehensive Cancer Center, University of Michigan Medical School, 1500 East Medical Center Drive – SPC 5312, Ann Arbor, MI 48109, USA
* Corresponding author.
E-mail address: cbradfor@med.umich.edu

Otolaryngol Clin N Am 50 (2017) 783–792
http://dx.doi.org/10.1016/j.otc.2017.03.014
0030-6665/17/© 2017 Elsevier Inc. All rights reserved.

oto.theclinics.com

significantly alter consideration of treatment modalities.[1] Squamous cell carcinoma is by far the most common type of cancer diagnosed in the head and neck,[2] but histology/location all affect the type of treatment available. Oncologic stage also significantly alters type of and modality (or modalities) of treatment.[3–5] In a rapidly advancing field and diversity among and between various tumors, decision making regarding management and treatment is difficult, particularly as most treatments lack strong level 1 evidence or a unified consensus.[2,6,7]

Patient characteristics and demographics also alter management and treatment. Although the standard of care regarding modality of treatment is largely established for each tumor type, many such algorithms allow multiple acceptable treatment options, and specific patient characteristics may lead to deviation from a standard. Comorbidities, such as severe heart disease, may impact perioperative risk and surgical candidacy; connective tissue disorders may represent a relative contraindication to radiotherapy; immunocompromised states limit consideration of immunotherapies; and renal insufficiency impacts cytotoxic chemotherapeutic options. Among patients with head and neck cancer, the presence of comorbidities is significant; in one study, 21% of patients with head and neck cancer had moderate or severe comorbidities, and the rate of death among these patients was decidedly higher than among those patients who were generally healthier.[8] Thus, carefully considered patient-centric choices must consider factors seemingly unrelated to the incident malignancy.

Importantly, a patient's priorities regarding functional outcome, perceived quality of life, and oncologic outcome may significantly affect decision making, as certain patients may opt for or against certain therapies depending on their perceptions regarding treatment and quality-of-life priorities.[9,10] The patient's decision regarding therapy is of utmost importance, and the care team's role is to help the patient make the most informed decision that is consistent with his or her life priorities.[10]

Finally, institutional abilities will impact management and treatment. The field of head and neck oncology is constantly evolving as new therapies are emerging, from surgical technologies, to refined radiation planning, to improvements in understanding the role of immunotherapy. Availability of these treatments and the highly trained providers required to administer them may differ between institutions, altering management and treatment. Additionally, many of the newest therapies and combinations thereof are currently in clinical trials not yet accessible to many institutions.

TEAM-BASED APPROACH

Given these layers of complexity, multidisciplinary care provided by surgical oncologists, pathologists, radiologists, radiation oncologists, medical oncologists, endocrinologists, and others working in concert represents the necessary standard of care.[11–13] Additionally, due to the involvement of many critical structures affecting function in head and neck cancer, treatment involves more than just a team of physicians. Many of these cancers and their treatment significantly affect quality of life, as they can lead to significant consequences involving socialization, speech, swallowing, taste, hearing, facial function, endocrine function, and cosmesis.[14] Furthermore, researchers in the field are making new advancements in the management and treatment of head and neck cancer, and new trials are constantly being opened, leading to a need for good communication between head and neck cancer researchers and clinicians. Therefore, in addition to the many physicians required to treat head and neck carcinoma, a comprehensive treatment team might include dedicated head and neck cancer researchers and study coordinators, speech language pathologists, audiologists, a dedicated nursing staff, nutritionists, dentists, and social workers, among others.

The multidisciplinary tumor board provides an opportunity for all of the various providers of a patient to discuss each individual patient's case, and develop a consensus regarding the recommended plan of care. This concept has been present in the literature and in clinical care for many years, with a discussion regarding the importance of a multidisciplinary tumor board in head and neck squamous cell carcinoma published as early as 1978.[15] Many studies have been performed regarding the impact of multidisciplinary tumor boards on head and neck cancer treatment, with suggested benefits including improved patient survival,[12,16] improved compliance with clinical practice guidelines,[6,17] improved staging accuracy,[13,18] increased access to clinical trials,[6,12] improved communication,[6] more timely access to care,[19] and improved clinician and patient satisfaction. In one of these studies, Wheless and colleagues[13] performed a prospective trial on the effect of a multidisciplinary head and neck tumor board on diagnosis and treatment, and found that 24% of all patients in the study had changes in treatment planning after presentation at tumor board. This has significant implications for the patient, as of those patients requiring change in treatment, most received recommendations for escalation of treatment after multidisciplinary discussion.

Herein, we review some of the various components of the multidisciplinary head and neck tumor board and their role in decision making for diagnosis and treatment, including the primacy of the patient's own involvement.

Role of the Surgical Oncologist

Many patients initially present to a surgical oncologist as their introduction to the multidisciplinary head and neck cancer care team. On presentation, a complete history and physical examination is performed, including comprehensive tumor staging/characterization, functional status, assessment of medical comorbidities that may affect treatment, health behaviors, and other related factors that impact treatment choices. Importantly, at the initial patient consultation, discussion regarding patient-centric goals of care and priorities should be introduced and explored. If a pathologic diagnosis has not yet been obtained, in-office, radiology-assisted, or operative biopsy might be considered and arranged. Additional imaging is frequently ordered and obtained.

It has been shown that many patients tend to follow the recommendations of the provider they encounter first regarding their care; additionally, many patients perceive that the first provider is the most involved in their care.[20] As a result, the surgical oncologist can play a critical and influential role in decision making. However, truly multidisciplinary care requires that treatment options be discussed by the surgical oncologist along with all other providers, to best reflect the input and consensus of other members of the team rather than simply one option or perspective.

During the multidisciplinary tumor board, the surgical oncologist has the greatest understanding about surgical options for treatment and reconstruction. If extirpative surgery is being considered, it is helpful to discuss among involved providers issues regarding the surgical approach, type/extent of surgery, resectability, and patient fitness for surgery, including an assessment of performance status as well as comorbidities that can alter perioperative planning, all of which benefit from multiple perspectives.

Role of the Medical Oncologist

The medical oncologist is critical to the discussion regarding diagnosis and treatment. Typically, this individual is most knowledgeable regarding systemic treatment options. With the increasing number of systemic therapies, combination therapies, and immunotherapies, as well as the diversity of cancer types in the head and neck requiring specific therapies, the medical oncologist's input is indispensable in recommending the correct treatment for a particular patient's cancer in the context of his or her performance status and comorbidities. Side effects are also a serious consideration when planning systemic treatment, and the medical oncologist is uniquely qualified to anticipate and mitigate both short-term and long-term side effects.

Medical oncology input to the multidisciplinary tumor board is critical to tailor treatment for the patient, and to discuss and recommend systemic treatment, should it be warranted. Their understanding of the various chemotherapeutic agents and mechanisms of action allow them to provide expert advice on the timing and coordination of systemic treatment with other modalities. For patients with recurrent or metastatic disease, their knowledge of existing clinical trials can provide additional options for patients, and can facilitate a patient's entry into these trials. For clinical trials that may be taking place in other institutions, the medical oncologist can also provide a referral to these institutions so patients have the option to participate in these trials as well. The medical oncologist also provides support to the patient and families throughout treatment, which is critical for patients during systemic treatment, particularly if the patient experiences complications from a side effect of treatment. Finally, the medical oncologist also is uniquely suited to provide supportive, palliative, and end-of-life care for patients with unresectable or untreatable carcinomas in concert with the rest of the team.[21]

Role of the Radiation Oncologist

Radiation oncologists are another core component of a multidisciplinary tumor board. With approximately half of all patients with cancer requiring radiotherapy as a component of their therapy, radiation oncologists play a critical role in oncologic care.[22] As the experts in planning and administering radiation as primary or adjuvant therapy for head and neck carcinoma, input from the radiation oncologist is critical to the multidisciplinary tumor board when deciding on initial treatment approaches. Candidacy for radiation therapy is distinct from candidacy for surgery or chemotherapy and requires additional expertise.[23–25] Determination and discussion of planned radiation fields is similarly nuanced and sometimes requires multidisciplinary discussion. If radiation fields are planned carefully, they can minimize significant side effects like xerostomia and irradiation of critical targets like the brain and spinal cord, while still maximizing the oncological effect.[26,27] Using techniques like intensity-modulated radiation therapy, therapeutic doses can be delivered effectively and safely to involved and at-risk fields.[25] Consideration of these fields at the tumor board with all of the various providers present ensures reasoned plans that incorporate radiologic nuance, operative findings/impressions, as well as the technical details from radiation physics.

For patients with second primary tumors, recurrent or persistent disease, decision making is frequently impacted by prior therapy, and options may be quite limited. The radiation oncologist can review previous treatments and determine if the patient is a candidate for re-irradiation, which may be effective,[28] but can result in significant side effects.[29] Re-irradiation is feasible and can be well-tolerated in previously radiated patients, and improved locoregional control can be achieved in patients using intensity-modulated radiation therapy; however, such decisions cannot be made lightly, as the risks are significant.[28,30,31] For patients who are not candidates for curative treatment, radiation therapy also can be used for palliative treatment, and planning and consideration thereof is similarly complex.[32–34]

Role of the Pathologist

The pathologist plays an important role in the diagnosis and staging of head and neck carcinoma, which plays an important role in treatment decision making. Ensuring the correct pathologic diagnosis is critical and frequently challenging.[35] As a result, studies have shown that a second opinion evaluation of pathology specimens is of great value when staging tumors, especially involving patient referral from community to tertiary care centers.[35,36] Kronz and colleagues[35] found that a second opinion on surgical pathology from a variety of subsites, including head and neck, resulted in a 1.4% rate of changed diagnosis. However, when evaluating head and neck neoplasms only, Westra and colleagues[36] found that secondary review of 814 head and neck pathology specimens resulted in an even more significant change in diagnosis in 7% of cases. Of those cases in which diagnosis was altered, 87% resulted in a change in treatment, and 56% resulted in a worse diagnosis. They thus concluded that secondary review, as is performed in conjunction with a multidisciplinary tumor board, is critical in head and neck neoplasms before decision making regarding treatment.[36]

Recently, it was discovered that human papilloma virus (HPV) is an etiology in a growing number of oropharyngeal carcinomas.[37] These HPV-related carcinomas have been found to be more sensitive to chemoradiation, with improved overall and disease-free survival.[38,39] However, there is currently no standard approach for HPV testing of clinical samples. Depending on institutional biases, tests differ in both design and detection targets.[40] Current targets include HPV DNA, HPV RNA, viral oncoproteins, p16 and other cellular proteins, and HPV-specific serum antibodies.[40] The pathologist plays a critical role in deciding the necessity for additional testing for the presence of HPV, which would significantly alter treatment-related decisions.

Thus, involvement of an experienced head and neck pathologist is a welcome and often critical member of the multidisciplinary team and tumor board discussion. The pathologist may assist in determining when more tissue or special staining can be helpful to better delineate an uncertain diagnosis; clinical details shared in a tumor board setting are often critical to making these nuanced decisions.

Perhaps most importantly, the pathologist also has the unique ability to weigh in on subtle but critical pathologic features that may affect treatment, such as how to interpret a "close" margin after resection, or how much perineural invasion was seen in a sample. This input is invaluable in the multidisciplinary tumor board, particularly when shades of gray dictate precisely how these pathologic features may impact a decision regarding delivery of adjuvant therapy.

Role of the Radiologist

A radiologist with specific experience in the head and neck is another indispensable contributor to the multidisciplinary tumor board, as imaging is often critical for correct staging of head and neck cancer. Like pathologic diagnosis, increased scrutiny of imaging improves cancer staging.[41–43] In a study by Lysack and colleagues,[41] there was a 56% discrepancy rate between cancer stages between the original radiology report and the second opinion radiology report. Of the discrepant cases, 91% of the changes resulted in upstaging of the patient's tumor, and management was changed in 38% of these patients. In those cases that had pathologic staging data, the second opinion report agreed with the pathologic stage 93% of the time, compared with only a 40% concordance with the primary report. Several other studies confirm the result that second opinions improve diagnostic interpretation and staging in patients with head and neck cancer, resulting in meaningful changes in treatment and prognosis[42,43]; one of these studies unearthed previously unseen distant metastases in

1.5% of cases.[42] Additionally, this study suggests that the multidisciplinary tumor board setting improves interpretation due to access to a full history and physical examination, which improves diagnostic precision.[42] This clearly results in a significant impact on patients and their management. As a result, it is suggested that review of all radiological studies occur on transfer or referral of all new patients.[41]

After review, additional studies may be warranted to facilitate metastatic workup, to better delineate tumor extension, or to better define targets for radiation therapy. Based on the information the tumor board is attempting to obtain, the radiologist can recommend the best additional studies required and facilitate their performance.

Role of Researchers and Research Coordinators

Exciting developments in the management and treatment of head and neck carcinoma are happening with increasing frequency, including how we manage the distinctive presentation of HPV, to the advent of next-generation sequencing studies.[44,45] With these advancements, our field is moving toward a more personalized approach toward treatment, and setting the stage for targeted treatment for patients in the future, guided by the genetic characteristics of a specific tumor.[44] With the development of new targeted therapies and therapeutic trials, the input of dedicated head and neck cancer researchers is important to discuss the role of possible therapeutic trials for patients at all disease stages. The multidisciplinary tumor board facilitates communication between researchers and clinicians, and discussion regarding the management of patients can lead to the development of new trials and new ideas for therapies. Additionally, communication between researchers, research trial coordinators, and clinicians can allow for better recruitment to studies for all patients,[6] particularly in cases in which discussion regarding the patient's history or physical may suggest concern for a unique mutational driver in a patient's tumor genetics. Like the medical oncologist, the research staff have extensive knowledge regarding the current clinical trials and can assist the treatment team in recommending and referring patients to institutions holding applicable clinical trials, facilitating a patient's involvement in these trials.

Role of the Patient

Patient decision making in head and neck cancer is difficult due to the significant morbidity that both the disease and treatment can engender. Patient priorities on quality-of-life–related outcomes are integral in the final decision regarding management and treatment of head and neck cancer.[46] Thus, patients may opt for more conservative or more aggressive therapy depending on their perception of quality of life and survival. In the treatment of head and neck carcinoma, patients and providers must navigate a delicate balance between quality of life and odds of survival when making a decision regarding which treatment modality to pursue. A study by Davies and colleagues[47] revealed that decision making in head and neck cancer does not fit the conventional model of decision making; although patients desire to maintain the final decision-making capacity, they also rely heavily on their trust in their physicians for information regarding which option to pursue. At the same time, other studies show that incorporation of patient perspectives directly impacts a patient's perspective on care.[20] Therefore, providers are tasked with the difficult job of guiding patients toward a decision that incorporates a patient's quality-of-life goals with their treatment goals. This, of course, requires a solid understanding of a patient's quality-of-life goals. Davies and colleagues[47] thus conclude that incorporation of all the necessary components of decision making into the multidisciplinary tumor board will likely be the most important factor that provides the most improvement in patient decision making.

Therefore, goals of care and priorities should be assessed at the initial consultation so that patient priorities can be presented during tumor board discussion and can then be taken into consideration when discussing management options.

Role of Support Staff

The multidisciplinary tumor board might also include a variety of support staff, including speech and language pathologists, audiologists, a dedicated nursing staff, nutritionists, dentists, and social workers, among others. For all modalities of treatment, patients can experience a number of side effects, including dysphagia, difficulty speaking, hearing loss, cranial nerve function loss, and/or depression.[48,49] Referral before treatment, as well as close monitoring throughout treatment and afterward is recommended,[50] and in a study on compliance, treatment by a multidisciplinary tumor board was the only significant factor associated with compliance with speech language pathology.[51]

CONVEYING AND IMPLEMENTING TREATMENT RECOMMENDATIONS

Discussion of a patient's case by the surgical oncologist, medical oncologist, radiation oncologist, pathologist, radiologist, and research staff, with patient preferences in mind, results in a management consensus that then must be conveyed to the patient. During this interaction, a report by Charles[52] suggests that this conversation should contain 4 components: sharing treatment benefits and risks, patient sharing of treatment goals, discussion of treatment options, and a formal agreement of an established plan. Determining how best to discuss and convey this can be difficult, and more than one physician may be required to participate.[17] Patients should be informed clearly in such a way that the patient understands the diagnosis, as well as the possible and recommended options for treatment.[17] If the patient preferences were included in the initial conversation and were considered at the multidisciplinary tumor board, the discussion can proceed with how the recommendations reflect or differ from the patient's preferences. The provider should ensure that the patient understands all of his or her options, and then a discussion between the patient and provider should ensue. Finally, there should be a formal summary of the agreed on plan.

Like the ensuing discussion regarding treatment, implementing the treatment consensus requires a concerted effort between the various providers and the patient. However, because the tumor board discussion takes place with all of the involved participants in treatment, patients can be started on treatment by the required providers shortly after the decision is made. Several studies have examined the frequency of which tumor board recommendations are implemented, and found that most recommendations are implemented.[53,54] In particular, one of these studies showed that of 344 cases, only 4% of cases deviated from the recommendations of the tumor board. Of these 4%, most deviations were due to patient refusal or due to poor medical status.[53] Although not addressed by this study, it is hoped that inclusion of patient preferences in discussion at tumor board will result in recommendations more concordant with patient preferences and thus fewer deviations from tumor board recommendations.

SUMMARY

In summary, the diagnosis and treatment of head and neck cancer is extremely complex due to the wide diversity of tumor types, the complex anatomy of the head and neck, the significant functional morbidity of tumors and treatment, the variability in patient preferences and quality-of-life outcomes, and the rapid development of new treatments and therapies. As a result, multiple medical providers are involved in a patient's care, and the multidisciplinary tumor boards provide a forum whereby they can share and discuss the intricacies of each individual patient's case. Patient-centric decision making requires a careful balance between quality of life and survival outcomes, and tends to rely heavily on professional recommendations. Thus, the treating oncology team should have a deep understanding of each individual patient's goals for care, and patient preferences should be incorporated in the discussion at the multidisciplinary tumor board. Finally, when recommendations are presented to the patient and decisions are to be finalized, the patient should benefit from the collective wisdom of a team of providers to achieve and implement a patient-centric and clinically sound consensus.

REFERENCES

1. Chin D, Boyle GM, Porceddu S, et al. Head and neck cancer: past, present, and future. Expert Rev Anticancer Ther 2006;6(7):1111–8.
2. Westin T, Stalfors J. Tumour boards/multidisciplinary head and neck cancer meetings: are they of value to patients, treating staff or a political additional drain on healthcare resources? Curr Opin Otolaryngol Head Neck Surg 2008;16(2):103–7.
3. Matzinger O, Zouhair A, Mirimanoff RO, et al. Radiochemotherapy in locally advanced squamous cell carcinomas of the head and neck. Clin Oncol 2009; 21(7):525–31.
4. Bonner JA, Harari PM, Giralt J, et al. Radiotherapy plus Cetuximab for squamous-cell carcinoma of the head and neck. N Engl J Med 2006;354(6):567–78.
5. Fletcher GH, Evers WT. Radiotherapeutic management of surgical recurrences and postoperative residuals in tumors of the head and neck. Radiology 1970; 95(1):185–8.
6. Giralt J, Benavente S, Arguis M. Optimizing approaches to head and neck cancer: strengths and weaknesses in multidisciplinary treatments of locally advanced disease. Ann Oncol 2008;19(Supplement 7):vii195–9.
7. Friedland PL, Bozic B, Dewar J, et al. Impact of multidisciplinary team management in head and neck cancer patients. Br J Cancer 2011;104(8):1246–8.
8. Piccirillo JF. Importance of comorbidity in head and neck cancer. Laryngoscope 2000;110(4):593–602.
9. McNeil BJ, Weichselbaum R, Pauker SG. Speech and survival: tradeoffs between quality and quantity of life in laryngeal cancer. N Engl J Med 1981;305(17):982–7.
10. Deber RB. What role do patients wish to play in treatment decision making? Arch Intern Med 1996;156(13):1414.
11. Stalfors J, Björholt I, Westin T. A cost analysis of participation via personal attendance versus telemedicine at a head and neck oncology multidisciplinary team meeting. J Telemed Telecare 2005;11(4):205–10.
12. Birchall MA, Bailey D, Lennon A. Performance and standards for the process of head and neck cancer care: south and west audit of head and neck cancer 1996–1997 (SWAHN I). Br J Cancer 2000;83(4):421–5.
13. Wheless SA, McKinney KA, Zanation AM. A prospective study of the clinical impact of a multidisciplinary head and neck tumor board. Otolaryngol Head Neck Surg 2010;143(5):650–4.
14. Stalfors J, Lundberg C, Westin T. Quality assessment of a multidisciplinary tumour meeting for patients with head and neck cancer. Acta Otolaryngol 2007;127(1):82–7.

15. Friedman E, Friedman C. Tumors of the head and neck. Int J Oral Surg 1978;7(4): 291–5.
16. Liao C-T, Kang C-J, Lee L-Y, et al. Association between multidisciplinary team care approach and survival rates in patients with oral cavity squamous cell carcinoma. Head Neck 2016;38(S1):E1544–53.
17. Kagan AR. The multidisciplinary clinic. Int J Radiat Oncol Biol Phys 2005;61(4): 967–8.
18. Davies AR, Deans DAC, Penman I, et al. The multidisciplinary team meeting improves staging accuracy and treatment selection for gastro-esophageal cancer. Dis Esophagus 2006;19(6):496–503.
19. Patil RD, Meinzen-Derr JK, Hendricks BL, et al. Improving access and timeliness of care for veterans with head and neck squamous cell carcinoma: a multidisciplinary team's approach. Laryngoscope 2015;126(3):627–31.
20. Shuman AG, Larkin K, Thomas D, et al. Patient Reflections on Decision Making for Laryngeal Cancer Treatment. Otolaryngol Head Neck Surg 2017;156(2):299–304.
21. Popescu RA, Schafer R, Califano R, et al. The current and future role of the medical oncologist in the professional care for cancer patients: a position paper by the European Society for Medical Oncology (ESMO). Ann Oncol 2013;25(1):9–15.
22. Delaney G, Jacob S, Featherstone C, et al. The role of radiotherapy in cancer treatment. Cancer 2005;104(6):1129–37.
23. Strojan P, Corry J, Eisbruch A, et al. Recurrent and second primary squamous cell carcinoma of the head and neck: when and how to reirradiate. Head Neck 2014; 37(1):134–50.
24. Eisbruch A, Dawson L. Re-irradiation of head and neck tumors. Hematol Oncol Clin North Am 1999;13(4):825–36.
25. Eisbruch A. Clinical aspects of IMRT for head-and-neck cancer. Med Dosim 2002;27(2):99–104.
26. David M, Eisbruch A. Delineating neck targets for intensity-modulated radiation therapy of head and neck cancer. Front Radiat Ther Oncol 2011;43:255–70.
27. David MB, Eisbruch A. Delineating neck targets for intensity-modulated radiation therapy of head and neck cancer. What we learned from marginal recurrences? Front Radiat Ther Oncol 2007;40:193–207.
28. Biagioli MC, Harvey M, Roman E, et al. Intensity-modulated radiotherapy with concurrent chemotherapy for previously irradiated, recurrent head and neck cancer. Int J Radiat Oncol Biol Phys 2007;69(4):1067–73.
29. Lee JY, Suresh K, Nguyen R, et al. Predictors of severe long-term toxicity after re-irradiation for head and neck cancer. Oral Oncol 2016;60:32–40.
30. Lee N, Chan K, Bekelman JE, et al. Salvage re-irradiation for recurrent head and neck cancer. Int J Radiat Oncol Biol Phys 2007;68(3):731–40.
31. Nagar YS. Chemo-reirradiation in persistent/recurrent head and neck cancers. Jpn J Clin Oncol 2004;34(2):61–8.
32. Corry J, Peters LJ, Costa ID, et al. The "QUAD SHOT"—a phase II study of palliative radiotherapy for incurable head and neck cancer. Radiother Oncol 2005; 77(2):137–42.
33. Fortin B, Khaouam N, Filion E, et al. Palliative radiation therapy for advanced head and neck carcinomas: a phase 2 study. Int J Radiat Oncol Biol Phys 2016;95(2):647–53.
34. Hodson D, Bruera E, Eapen L, et al. The role of palliative radiotherapy in advanced head and neck cancer. Can J Oncol 1996;6(Supp 1):54–60.
35. Kronz JD, Westra WH, Epstein JI. Mandatory second opinion surgical pathology at a large referral hospital. Cancer 1999;86(11):2426–35.

36. Westra WH, Kronz JD, Eisele DW. The impact of second opinion surgical pathology on the practice of head and neck surgery: a decade experience at a large referral hospital. Head Neck 2002;24(7):684–93.

37. Gillison ML. Human papillomavirus-associated head and neck cancer is a distinct epidemiologic, clinical, and molecular entity. Semin Oncol 2004;31(6):744–54.

38. Fakhry C, Westra WH, Li S, et al. Improved survival of patients with human papillomavirus-positive head and neck squamous cell carcinoma in a prospective clinical trial. J Natl Cancer Inst 2008;100(4):261–9.

39. Ang KK, Harris J, Wheeler R, et al. Human papillomavirus and survival of patients with oropharyngeal cancer. N Engl J Med 2010;363(1):24–35.

40. Bishop JA, Ma X-J, Wang H, et al. Detection of transcriptionally active high-risk HPV in patients with head and neck squamous cell carcinoma as visualized by a novel E6/E7 mRNA in situ hybridization method. Am J Surg Pathol 2012;36(12):1874–82.

41. Lysack JT, Hoy M, Hudon ME, et al. Impact of neuroradiologist second opinion on staging and management of head and neck cancer. J Otolaryngol Head Neck Surg 2013;42(1):39.

42. Loevner L, Sonners A, Schulman B, et al. Reinterpretation of cross-sectional images in patients with head and neck cancer in the setting of a multidisciplinary cancer center. AJNR Am J Neuroradiol 2002;23(10):1622–6.

43. Hatzoglou V, Omuro AM, Haque S, et al. Second-opinion interpretations of neuro-imaging studies by oncologic neuroradiologists can help reduce errors in cancer care. Cancer 2016;122(17):2708–14.

44. Michmerhuizen NL, Birkeland AC, Bradford CR, et al. Genetic determinants in head and neck squamous cell carcinoma and their influence on global personalized medicine. Genes Cancer 2016;7(5–6):182–200.

45. Walline HM, Komarck CM, McHugh JB, et al. Genomic integration of high-risk HPV alters gene expression in oropharyngeal squamous cell carcinoma. Mol Cancer Res 2016;14:941–52.

46. Plante DA, Piccirillo JF, Sofferman RA. Decision analysis of treatment options in pyriform sinus carcinoma. Med Decis Making 1987;7(2):74–83.

47. Davies L, Rhodes LA, Grossman DC, et al. Decision making in head and neck cancer care. Laryngoscope 2010;120(12):2434–45.

48. Dingman C, Hegedus PD, Likes C, et al. A coordinated, multidisciplinary approach to caring for the patient with head and neck cancer. J Support Oncol 2008;6:125–31.

49. Improving outcomes in head and neck cancers. National Institute for Clinical excellence. Available at: www.nice.org.uk. Accessed September 9, 2016.

50. Licitra L, Keilholz U, Tahara M, et al. Evaluation of the benefit and use of multidisciplinary teams in the treatment of head and neck cancer. Oral Oncol 2016;59:73–9.

51. Starmer H, Sanguineti G, Marur S, et al. Multidisciplinary head and neck cancer clinic and adherence with speech pathology. Laryngoscope 2011;121(10):2131–5.

52. Charles CA. Shared treatment decision making: what does it mean to physicians? J Clin Oncol 2003;21(5):932–6.

53. Leo F, Venissac N, Poudenx M, et al. Multidisciplinary management of lung cancer: how to test its efficacy? J Thorac Oncol 2007;2(1):69–72.

54. Petty JK, Vetto JT. Beyond doughnuts: tumor board recommendations influence patient care. J Cancer Educ 2002;17:97–100.

Head and Neck Cancer Pain

Jakun W. Ing, MD, MPH

KEYWORDS

- Head and neck cancer pain • Multimodal therapy • Opioid management
- Neuropathic pain • Mucositis • Acute postsurgical pain

KEY POINTS

- Head and neck cancer pain is multifactorial and patient care benefits from a multimodal approach.
- A strong understanding of pharmacotherapy is essential for management of cancer pain.
- Opioid therapy is a mainstay of head and neck cancer pain management, but the risks and benefits of this therapy should still be evaluated on a constant basis.
- Treatments, such as radiation therapy and surgery, may result in significant acute pain that should be managed aggressively to avoid significant decrease in quality of life and compliance with treatment regimens.

INTRODUCTION

Head and neck cancer, treated or untreated, can cause significant morbidity and mortality. Patients can experience severe impairments, both from the cancer and the treatments. Of all the causes of morbidity in head and neck cancer, however, pain is one of the most significant.[1–3]

Pain from head and neck cancer, as with other cancers, is generally the result of multiple generators.[4] One important source of pain is nociceptive pain, which is defined as pain from noxious stimuli.[5] Nociceptive pain may be further differentiated into somatic pain and visceral pain. Somatic pain is generally characterized as well-localized pain and is often described and sharp and throbbing. Visceral pain, caused by organ injury and mediated by the sympathetic nervous system, is often characterized as dull and difficult to localize. Visceral pain may also result in referred pain to other parts of the body. Another type of pain is inflammatory pain, caused by tissue injury, although some investigators consider this a type of nociceptive pain.[5] Also, bone pain may be a significant consequence of metastatic cancer, although its mechanism is unknown.[6]

Disclosure Statement: In accordance with UCLA policies and procedures and the author's ethical obligation as a researcher, the author is reporting that he has no financial conflicts of interest and has not received any additional funding sources.
University of California Los Angeles, Comprehensive Pain Center, 1245 16th Street, Suite 225, Santa Monica, CA 90404, USA
E-mail address: jing@mednet.ucla.edu

Otolaryngol Clin N Am 50 (2017) 793–806
http://dx.doi.org/10.1016/j.otc.2017.04.001
0030-6665/17/© 2017 Elsevier Inc. All rights reserved.

Neuropathic pain is defined as pain after neural injury.[5] Neuropathic pain may be a result of overt injury to large nerve structures, but it may also result from unseen damage to peripheral nerve structures. Neuropathic pain is often described as burning and tingling in nature. Head and neck cancer or its treatment may involve any number of cranial nerves or upper cervical nerves. Neuropathic pain often does not respond well to typical treatments for nociceptive pain and requires a different therapeutic modality.[7]

Pain in the head and neck cancer patient may be acute or chronic. Chronic pain is generally defined as pain lasting longer than 3 months.[8] A head and neck patient is most likely to suffer from episodes of acute pain overlying chronic pain throughout the duration of the illness.[9]

Pain may be the result of the primary tumor or from malignancy.[4,8,10] Pain may be the result of treatments of head and neck cancer.[10] Pain after treatment is generally multifactorial as well. Radiation therapy and chemotherapy, important first-line therapies for many head and neck cancers, may result in significant pain, with mucositis an important painful adverse effect.[11] Surgery clearly has the potential to cause significant acute and chronic pain.[12–14]

The World Health Organization (WHO) has established guidelines for the treatment of cancer pain.[15] These guidelines take the form of a 3-step tiered ladder, which emphasizes nonopioid treatment on the first tier, followed by more potent opioids in the second and third tiers (**Fig. 1**). The WHO established these guidelines as a method of treating cancer-related pain in a cost-effective and efficient manner.[16] Although the efficacy of these guidelines is contested, they still serve as a useful baseline for establishing treatment options for patients with head and neck cancer pain.[17]

PHARMACOTHERAPY

The mainstay of cancer pain treatment is pharmacotherapy. Given that cancer-related pain is multifactorial, it logically follows that patients may derive benefit from multimodal pharmacotherapy or the treatment of pain using medications from different classes and with different mechanisms of action.[18]

Any treatment of pain in a head and neck cancer patient must take into account the possibility that a patient may have difficulty with administration.[19] A patient's ability to swallow medication may be compromised by the cancer or the treatment. Radical surgery may result in significant structural abnormalities or the resection of important parts of the swallowing mechanism.[12] Some patients may only be able to have

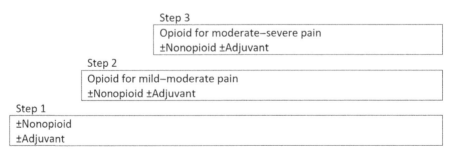

Fig. 1. World Health Organization 3-step ladder for cancer pain management. (*Adapted from* World Health Organization. The World Health Organization's cancer pain ladder for adults. Available at: http://www.who.int/cancer/palliative/painladder/en/. Accessed September 25, 2016; with permission.)

medications administered through a gastric tube. This, therefore, requires that enteral medications be crushed and may preclude the use of sustained-release medications.

OPIOIDS

Opioids are a mainstay of treatment of cancer-related nociceptive pain. Opioids are potent, versatile, and effective. They are available in many different formulations and modes of administration. The oral administration tends to be well tolerated and highly effective, although, as described previously, may not be suitable for all head and neck cancer patients.

Opioids act on mu (μ), delta (δ), and kappa (κ) receptors in the central and peripheral nervous system. Receptor binding, while resulting in analgesia, may also cause a host of undesired side effects, including nausea, vomiting, constipation, sedation, pruritus, and respiratory depression. Chronic opioid use may also result in tolerance, dependence, and hyperalgesia. A strong understanding of the pharmacology of these medications as well as their side effects is essential for safe opioid therapy. Some side effects, in particular constipation, should be treated aggressively because they can pose significant morbidity.

Opioid rotation is a viable option for maintaining analgesic efficacy.[20] This may be accomplished by changing the prescribed opioid as often as every several months. Due to a phenomenon known as incomplete cross-tolerance, a new drug should be dosed below the equianalgesic dose.[21,22] Equianalgesic doses are described in **Table 1**. If short-acting opioids do not provide sufficient duration of relief or a patient is requiring them around the clock, long-acting or sustained-release formulations should be considered.

There has been considerable recent scrutiny regarding opioid prescriptions in the United States. Although this is more applicable to treatment of noncancer pain, any provider must still be vigilant in monitoring for abuse and diversion of these medications and constantly weigh the benefits and risks of maintaining opioid therapy. Most states have online databases that track controlled medication prescriptions, and random urine screening is highly recommended.

Tramadol

Tramadol is a commonly prescribed analgesic that combines weak μ-receptor activity along with serotonin and norepinephrine reuptake inhibition. Given this activity, it may be an effective medication treating neuropathic pain.[17]

Table 1
Equianalgesic dosing of opioids

Drug	Equianalgesic Dose (mg)		Usual Starting Dose	
	Parenteral	Oral	Parenteral	Oral
Codeine	100–130	200	10 mg q3–4h	15–30 mg q4–12h
Hydrocodone	N/A	30–45	N/A	5–10 mg q4–6h
Hydromorphone	1.5	7.5	0.2 mg IV q2-3h	2 mg q4–8h
Morphine	10	30	2.5 mg q4h	10 mg q4h
Oxycodone	N/A	20–30	N/A	5 mg q4–6h

Data from Therapeutic Research Center. Equianalgesic dosing of opioids for pain management. Pharmacist's Letter/Prescriber's Letter. 2012. Available at: https://www.nhms.org/sites/default/files/Pdfs/Opioid-Comparison-Chart-Prescriber-Letter-2012.pdf. Accessed on September 25, 2016.

Providers should be aware that tramadol may interact with certain medications. One of the most significant interactions is serotonin syndrome, characterized by hyperpyrexia, hyperreflexia, tremor, agitation, and diarrhea. Tramadol should not be given to a patient taking monoamine oxidase inhibitors, and there is a theoretic risk with selective serotonin reuptake inhibitors as well.[8] Also, tramadol may lower seizure threshold and should be avoided in patients on antiepileptic medications.

Tramadol is a schedule IV medication and prescribers may call in this medication to the pharmacy. It is still advisable to assess patients in person prior to any refills, especially if there is a change in medication or dosing.

Codeine

Codeine is a widely used opioid and is often prescribed both as an analgesic and a cough expectorant. Codeine has weak μ-receptor activity compared with other opioids. Codeine is dependent on cytochrome P450 (CYP) 2D6 for conversion to its active metabolite, morphine. Genetic polymorphism of CYP2D6 or medications that interfere with CYP2D6's activity may explain its variable effect, especially among white patients.[5]

Codeine is available in multiple routes of administration, but the most commonly used form is in combination with acetaminophen. As with all compound drugs containing acetaminophen, the total amount of daily acetaminophen must be observed.

Morphine

Morphine is a powerful and versatile opioid that often serves as a basis of comparison for other opioids. Derived from opium, morphine is hydrophilic, which limits movement across the blood-brain barrier.[8]

Morphine is available in oral immediate-release and sustained-release formulations, and an elixir form is available as well. Morphine has limited oral bioavailability (approximately 33%) given first-pass metabolism.[17] It may also be given through suppository, intramuscular (IM), subcutaneous, intravenous (IV), epidural, or intrathecal administration. The IV route is commonly used in the hospital and provides greater potency and faster time of onset.

Morphine is metabolized through the glucuronidation pathway into morphine 3-glucuronide and morphine 6-glucuronide. These metabolites are excreted renally, so renal insufficiency or failure may result in metabolite accumulation.[23] In patients with renal failure, morphine should be substituted for a different opioid.

Hydrocodone

Hydrocodone is commonly prescribed in combination with acetaminophen. Hydrocodone by itself has weak analgesic effect. Hydrocodone is metabolized via CYP2D6 into hydromorphone, which is far more potent.[17] As with codeine, variable expression as well as interaction with medications can affect the potency of this medication.

Historically, of the most popular opioids prescribed, hydrocodone is now a schedule II medication and cannot be called into a pharmacy.

Oxycodone

Oxycodone is another commonly prescribed opioid. Oxycodone is available in oral immediate-release or sustained-release formulations, and it may be given in combination with acetaminophen. Oxycodone is not as potent as morphine but has superior oral bioavailability.[8]

Oxycodone is metabolized via CYP2D6 into oxymorphone, which is far more potent than oxycodone and is responsible for most of its overall analgesic effect.[17] As with hydrocodone and codeine, CYP2D6 activity may modify its analgesic effect.

Hydromorphone

Hydromorphone is a derivative of morphine. It is significantly more potent than morphine and has high oral bioavailability. Like morphine, it is highly versatile, with multiple formulations for different modes of administration. The parenteral form of hydromorphone is commonly used in the acute hospital setting. Oral and suppository formulations are also available. Sustained-release versions of hydromorphone are available but tend to be less accessible than similar versions of morphine.

Hydromorphone, like morphine, is metabolized via the glucuronidation pathway. Hydromorphone's chief metabolite, hydromorphone 3-glucuronide, however, is generally not highly active, and hydromorphone is a good choice for a patient with significant renal insufficiency.[8]

Fentanyl

Fentanyl is a potent opioid generally known for its rapid effect and short duration. It is far more potent than hydromorphone or morphine and must be dosed accordingly.

Fentanyl is available in many different formulations, but the most widely used versions are IV and transdermal. IV fentanyl is useful for acute pain associated with surgeries, but its potency and brief duration restrict its use to highly monitored settings, such as the postanesthesia care unit or the intensive care unit. Its rapid offset is due to redistribution and not due to short half-life.[8] In practice, fentanyl may accumulate over a period of time with continuous infusions, such as in the intensive care setting. IV fentanyl is generally not a good choice for the treatment of chronic pain.

Transdermal fentanyl, in contrast, is a sustained-release formulation and is often appropriate for the management of cancer pain.[24] Its effect depends on its ability to release fentanyl in the subcutaneous fat. Transdermal fentanyl, therefore, takes a fair amount of time for effect (at least 12 hours), whereas on removal of the patch, serum fentanyl levels fall to 50% at approximately 13 hours to 22 hours.[25] Like any other opioid, transdermal fentanyl has significant abuse potential and its use must be strictly monitored. Patients should avoid placement of heat or damage to the patch to prevent inadvertently increased release of the medication.[26]

Fentanyl has also been recently formulated into lollipops, lozenges, intranasal sprays, and other rapid-acting formulations. These medications, in effect, allow for breakthrough pain control outside the hospital. They are often significantly expensive and may be restricted to use with cancer pain only.

Methadone

Methadone is an effective, long-acting opioid for cancer pain,[27,28] and it is also commonly used in maintenance therapy for opioid addiction. It is not a sustained-release medication, however, and, therefore, behaves differently. Methadone has significant activity with multiple opioid receptors. Methadone is also an N-methyl-D-aspartate (NMDA) receptor antagonist, which may explain its effectiveness in treating neuropathic pain.[29]

Methadone has excellent oral bioavailability and a long half-life. Its analgesic duration is approximately 6 hours to 8 hours. Its elimination half-life, however, is much longer.[8] Therefore, methadone for cancer pain should be dosed 3 times a day, whereas it may be given only once daily for maintenance therapy for opioid addiction.

In addition to pill formulation, methadone is available as an elixir and may also be administered IV.

Methadone does not have any active metabolites, making it an ideal opioid for use with liver and renal failure. There is a risk for QT prolongation, however, and any patient on methadone therapy should have periodic ECGs to monitor QTc interval.

Tapentadol

Tapentadol is a newer opioid approved for acute pain by the Food and Drug Administration (FDA) in 2008. It combines μ-receptor activity along with norepinephrine reuptake inhibition. It is most often compared with tramadol but with much stronger μ-receptor activity and no serotonin activity. Like tramadol, its dual mechanism makes it useful for conditions, such as neuropathic pain. It does not seem to have the same risk of serotonin syndrome. Tapentadol is excreted renally and its safety in the setting of renal or hepatic failure has not been studied.[30]

NONSTEROIDAL ANTI-INFLAMMATORY DRUGS

Anti-inflammatories have been a mainstay of pain treatment for centuries, given their analgesic, antipyretic, and anti-inflammatory properties. **Table 2** lists suggested dosages for common nonsteroidal anti-inflammatory drugs (NSAIDs). NSAIDs exert their effect through peripheral inhibition of the cyclooxygenase (COX) enzyme, which then blocks the production of prostacyclin. COX-1 maintains platelet function and gastric mucosa, whereas COX-2 seems to play a role in the inflammatory response.[17]

NSAIDs may be a useful adjunct for the treatment of cancer-related pain.[31] NSAIDs are considered a first-step medication in this regard. NSAIDs may also have a role in multimodal therapy for more severe cancer-related pain.[31]

NSAIDs unfortunately cause a variety of side effects that may limit their use in the head and neck cancer population. NSAIDs are commonly associated with adverse gastrointestinal effects, including dyspepsia and peptic ulcer disease. These are likely the result of inhibition of prostaglandins, which maintain gastrointestinal mucosal lining.[8]

NSAIDs may cause renal insufficiency or even renal failure. The mechanism is likely the effect of renal vasoconstriction due to inhibition of prostaglandins, which normally

Table 2 Nonsteroidal anti-inflammatory drugs				
	Oral Analgesic Dose (mg)	Dose Interval (h)	Maximum Daily Dose (mg)	Comments
Aspirin	500–1000	4–6	4000	Rectal suppository available
Celecoxib	200–400	12–24	400	Only COX-2 selective on the US market
Ibuprofen	200–400	4–6	2400	Widely available
Ketorolac	30–60 (15–30 IV/IM)	6	150	IM/IV preparations available; limit to 5 d
Meloxicam	7.5–15	24	15	Highly selective for COX-2 compared to COX-1
Naproxen	250–500	6–8	1500	

Data from Waldman SD. Pain management. 2nd edition. Philadelphia: Elsevier; 2011. p. 887.

leads to renal vasodilation. Acute kidney injury is usually reversible after discontinuation of the NSAID and conservative therapy.[8]

NSAIDs may also cause platelet dysfunction through the inhibition of platelet COX-1 activity. Acetylsalicylic acid is an irreversible platelet inhibitor, suggesting at least 1 week of effect until new platelets are formed.[5] Other NSAIDs are reversible inhibitors and platelets may require less time to regain function.

All NSAIDs may increase the risk of adverse cardiac events, especially in patients with preexisting cardiac disease or multiple risk factors.[32,33] The US FDA now requires labeling that specifies the cardiac risk in all NSAIDs.

SELECTIVE CYCLOOXYGENASE 2 INHIBITORS

A majority of NSAIDs are nonselective. COX-2 inhibitors preferentially block COX-2 activity. Given the housekeeping function of COX-1, selective COX-2 inhibitors should theoretically have anti-inflammatory properties without some of the more damaging side effects of other NSAIDs.

COX-2 therapy compared with nonselective COX therapy seems associated with a reduction of gastroduodenal toxicity and platelet effect.[34] Selective COX-2 inhibitors, however, may still increase risk of renal failure[35] and adverse cardiac events.[36]

ACETAMINOPHEN

Acetaminophen is a widely used and versatile analgesic either taken separately or in combination with other medications, in particular opioids. It is available in different formulations and may be administered by oral, suppository, or IV formulations and is considered a step 1 medication on the WHO ladder.

Acetaminophen is an effective antipyretic and analgesic, but unlike NSAIDs, it has no anti-inflammatory property. Acetaminophen's mechanism is not clearly understood, but it is thought to act on central prostaglandin formation.[37]

Acetaminophen has few side effects or drug interactions, but its potential to cause hepatotoxicity is clearly an important issue. Acetaminophen is metabolized by the liver mainly by conjugation, but a small amount is metabolized by CYP into N-acetyl-p-benzoquinone imine (NAPQI). This metabolite may accumulate in high doses or preexisting liver failure and cause extensive liver damage. There seems to be no precise consensus for a safe maximum daily amount of acetaminophen,[38] with suggestions of 3 g to 4 g, and less in preexisting liver failure.

When administered with opioids, acetaminophen may have an opioid-sparing effect.[17] It is, therefore, commonly compounded with opioids, such as codeine, tramadol, hydrocodone, and oxycodone. Patients should be acutely aware of their total acetaminophen intake, including separately administered acetaminophen and any acetaminophen in compounded medications.

IV acetaminophen is an intriguing adjunct for acute cancer-related pain or perioperative pain or in circumstances where a patient cannot take enteral or suppository medications. IV acetaminophen has faster onset when compared with oral acetaminophen and seems to lack the effect of first-pass metabolism by the liver, increasing its safety profile.[39] The use of IV acetaminophen is limited by its high price and IV route of administration.

ANTICONVULSANTS

Certain anticonvulsant medications are effective for neuropathic pain. Gabapentin is the most widely used anticonvulsant for neuropathic pain given its efficacy, low cost, and side-effect profile. Gabapentin binds voltage-gated calcium channels, which decreases neuronal activity.

Gabapentin has few drug interactions but may cause side effects, such as dizziness, sedation, and weight gain. Gabapentin should usually be titrated slowly, and patients should ideally take the medication 3 times daily for full effect. Gabapentin is excreted renally, so its dose must be adjusted in renal failure (**Table 3**).

Pregabalin also binds voltage-gated calcium channels and has similar effect. Pregabalin may be titrated more quickly than gabapentin. Pregabalin has similar side effects to gabapentin. Pregabalin is excreted renally, so, as in gabapentin, its dose must be adjusted in renal failure (see **Table 3**). Pregabalin is also a schedule V controlled substance.

ANTIDEPRESSANTS

Certain antidepressant medications seem to have an impact on neuropathic pain and, therefore, are useful adjuncts in cancer pain management.

Tricyclic antidepressants (TCAs) inhibit serotonin and noradrenergic reuptake. They are cost effective and dosed once daily, unlike gabapentin or pregabalin. They are useful for a wide range of pain syndromes and may also have an opioid-sparing effect.[5]

TCAs inhibit serotonin and noradrenergic reuptake, but they may also have NMDA receptors antagonism as well as sodium channel blockade, increasing their effectiveness.[5] Analgesic dosing is typically lower than antidepressant dosing. They unfortunately have several side effects, the most significant including sedation, weight gain, and a host of anticholinergic effects (dry mouth, tachycardia, blurry vision, urinary retention, and confusion). They also increase the risk of arrhythmias.

Duloxetine is a serotonin-norepinephrine reuptake inhibitor and is approved to treat both pain and psychiatric conditions.[8] Major side effects include dry mouth, dizziness, nausea, and sedation. Duloxetine should be avoided in liver and renal failure.

SKELETAL MUSCLE RELAXANTS

Skeletal muscle relaxants belong to a broad category of medications with different pharmacologic mechanisms. **Table 4** suggests dosages for commonly used muscle relaxants. The mechanisms of these medications are generally not well understood but are thought to act via the central nervous system. Skeletal muscle relaxants are effective for myofascial pain and are often part of multimodal therapy for cancer-related pain.[40]

Baclofen is a γ-aminobutyric acid (GABA)-receptor agonist that inhibits excitatory neurotransmitter release and may also inhibit release of substance P. Baclofen is frequently used to treat spasticity. Baclofen can cause significant drowsiness. Abrupt discontinuation of baclofen can lead to withdrawal, and patients should be weaned off medication instead.[17]

Table 3 Adjustment of anticonvulsant dosage based on renal function				
Creatinine clearance	$\geq$60	30–59	15–29	<15
Gabapentin total daily dose (mg/d)	900–3600	400–1400	200–700	100–300
Pregabalin total daily dose (mg/d)	150–600	75–300	25–150	25–75

Data from Neurontin [package insert]. Parke-Davis (NY); 2010; and Lyrica [package insert]. Parke-Davis (NY); 2011.

Table 4
Skeletal muscle relaxants

Drug	Common Starting Dosage (mg)	Half-Life (h)	Side Effects
Baclofen	5 mg tid	5.5	Drowsiness, hypotension, constipation, urinary retention
Carisoprodol	350 mg po QID	2.4	Drowsiness, nausea/vomiting, dizziness, ataxia; withdrawal potential
Cyclobenzaprine	5 mg daily	18	Drowsiness, dizziness, dry mouth, headache, diarrhea, constipation
Methocarbamol	750 mg po qid	1–2	Dizziness, blurred vision, drowsiness, nausea, headache
Tizanidine	2 mg qid	2.5	Drowsiness, dry mouth, dizziness, hypotension, constipation

Data from Benzon H, Raja SN, Fishman SE, et al. Essentials of pain medicine. Philadelphia: Elsevier; 2011. p. 144.

Carisoprodol is a central-acting muscle relaxant that may inhibit the descending reticular activating system. It unfortunately has significant potential for dependence, and the other muscle relaxants are generally better choices.

Cyclobenzaprine is structurally similar to TCAs and seems to block descending serotonergic pathways in the spinal cord.[17] It may cause significant sedation and anticholinergic side effects similar to the TCAs.

Methocarbamol is a central-acting muscle relaxant. It may be administered in either oral or IV formulation. The oral formulation seems well tolerated in hepatic or renal failure, although the IV formulation should be avoided in renal failure due to the addition of polyethylene glycol.[41] Side effects include drowsiness, nausea, and headache.

Tizanidine is an α_2-adrenergic receptor agonist. Tizanidine may be used to treat spasticity. Side effects include sedation and hypotension.

PROCEDURES

Interventional pain procedures may be useful adjuncts to complement pharmacologic therapy for head and neck cancer pain. Procedures may help decrease opioid intake or offer an alternative treatment of pain resistant to pharmacologic therapy.

Nerve blocks may be considered if a patient seems to be suffering from pain related to a specific nerve, such as the trigeminal nerve or glossopharyngeal nerve.[40] Should a nerve block be successful, a neurolytic block may offer extended relief. Neurolytic blocks may be indicated with severe pain persisting with less invasive techniques, although benefits must be weighed against the risks of serious complications, such as profound loss of motor control.[5]

Sympathectomy may be considered for visceral pain associated with head and neck cancer. A stellate ganglion block may be the most suitable sympathetic block for a head and neck cancer patient, given the general location of the lesions. Other sympathetic blocks may be appropriate, however, for malignant growths in other parts of the body. A celiac plexus block, for example, may be used for metastasis into the abdominal cavity.

Certain patients may be candidates for intrathecal pump implantation, which allows for constant administration of intrathecal opioid by itself or in combination with other adjunct pain medications. A good candidate for intrathecal therapy should have at least a 3-month life expectancy and have pain intractable to more conservative therapies or difficulty with oral opioid intake, whether due to dysphagia, gastric tube requirement, or severe nausea.[8]

COMPLEMENTARY AND ALTERNATIVE MEDICINE

Complementary and alternative medicine has not been well studied in the head and neck cancer population but may provide alternatives for patients looking for nonpharmacologic therapies.[42] Modalities vary widely, and treatments are often not covered by insurance.

Psychotherapy may offer coping strategies and mechanisms for patients afflicted by cancer-related pain through insight-oriented therapy or behavior therapy.[5] Cognitive behavior therapy relies on identification and modification of behaviors that may be contributing to the patient's overall pain. Biofeedback is another approach that trains patients to control physiologic processes. Other modalities include hypnosis and meditation.

Acupuncture, well-known to Eastern medicine, is another popular medicinal methodology that may be used for this population.[40] Acupuncture involves the stimulation of well-established points, known as meridians, using very fine needles, which may result in symptom relief (pain, nausea, anxiety, and so forth). Acupressure may be used to stimulate the same meridians without needles and can be performed by patients at home.

PAIN SECONDARY TO TREATMENT

Not surprisingly, many treatments for head and neck cancer result in significant pain. Pain from these conditions may dramatically interfere with quality of life and decrease compliance with treatment and, therefore, should be treated aggressively.[43]

Radiation Therapy and Mucositis

Radiation therapy results in acute and long-term complications, including significant pain.[44,45] Pain from radiation therapy usually escalates around the third week of treatment and persists for weeks.[46] Radiation therapy may also result in mucositis, discussed later, as well as odynophagia and dysphagia, which may lower quality of life and compliance with treatment.[44]

Radiation therapy seems to cause pain through damage of normal tissues, resulting in inflammation, epithelial thinning, and ulceration.[47] There is often a strong neuropathic component in addition to nociceptive pain,[48] which suggests that robust multimodal therapy must include neuropathic pain medications, such as gabapentin.

Mucositis is a well-known condition associated with the treatment of head and neck cancer and may challenge practitioners already treating a patient's chronic pain related to head and neck cancer. It is characterized by painful lesions in the oropharynx and is most common when chemotherapy is combined with radiation therapy.[49] Mucositis not only impairs quality of life by impairing activities of daily living, such as eating and drinking, but also may increase the risk of hospitalization and interrupt or otherwise decrease compliance with the treatment regimen.[50] Pain with swallowing may also limit the types of medications that can be administered.

Mucositis may be best treated with IV opioids via PCA until it resolves or improves. Patients may also obtain relief from transdermal fentanyl.[51] As the lesions heal and improve, patients may be able to tolerate oral pain medications as well. Like other cancer-related pain, a multimodal regimen may be preferable to single drug therapy. Neuropathic pain medications, such as gabapentin and pregabalin, may prove

| Table 5 | | |
| Suggested starting dosages for patient-controlled analgesia | | |
Drug	Demand (Bolus) Dose	Lockout Time (min)
Hydromorphone	2–3 μg/kg	5–15
Morphine	0.01–0.02 mg/kg	5–15

Data from Benzon H, Raja SN, Fishman SE, et al. Essentials of pain medicine. Philadelphia: Elsevier; 2011. p. 241.

beneficial.[52] Viscous lidocaine may be used as a topical analgesic, although it has been associated with systemic toxicity and may impair gag reflex as well as taste sensation.[40]

Postsurgical Pain

Postsurgical pain in head and neck cancer patients may be challenging to manage. Many of these patients are already on significant amounts of opioid, increasing the risk of hyperalgesia. Postsurgical pain also has multiple sources, not only from tissue damage and inflammation but also from nerve damage.[53] Postsurgical pain may also be worsened by common activities, such as talking and swallowing.

As with other cancer-related pain, aggressive multimodal therapy may be necessary after surgery.[43] Opioid therapy is generally necessary, and an increase from the patients' baseline regimen may be required. Resumption of enteral pain medications is recommended as soon as possible, although patients may benefit from a short course of IV opioid via PCA until the pain is better controlled.[13] **Table 5** suggests starting setting for the PCA. Practitioners should avoid basal infusions to minimize the risk of overmedication with the PCA.

For patients who cannot take oral medications postoperatively due to surgical changes, practitioners may administer opioid elixirs through the gastric tube. Most sustained-release opioid formulations cannot be administered through this route, although patients with a previous sustained-release opioid requirement may be transitioned to a fentanyl patch or methadone. Suppository formulations are also available although many patients understandably are reluctant to consider this route.

Multimodal adjuncts may include gabapentin, acetaminophen, muscle relaxants, and NSAIDs. Gabapentin and pregabalin may be useful in the preoperative setting for decreasing postoperative pain and, therefore, should be considered for any head and neck cancer patient about to undergo surgery.[54] Acetaminophen may be an effective adjunct, especially in the IV formulation, as described previously, although enteral formulations may still provide an opioid-sparing effect. NSAIDs are potentially effective for postsurgical pain,[13] although most surgeons are reluctant to administer NSAIDs in the postsurgical setting due to increased risk of bleeding.

For patients already on chronic high-dose opioids, ketamine may be a reasonable addition to multimodal therapy. Ketamine is an NMDA receptor antagonist that serves as a dissociative anesthetic at high doses but seems to have analgesic properties and an opioid-sparing effect at low-dose infusions as well.[8] Ketamine use should be directed by an experienced pain management provider.

SUMMARY

Chronic pain in head and neck cancer patients is a difficult medical condition with significant implications to a patient's overall health and quality of life. The treatment of this pain may require a specific plan tailored to individuals, with the understanding that head and neck cancer is a dynamic process that may cause a patient's pain to vary dramatically from one moment to another.

Any practitioner caring for a head and neck cancer patient should be familiar with all the treatment options available for pain management, including multiple classes of pain medications, each of which may have a role in the alleviation a patient's pain, with full understanding of the limitations of side effects of all these medications and including multidisciplinary therapy as appropriate. Practitioners should not hesitate to consult with pain management colleagues regarding the management of these patients, especially if a patient requires significant escalation of medications or the practitioner anticipates a major upcoming event that may cause acute-on-chronic pain.

REFERENCES

1. Carrillo JF, Carrillo LC, Ramirez-Ortega MC, et al. The impact of treatment on quality of life of patients with head and neck cancer and its association with prognosis. Eur J Surg Oncol 2016;42(10):1614–21.
2. Chua KS, Reddy SK, Lee MC, et al. Pain and loss of function in head and neck cancer survivors. J Pain Symptom Manage 1999;18(3):193–202.
3. Funk GF, Karnell LH, Christensen AJ. Long-term health-related quality of life in survivors of head and neck cancer. Arch Otolaryngol Head Neck Surg 2012; 138(2):123–33.
4. Benoliel R, Epstein J, Eliav E, et al. Orofacial pain in cancer: part I–mechanisms. J Dent Res 2007;86(6):491–505.
5. Benzon HT, Rathmell JP, Turk DC, et al. Raj's practical management of pain. 4th edition. Philadelphia: Elsevier Health Services; 2008.
6. Rosier R. Bone pain. Am J Hosp Palliat Care 1992;9(6):37.
7. Kanner R. Diagnosis and management of neuropathic pain in patients with cancer. Cancer Invest 2001;19(3):324–33.
8. Benzon H, Raja SN, Fishman SE, et al. Essentials of pain medicine. Philadelphia: Elsevier Health Sciences; 2011.
9. Chaplin JM, Morton RP. A prospective, longitudinal study of pain in head and neck cancer patients. Head Neck 1999;21(6):531–7.
10. Chen SC, Liao CT, Chang JT. Orofacial pain and predictors in oral squamous cell carcinoma patients receiving treatment. Oral Oncol 2011;47(2):131–5.
11. Trotti A, Bellm LA, Epstein JB, et al. Mucositis incidence, severity and associated outcomes in patients with head and neck cancer receiving radiotherapy with or without chemotherapy: a systematic literature review. Radiother Oncol 2003; 66(3):253–62.
12. Gellrich NC, Schimming R, Schramm A, et al. Pain, function, and psychologic outcome before, during, and after intraoral tumor resection. J Oral Maxillofac Surg 2002;60(7):772–7.
13. Gil Z, Smith DB, Marouani N, et al. Treatment of pain after head and neck surgeries: control of acute pain after head and neck oncological surgeries. Otolaryngol Head Neck Surg 2006;135(2):182–8.
14. Inhestern J, Schuerer J, Illge C, et al. Pain on the first postoperative day after head and neck cancer surgery. Eur Arch Otorhinolaryngol 2015;272(11):3401–9.
15. World Health Organization's cancer pain ladder for adults. Available at: http://www.who.int/cancer/palliative/painladder/en/. Accessed September 25, 2016.
16. Meuser T, Pietruck C, Radbruch L, et al. Symptoms during cancer pain treatment following WHO-guidelines: a longitudinal follow-up study of symptom prevalence, severity and etiology. Pain 2001;93(3):247–57.

17. Waldman SD. Pain management. 2nd edition. Philadelphia: Elsevier Health Sciences; 2011.
18. Olsen KD, Creagan ET. Pain management in advanced carcinoma of the head and neck. Am J Otol 1991;12(3):154–60.
19. Modi BJ, Knab B, Feldman LE, et al. Review of current treatment practices for carcinoma of the head and neck. Expert Opin Pharmacother 2005;6(7):1143–55.
20. Bruera E, Pereira J, Watanabe S, et al. Opioid rotation in patients with cancer pain. A retrospective comparison of dose ratios between methadone, hydromorphone, and morphine. Cancer 1996;78(4):852–7.
21. Barnett M. Alternative opioids to morphine in palliative care: a review of current practice and evidence. Postgrad Med J 2001;77(908):371–8.
22. Mercadante S, Bruera E. Opioid switching: a systematic and critical review. Cancer Treat Rev 2006;32(4):304–15.
23. Penson RT, Joel SP, Gloyne A, et al. Morphine analgesia in cancer pain: role of the glucuronides. J Opioid Manag 2005;1(2):83–90.
24. Muijsers RB, Wagstaff AJ. Transdermal fentanyl: an updated review of its pharmacological properties and therapeutic efficacy in chronic cancer pain control. Drugs 2001;61(15):2289–307.
25. Duragesic(R) [package insert]. Janssen Pharmaceutica Products, L.P. Titusville (NJ). 2003. Available at: https://www.accessdata.fda.gov/drugsatfda_docs/label/2005/19813s039lbl.pdf. Accessed September 25, 2016.
26. FDA Patient Safety News. Preventing Patient Deaths from Fentanyl Patches. 2007. Available at: http://www.fda.gov/downloads/safety/fdapatientsafetynews/ucm417877.pdf. Accessed September 25, 2016.
27. Nicholson AB. Methadone for cancer pain. Cochrane Database Syst Rev 2007;(4):CD003971.
28. Mercadante S, Porzio G, Ferrera P, et al. Sustained-release oral morphine versus transdermal fentanyl and oral methadone in cancer pain management. Eur J pain 2008;12(8):1040–6.
29. Haumann J, Geurts JW, van Kuijk SM, et al. Methadone is superior to fentanyl in treating neuropathic pain in patients with head-and-neck cancer. Eur J Cancer 2016;65:121–9.
30. Nucynta(R) [package insert]. Janssen Ortho, LLC. Gurabo (PR). 2010. Available at: http://www.accessdata.fda.gov/drugsatfda_docs/label/2010/022304s003lbl.pdf. Accessed September 25, 2016.
31. McNicol E, Strassels S, Goudas L, et al. Nonsteroidal anti-inflammatory drugs, alone or combined with opioids, for cancer pain: a systematic review. J Clin Oncol 2004;22(10):1975–92.
32. Schjerning Olsen AM, Fosbol EL, Lindhardsen J, et al. Duration of treatment with nonsteroidal anti-inflammatory drugs and impact on risk of death and recurrent myocardial infarction in patients with prior myocardial infarction: a nationwide cohort study. Circulation 2011;123(20):2226–35.
33. Ray WA, Varas-Lorenzo C, Chung CP, et al. Cardiovascular risks of nonsteroidal antiinflammatory drugs in patients after hospitalization for serious coronary heart disease. Circ Cardiovasc Qual Outcomes 2009;2(3):155–63.
34. Simon LS, Weaver AL, Graham DY, et al. Anti-inflammatory and upper gastrointestinal effects of celecoxib in rheumatoid arthritis: a randomized controlled trial. JAMA 1999;282(20):1921–8.
35. Perazella MA, Tray K. Selective cyclooxygenase-2 inhibitors: a pattern of nephrotoxicity similar to traditional nonsteroidal anti-inflammatory drugs. Am J Med 2001;111(1):64–7.

36. White WB, Faich G, Borer JS, et al. Cardiovascular thrombotic events in arthritis trials of the cyclooxygenase-2 inhibitor celecoxib. Am J Cardiol 2003;92(4):411–8.
37. Lucas R, Warner TD, Vojnovic I, et al. Cellular mechanisms of acetaminophen: role of cyclo-oxygenase. FASEB J 2005;19(6):635–7.
38. Chandok N, Watt KD. Pain management in the cirrhotic patient: the clinical challenge. Mayo Clin Proc 2010;85(5):451–8.
39. Jahr JS, Lee VK. Intravenous acetaminophen. Anesthesiol Clin 2010;28(4):619–45.
40. Epstein JB, Schubert MM. Management of orofacial pain in cancer patients. Eur J Cancer B Oral Oncol 1993;29b(4):243–50.
41. Robaxin(R) [package insert]. Baxter Healthcare Corporation. 2003. http://www.accessdata.fda.gov/drugsatfda_docs/label/2004/11790slr046_robaxin_lbl.pdf. Accessed September 25, 2016.
42. Pan CX, Morrison RS, Ness J, et al. Complementary and alternative medicine in the management of pain, dyspnea, and nausea and vomiting near the end of life. A systematic review. J Pain Symptom Manage 2000;20(5):374–87.
43. Bianchini C, Malago M, Crema L, et al. Post-operative pain management in head and neck cancer patients: predictive factors and efficacy of therapy. Acta Otorhinolaryngol Ital 2016;36(2):91–6.
44. Chang JT, Lin CY, Lin JC, et al. Transdermal fentanyl for pain caused by radiotherapy in head and neck cancer patients treated in an outpatient setting: a multicenter trial in Taiwan. Jpn J Clin Oncol 2010;40(4):307–12.
45. Meyer F, Fortin A, Gelinas M, et al. Health-related quality of life as a survival predictor for patients with localized head and neck cancer treated with radiation therapy. J Clin Oncol 2009;27(18):2970–6.
46. Epstein JB, Elad S, Eliav E, et al. Orofacial pain in cancer: part II–clinical perspectives and management. J Dent Res 2007;86(6):506–18.
47. Epstein JB, Stewart KH. Radiation therapy and pain in patients with head and neck cancer. Eur J Cancer B Oral Oncol 1993;29b(3):191–9.
48. Epstein JB, Wilkie DJ, Fischer DJ, et al. Neuropathic and nociceptive pain in head and neck cancer patients receiving radiation therapy. Head Neck Oncol 2009;1:26.
49. Elting LS, Keefe DM, Sonis ST, et al. Patient-reported measurements of oral mucositis in head and neck cancer patients treated with radiotherapy with or without chemotherapy: demonstration of increased frequency, severity, resistance to palliation, and impact on quality of life. Cancer 2008;113(10):2704–13.
50. Alfieri S, Ripamonti CI, Marceglia S, et al. Temporal course and predictive factors of analgesic opioid requirement for chemoradiation-induced oral mucositis in oropharyngeal cancer. Head Neck 2016;38(Suppl 1):E1521–7.
51. Cai Q, Huang H, Sun X, et al. Efficacy and safety of transdermal fentanyl for treatment of oral mucositis pain caused by chemotherapy. Expert Opin Pharmacother 2008;9(18):3137–44.
52. Epstein JB, Schubert MM. Oropharyngeal mucositis in cancer therapy. Review of pathogenesis, diagnosis, and management. Oncology (Williston Park, NY) 2003; 17(12):1767–79 [discussion: 1779–82, 1791–2].
53. Hoppenfeld JD. Fundamentals of pain medicine: how to diagnose and treat your patients. Philadelphia: Wolters Kluwer Health; 2014.
54. de Wit R, van Dam F, Loonstra S, et al. The Amsterdam Pain Management Index compared to eight frequently used outcome measures to evaluate the adequacy of pain treatment in cancer patients with chronic pain. Pain 2001;91(3):339–49.

Psychosocial Distress and Distress Screening in Multidisciplinary Head and Neck Cancer Treatment

Charlene Williams, PhD

KEYWORDS

- Psychosocial distress screening • Depression • Anxiety • Head and neck cancer
- Multidisciplinary • Quality of life (QOL) • Cognitive behavioral therapy (CBT)
- Behavioral medicine • Patient-centered

KEY POINTS

- Psychosocial distress is an important indicator of suffering, and a risk factor for negative psychological, quality-of-life, and medical outcomes.
- Patients with head and neck cancer (HNC) evidence high rates of psychosocial distress, yet distress is often not recognized in oncology treatment settings.
- Although untreated distress is associated with negative psychological and medical outcomes, distress is highly responsive to treatment, with resultant improvements in psychosocial and medical outcomes.
- Screening and referral for psychosocial distress is rapidly becoming the standard of care, and is now required of cancer centers to retain accreditation with the American College of Surgeons. Distress screening guidelines are available to help HNC centers implement effective psychosocial distress screening programs.
- Multidisciplinary HNC treatment can provide a solid foundation from which to implement psychosocial distress screening clinical intervention and research. Integrative cognitive behavioral (CBT)-behavioral medicine intervention may be of particular benefit in this population.

INTRODUCTION

Multidisciplinary cancer care involves assessment, diagnosis, and treatment of the significant variables impacting patients' health and well-being. Traditionally, the field of medicine and head and neck cancer (HNC) treatment has focused on diagnosis and treatment of physical symptoms and disorders to the exclusion of psychological

Disclosure Statement: The author has nothing to disclose.
UCLA Department of Head and Neck Surgery, Head and Neck Cancer Program, 200 UCLA Medical Plaza, Suite 550, Los Angeles, CA 90095-6959, USA
E-mail address: cwilliams@mednet.ucla.edu

Otolaryngol Clin N Am 50 (2017) 807–823
http://dx.doi.org/10.1016/j.otc.2017.04.002
0030-6665/17/© 2017 Elsevier Inc. All rights reserved.

oto.theclinics.com

variables. This paradigm led to cancer treatment that may be described as reductionist (or mechanistic), treating patients as physical "cases," rather than whole persons who experience physical and psychological responses to cancer and cancer treatment.

As cancer and HNC treatment has evolved, the field has progressed toward what is referred to as "whole-patient" or "patient-centered" care. Fundamental to this shift is the increasing recognition of psychosocial factors and psychological well-being as inherently important aspects of patients' health, in addition to their impact on quality-of-life (QOL) and medical outcomes. Accordingly, HNC research has increasingly included a focus on QOL outcomes, concurrent with the development of surgical procedures designed to maximize organ and functional preservation and improve cosmesis, as well as de-intensification of radiation treatment protocols. However, routine inclusion of psychosocial assessment and intervention into HNC treatment has lagged behind, largely due to the mismatch between busy HNC settings and obstacles to implementation (perceived time burden, incomplete understanding of negative impacts of psychosocial variables, medical/HNC subculture norms).

Psychosocial distress screening (DS) originated as an effort to legitimize and facilitate the recognition, measurement, and treatment of psychosocial aspects of cancer care. This early work led to the creation of a concise DS instrument, the Distress Thermometer (DT), that could be rapidly administered, and would therefore be likely to be used in busy oncology settings.[1,2]

Patients with HNC experience significantly elevated rates of psychosocial distress, with 20% to 60% reporting distress at various points throughout the treatment trajectory.[3–5] Despite the high frequency of clinically significant distress in oncology patients, medical professionals frequently fail to recognize distress in their patients.[6] This is particularly concerning in that although distress is very responsive to treatment, untreated distress is associated with significantly worse psychosocial and medical outcomes.[3,7]

To address these concerns, routine DS and appropriate referral of all patients with cancer is now considered the standard of care by the American College of Surgeons (ACoS) Commission on Cancer,[8] the National Comprehensive Cancer Network[9] (NCCN), and the Institute of Medicine.[10] In accord with this position, DS and referral have been required of cancer centers since 2015 to maintain accreditation with the ACoS. To facilitate the adoption of DS programs, the ACoS, NCCN, American Psychosocial Oncology Society, and other major psycho-oncology professional associations have published standards and guidelines for implementation.[3,8,11–13]

In this article, the characteristics and impacts of psychosocial distress in patients with HNC are examined and guidelines for HNC DS programs are presented. Successful implementation requires understanding the essential components of DS, common challenges, and effective strategies needed to initiate and sustain DS programs. Multidisciplinary HNC treatment that includes a psychosocial component can provide an ideal foundation for the implementation of DS, and facilitate integrative HNC treatment and research that serves the whole patient.

PSYCHOSOCIAL DISTRESS

Psychosocial distress is defined by the NCCN as an "unpleasant emotional experience of a psychological (cognitive, behavioral, emotional), social, and/or spiritual nature that may interfere with the ability to cope with cancer, its physical symptoms and its treatment."[14(p6)] Although distress shares significant overlap with depression, anxiety, and other psychosocial symptomatology, the term was designed to be broadly inclusive rather than diagnostic, readily understandable to patients and medical staff, and relatively free of the stigma associated with psychiatric labels or diagnoses.

Early workers in DS strove to create a measure that would be familiar to patients and medical professionals, and brief enough to be routinely implemented into busy oncology practices.[2] This effort resulted in the Distress Thermometer (DT),[1] a combined visual analogue/numerical rating scale modeled after the well-known pain scale (with pain rated 0–10).[15] The DT reflects the conceptualization of psychosocial distress as an indicator of suffering, with distress referred to as "the sixth vital sign" (in addition to pulse, respiration, blood pressure, temperature, and pain).[2,16]

The DT continues to be one of the most widely used self-report measures of psychosocial distress, although distress is also frequently assessed by other self-report questionnaires measuring anxiety and depressive symptoms that yield, or are viewed as, proximal measures of distress (Hospital Anxiety and Depression Scale [HADS][17]; Brief Symptom Inventory-18 [BSI-18][18]).[3,12,13,19]

CHARACTERISTICS OF PSYCHOSOCIAL DISTRESS IN PATIENTS WITH HEAD AND NECK CANCER
Distress Rates in Patients with Head and Neck Cancer

Patients with HNC demonstrate significantly heightened rates of psychological distress, ranging from 20% to 60%,[4,20–23] with elevations noted when patients undergo treatments with significant side effects (surgery, radiation, chemoradiation), and associated with functional losses, particularly impairments in swallowing or speaking,[24–27] as well as disfigurement, fatigue, and pain.[28–31] Additional risk factors for distress in patients with HNC include pretreatment mental status (depression, distress),[20,32,33] lack of perceived social support,[34–36] smoking and alcohol use disorders,[37–39] and avoidant coping.[40–44]

In addition to distress, patients with HNC also evidence among the highest rates of depression compared with other cancer populations, as well as significantly elevated rates of anxiety.[21,45–47] Although levels of distress, depression, and anxiety diminish for most patients after conclusion of treatment, a substantial proportion of patients with HNC continue to demonstrate heightened rates of psychosocial distress and depression even long after treatment has ended.[29,48] Of significant concern, patients with HNC are at markedly elevated risk of suicide, with a suicide rate 4 times that of the general population, and one of the highest suicide rates of all cancer populations.[49–52]

Head and Neck Cancer Distress Rates: Functional Losses and Tumor Site

Among patients with HNC, certain subgroups are at significantly greater risk of psychological impacts, including severe distress, clinical depression, and suicide.[45,49–52] These subpopulations can be identified by functional losses and/or by tumor site. It is well known that distress and related negative psychological impacts are significantly greater in HNC patients in whom the function of swallowing is impaired.[24,25,53] Patients who are likely to experience these functional losses typically have head and neck cancers of the upper aerodigestive tract (eg, oropharyngeal, hypopharyngeal). In addition, speech impairment or loss is strongly predictive of distress and negative psychological outcomes in patients with HNC.[26,27]

Recent research has found that HNC patients with upper aerodigestive tract cancer have a significantly elevated risk of suicide compared with other HNC patients, and patients with cancer overall. Specifically, Kam and colleagues[49] found that patients with hypopharyngeal, laryngeal, oropharyngeal and oral cavity, and nasopharyngeal cancers are at markedly greater risk of suicide. Disturbingly, incidence of suicide was increased 12-fold in patients with hypopharyngeal cancer and 5-fold in patients with laryngeal cancer.[49]

Distress Through the Treatment Trajectory

The nature of distress throughout the treatment trajectory can vary dependent on a number of factors, including treatment modality and morbidity. HNC treatment is often multimodal, with patients frequently undergoing sequential and/or combined treatment modalities (surgery, radiation, chemotherapy, and immunotherapy). Some combined treatment regimens, such as chemoradiation, can result in significantly greater side effects and aftereffects (eg, swallowing and eating difficulties, nutritional deficits, distress, and depression).

The components of distress (anxiety and depression) tend to vary throughout the arc of treatment. Typically, higher rates of anxiety are observed at or near the beginning of treatment, or when shifting to a new treatment mode. The incidence of anxiety typically decreases as patients progress through treatment and immediately after completing treatment.[54,55] However, some reports indicate the incidence of anxiety may increase long after treatment has ended.[56]

In contrast, the incidence of depressive symptoms appears to increase as patients move into and through the active phase of HNC treatment, as they experience increasing side effects and morbidity due to treatment and/or the cancer itself.[4,45] Although the incidence of depression is found to typically decrease after treatment has been completed, a significant proportion of patients with HNC evidence heightened levels of depressive symptoms long after treatment has ended, particularly when patients must contend with enduring deficits in swallowing, speech, disfigurement, and related social withdrawal and isolation.[26,27,29,48,53,57]

PSYCHOLOGICAL AND MEDICAL OUTCOMES OF DISTRESS IN PATIENTS WITH HEAD AND NECK CANCER

Psychosocial distress has been found to be associated with significantly worse psychological and medical outcomes. When studied prospectively, psychosocial distress at baseline, or at the beginning of HNC treatment, is predictive of heightened distress at later time points.[4,32,56,58] In addition, psychosocial distress has been found to be both associated with, and a predictor of, depression, anxiety, and lower QOL in patients with HNC throughout the treatment trajectory.[27,56,58,59]

In addition to impacting psychological variables, psychosocial distress has been found to predict multiple negative medical outcomes, including negative health-related behaviors, delays in seeking treatment, poor treatment adherence, and survival.[37,44,60,61] Further, in a recent study of patients with HNC, Aarstad and colleagues[7] found that psychosocial distress was an independent predictor of survival, even after statistically controlling for multiple factors (eg, physical morbidities, smoking and alcohol use).

PSYCHOSOCIAL DISTRESS SCREENING: GUIDELINES AND CHALLENGES

Given the high rate of psychosocial distress in patients with HNC, the multiple, often severe negative outcomes of untreated distress, and the fact that distress is highly responsive to treatment, it is increasingly evident that the inclusion of DS in HNC treatment comprises an essential component of best practice. Successful implementation of an effective DS program is a challenging task for any HNC center, and is greatly facilitated by using the criteria and guidelines established by key medical and oncology organizations.[8,9,11–13] Crucial guidance regarding challenges faced by

Table 1	
Head and neck cancer psychosocial distress screening programs: required components	
1. Establish multidisciplinary cancer committee	• Should include all disciplines, including head and neck cancer physician • Must include psychosocial representation
2. Screening	• Validated distress measure assessing ≥2 areas of distress ○ Recommended: include depression measure • Sensitivity and specificity of distress measure must be adequate • Administered at ≥1 pivotal visit
3. Follow-up assessment/ evaluation	• Establish algorithm for distress screening follow-up ○ Use established distress cutoff scores ○ Follow-up with validated depression and anxiety measures, clinical interview
4. Referral/treatment and follow-up	• Referral for psychosocial intervention • Follow-up with patient, oncology team, and family caregivers (as appropriate)
5. Documentation	• Documentation of distress screening results, further assessment, referrals/treatment, and follow-up • Can be used for quality assurance and research

oncology centers in implementing DS may be found in excellent "lessons learned" articles that describe common obstacles and effective strategies to facilitate DS.[3,62] Core components of DS implementation for HNC centers are outlined in the next section and in **Table 1**.

IMPLEMENTING BEST PRACTICE HEAD AND NECK CANCER PSYCHOSOCIAL DISTRESS SCREENING: PROACTIVELY MEETING CHALLENGES AND AVOIDING PITFALLS
Establish Multidisciplinary Head and Neck Cancer Distress Screening Committee

The first step in initiating HNC DS programs is to establish a multidisciplinary HNC committee with representation from all stakeholders (surgery, radiation, and medical oncology physicians, mental health professionals, HNC specialist providers such as swallowing/speech therapists and maxillofacial prosthodontics, nurses, and key administrative personnel). Inclusion of psychosocial representation is mandatory. Consistent with a patient-centered approach, an important point made in the literature is the recommendation to systematically include patient feedback as DS is implemented, so as to more completely include input from all stakeholders.[11,12,62]

Using a multidisciplinary approach in formulating, refining, and further development of HNC distress screening facilitates implementation of an effective DS program tailored to the needs and concerns of all stakeholders. Further, this increases buy-in and avoids the potential pitfalls of staff overload, resentment, and burnout. Communication with, and inclusion of, higher-level administrators of the medical/HNC center in the development and implementation of the DS program is essential to its success, and serves to proactively develop support for the resources needed, and results obtained.

Guidelines for implementation of DS increasingly emphasize the necessity of prioritizing development of the referral/treatment component.[11,12,62] Only when screening for distress is combined with appropriate referral and treatment are patients' psychological and medical outcomes improved.[3,11,63] It is strongly recommended that the committee develop and have referrals and/or treatment well in place before beginning actual screening, as significant resources are required to develop and manage this essential component.

Screening

Timing of screening

DS should be initiated at one or more "pivotal medical visits"[9] to be in compliance with best care practice and ACoS requirements. Pivotal medical visits refer to those medical visits or encounters at which patients may be expected to be at higher risk of (or more vulnerable to) experiencing distress. Examples include the initial or second visit, time of diagnosis, beginning or ending treatment, changes in treatment modality, changes in HNC disease status (recurrence, progression), and when transitioning to palliative care.[9,12]

Of note, there is some disagreement in the literature as to whether the initial screening should be administered at the first versus the second visit. Although the NCCN has recommended screening on the first visit, other experts raise the issue that often patients do not yet know crucial information, such as whether they in fact have a diagnosis of cancer, let alone potential treatment recommendations.[9,12] Consequently, distress scores at the first visit for initial patients with HNC may reflect the distress related to not yet knowing their disease status, rather than distress due to cancer diagnosis and treatment recommendations. Thus, it may be important to consider screening initial patients with HNC at the second visit, when distress scores are more likely to reflect patients' increased knowledge and reactions to diagnostic and treatment information.

Timing and frequency of DS should be tailored to the relative risk of distress in the HNC patient population throughout the treatment trajectory. Initial DS at the first or second visit should be augmented by screening at pivotal medical visits, and when HNC patients may be at higher risk for distress related to adverse HNC treatment effects and morbidities, such as swallowing or speech deficits, disfigurement, pain, fatigue, and nutritional deficits.

In addition, psychosocial factors associated with higher risk for distress, poor QOL, and negative medical outcomes in patients with HNC may affect timing and frequency of screening in this population, such as low perceived social support,[35,64] pretreatment mental status (depression, distress),[27,48] and avoidant coping style.[40,44,58,65] For example, patients with HNC with a predominantly avoidant coping style may appear less distressed at initial visits, but be particularly susceptible to distress and negative psychological and medical outcomes as they progress further into treatment, when their avoidance coping is more likely to falter in the face of adverse treatment effects or HNC progression.[58] Thus, it is important that the timing of DS be tailored to the unique vulnerabilities and multiple risk points for patients with HNC throughout the treatment trajectory (**Table 2**).

Screening tools

Excellent reviews offer guidance in selecting DS measures, information concerning validity, reliability, sensitivity and specificity, and recommended cutoff scores.[3,12,19,66,67] One of the most commonly used DS questionnaires is the NCCN DT,[1] usually administered with its modifiable Problem Checklist. Other well-regarded DS measures also have been frequently used with patients with cancer, including the HADS[17] and the BSI-18.[18] Three of the most commonly used DS instruments with patients with HNC are listed in **Table 3**. Alternatively, distress may be assessed by clinical interview, although validity and reliability are not ensured unless a validated structured or semi-structured interview format is used.[12,19]

In selecting DS measures, careful consideration must be given to balancing time demands (patients' "response burden" and staff time) with the quality and quantity of the information obtained. Selection of DS measures should be guided by not only the

Table 2
Distress screening for patients with head and neck cancer: time periods and risk factors associated with increased distress

Time Period/Risk Factor	Factors Contributing to Distress Risk
Initial or second visit	Symptoms, diagnosis, treatment planning
Changes in treatment modality	Surgery, radiation, chemotherapy, chemoradiation, immunotherapy
Change in head and neck cancer status	Cancer stage (progression, recurrence)
Shift to palliative care	Increased morbidity Fear of dying/death
Functional losses	Swallowing Speech Disfigurement
Biopsychosocial factors	Pain Fatigue Nutritional deficits/malnutrition Low perceived social support, social isolation Avoidant coping style Smoking/alcohol use disorders Pretreatment history of depression

brevity/rapidity, but also the validity and sensitivity of the measure. Validity has multiple components, but here we are primarily referring to (1) construct validity: does the scale measure what it claims to measure, and (2) predictive validity: do scores accurately predict important outcomes. Sensitivity, in the case of DS, refers to the likelihood that the measure will correctly identify distressed patients as, in fact, distressed (true-positive). Screening measures must have a high sensitivity to achieve their primary goal of being able to correctly identify distress when it is present, as well as moderate to good specificity to correctly identify nondistressed patients as not distressed (true-negative).

The NCCN DT measure meets criteria for brevity, as a 1-item measure (usually given in tandem with a Problem Checklist modifiable to the population being assessed). The DT has been found to have acceptable validity and sensitivity, and compares favorably with longer distress measures, including the HADS (considered a "criterion measure" of distress) and the BSI-18.[66] It is strongly recommended that the DT be administered

Table 3
Validated distress screening measures frequently used with patients with head and neck cancer

Distress Screening Measure	Description of Distress Screening Measure
• Distress Thermometer (DT) (usually administered with Problem Checklist)	• 1-item DT, and modifiable Problem Checklist • Recommended: administer in combination with validated depression measure (eg, Patient Health Questionnaire-4)
• Hospital Anxiety and Depression Scale (HADS)	• HADS-Total = 14 items • HADS-Depression = 7 items • HADS-Anxiety = 7 items
• Brief Symptom Inventory-18	• 18-items; Global Severity Index • Subscales: Depression, Anxiety, Somatization

in combination with a validated depression screening measure, given the high incidence of depression in patients with cancer overall,[68] a concern even more pronounced in patients with HNC due to markedly elevated rates of depression and suicide in the HNC patient population.[5,21,46,47,49] Both the Patient Health Questionnaire-4 (PHQ-4)[69] and the Patient Health Questionnaire-2 (PHQ-2)[70] are excellent brief depression measures frequently used for this purpose.[68]

It is important that HNC centers using DS measures choose cutoff scores based on previous empirical research, rather than due to a felt need to limit the volume of patients identified and referred for distress.[12,66] With regard to the DT, much of the research suggests a cutoff score of 4 offers optimal sensitivity/specificity (true-positive/true-negative) for accurately identifying distressed cancer patients.[66] However, other literature cautions that a cutoff score of 4 may be too high, causing too many distressed patients to be missed.[11,71] This may be particularly pertinent for the HNC population, given the heightened risk of depression and suicide. Distress cutoff scores for the HADS and the BSI-18 are also available in the literature.[12,13]

Screening may be administered via either paper-and-pencil questionnaires or electronic/online self-report measures. Several electronic versions of DS are available.[22,68,72] Many cancer centers also create paper or electronic versions of DS measures tailored to their patient population, although the format and wording of empirically validated measures must be replicated precisely to ensure validity.

Follow-up Assessment/Evaluation

As part of the DS algorithm, when patients exceed the preestablished cutoff scores for distress, further evaluation should be rapidly implemented. Review of the initial DS measure may provide information as to the severity and causes of distress (depressed or anxious mood, social, spiritual, or other areas of distress). Follow-up evaluation may include self-report measures such as the HADS, Patient Health Questionnaire-9 (PHQ-9),[73] Generalized Anxiety Disorder-7 (GAD-7),[74] and/or clinical interview with a mental health professional, or clinical staff member sufficiently trained in the initial evaluation of DS results (**Table 4**).

Evaluation of patients who score above the established distress cutoff criteria should include follow-up assessment concerning depression, anxiety, other biopsychosocial problems, and potential suicidal ideation (if depression or suicidal ideation are indicated). If suicidal ideation is present, immediate follow-up evaluation by a mental health professional is mandatory (or a physician or nurse appropriately well-trained in suicide risk assessment), with treatment and/or referral appropriate to the level of risk.

Referral/Treatment

Referral and treatment are increasingly recognized as a critical component of DS, although one of the more challenging, planning-intensive aspects.[62] It is essential that HNC DS programs develop an integrated referral network of mental health specialists, social work, multidisciplinary health providers (eg, swallowing/speech therapists, maxillofacial prosthodontics, nutritionists) and administrative personnel, all of whom have expertise in helping distressed patients with HNC with a range of biopsychosocial concerns (**Box 1**).

Although the literature evaluating psychosocial interventions for patients with HNC is not yet well developed, preliminary evidence suggests there may be significant potential benefit for patients with HNC.[36,38,75–82] In addition, there is considerable evidence for the effectiveness of several psychosocial interventions with patients with cancer that may well be applicable to the HNC population.[83–89]

Table 4
Follow-up assessment/evaluation: psychosocial measures

Measurement Tool	Domains Assessed	Special Considerations
Patient Health Questionnaire-9 (PHQ-9)	Depression (9 items total) Suicidal ideation (1 item)	• When suicidal ideation present, immediate clinical response is mandatory
Hospital Anxiety and Depression Scale (HADS)	HADS-T = Distress HADS-D = Depression HADS-A = Anxiety	• HADS-T score increasingly used as measure of distress, although not intended by original authors of scale • HADS-D considered more reliable than HADS-A
Generalized Anxiety Disorder-7 (GAD-7)	Anxiety	• Considered more reliable than HADS-A
Clinical interview	Distress, depression, anxiety, other psychosocial distress, suicidal ideation/intent (if indicated)	• Should be conducted by mental health professional, or well-trained clinical staff • Suicidal ideation/intent must be evaluated by mental health professional

Management of psychosocial distress includes referrals to mental health professionals, and can involve nurses and allied clinical staff trained in psychoeducational interventions. Some investigators recommend a flexible "stepped care" algorithm based on matching distress severity and characteristics to level and type of intervention.[76]

Box 1
Common biopsychosocial problems in patients with head and neck cancer (HNC)

• Distress

• Mood disorders (depression, anxiety)

• Swallowing impairment

• Nutritional deficits/malnutrition

• Speech impairment

• Disfigurement

• Pain

• Fatigue

• Low perceived social support, social isolation

• Avoidant coping, maladaptive coping

• Smoking and/or alcohol use disorders

• Fear of recurrence

• Death and dying (fear, depression, coping)

• Spiritual/religious concerns

• Financial difficulties, insurance difficulties

• Work-related problems (secondary to effects of HNC and treatment)

More intensive treatment of psychosocial distress should include in-house and outside referrals to mental health professionals with experience in treating cancer and patients with HNC, and optimally with behavioral medicine and/or medical hypnosis expertise.

A burgeoning body of research offers substantial evidence for the efficacy of integrative cognitive behavioral therapy (CBT)–behavioral medicine, medical hypnosis, and mindfulness-based treatments for many cancer populations in reducing many of the aftereffects of cancer and cancer treatments (surgery, radiation, chemotherapy, immunotherapy)[84–86,88,89] that are relevant to HNC patients' experience, as listed in **Box 2**.

Empirical investigations of integrative CBT-behavioral medicine, medical hypnosis, and mindfulness, or mindfulness-based stress reduction (MBSR), treatments with patients with HNC are in the initial stages, with preliminary evidence suggesting that HNC patients may derive significant benefit from such interventions.[36,79–81,90] Psychosocial and behavioral medicine interventions that have demonstrated efficacy with cancer/HNC patients, or promising initial evidence with patients with HNC are listed in **Box 3**.

In devising treatment tailored to the HNC population, it is important to note that some reports indicate that many patients with HNC appear to prefer individualized treatment, as opposed to group treatment, and are more likely to accept and adhere to individualized treatment tailored to their specific needs, particularly when treatment is focused on reducing and/or coping with side effects or aftereffects of HNC treatment (pain, fatigue, nausea), coping with presurgical anxiety, or related HNC challenges.[91]

Documentation

Documentation is an essential component of DS, and should include screening measures used, patient distress score, clinical interpretation of distress score, further evaluation, suicidal ideation (if present, and intervention for same), referrals for treatment, and plan for follow-up, if needed. If patients refuse treatment referrals, this should also be documented. Note that when suicidal ideation is present, if results of immediate evaluation indicate significant risk, patients may not have the right to refuse care due to safety concerns.

Effective documentation provides multiple benefits, including improving patient care, quality assurance, and developing a baseline of initial data on patients' psychosocial distress that serve as a foundation for clinical intervention and research

---

Box 2
Therapeutic targets of integrative cognitive behavioral therapy (CBT)–behavioral medicine for patients with HNC

- Pain
- Fatigue (secondary to radiation, or other HNC treatment)
- Nausea (secondary to chemotherapy, postsurgical)
- Malnutrition/difficulties with eating
- Smoking cessation
- Distress
- Anxiety
- Depression

Box 3
Psychosocial treatments for patients with HNC and other cancers

- CBT treatment[77,78,83,92]

- Integrative CBT-behavioral medicine[36,86]

- Behavioral medicine (may include hypnosis, relaxation training, mindfulness and/or mindfulness-based stress reduction techniques, pain management)[36,79–81,84,87,90]

- Smoking cessation, alcohol cessation/reduction[38]

- Psychoeducational interventions[77,93]

- Coping and social skills interventions[82,94]

(distress, QOL, psychological and medical outcomes). Using this information will allow HNC centers to evaluate the effectiveness of their DS programs, which can facilitate provision of support from hospital administration, and aid in the development of whole-patient HNC care.

SUMMARY AND FUTURE DIRECTIONS

The provision of DS and referral routinely for patients with HNC is appropriately and rapidly becoming the standard of care. DS is of particular importance for patients with HNC, given their heightened incidence of distress, depression, and suicide, and the impact of psychosocial distress on QOL and medical outcomes. In the absence of formalized DS, psychosocial distress is frequently missed in HNC settings. However, once identified, distress is highly responsive to treatment.

Multidisciplinary HNC teams are uniquely positioned to implement effective psychosocial DS programs preventively to identify and treat distress that, left untreated, frequently leads to worsening psychological status, lower QOL, and negative medical outcomes. Further, multidisciplinary HNC teams can combine their expertise to tailor DS to the unique medical and psychological vulnerabilities of patients with HNC, using their shared understanding of the factors associated with increased risk for distress in this population.

Although research on psychosocial distress in cancer is burgeoning, more information is critically needed regarding distress in patients with HNC, the impact of distress on QOL and medical outcomes, and effective clinical interventions. To meet this need, it is essential that HNC centers implement DS routinely, using validated instruments, and follow through with referrals for treatment. Documentation of results is crucial, and can serve to inform clinical intervention and research.

Clinical interventions targeting common causes of distress in the HNC population are critically needed. Behavioral medicine (including medical hypnosis and mindfulness) is a promising area of specialization in mental health provision that has demonstrated efficacy with patients with cancer in reducing negative aftereffects of treatment and biopsychosocial problems similar to those faced by patients with HNC. Integrative CBT-behavioral medicine approaches have been found to be particularly effective. Tailoring treatment to the HNC population will be essential.

As the field of HNC moves beyond a reductionist medical model, narrowly focused on survival, and increasingly recognizes the importance of patients' psychological well-being and QOL, DS will provide an essential methodology and algorithm to aid the evolution toward whole-patient care. HNC centers can use DS to establish baseline data regarding patients' risk for distress, related negative impacts on QOL, psychological and medical outcomes, and use this information to improve clinical intervention and research. Multidisciplinary HNC teams offer a foundation from which to fulfill the original purpose of DS, to provide whole-patient care that targets and effectively meets the real needs of HNC patients to relieve suffering and improve well-being as they traverse the treatment trajectory.

ACKNOWLEDGMENTS

The author thanks Elizabeth Ercolano, DNSc for her very helpful comments on this article.

REFERENCES

1. Roth AJ, Kornblith AB, Batel-Copel L, et al. Rapid screening for psychologic distress in men with prostate carcinoma. Cancer 1998;82(10):1904–8.
2. Holland JC, Bultz BD. The NCCN guideline for distress management: a case for making distress the sixth vital sign. J Natl Compr Canc Netw 2007;5(1):3–7.
3. Carlson LE, Waller A, Mitchell AJ. Screening for distress and unmet needs in patients with cancer: review and recommendations. J Clin Oncol 2012;30(11): 1160–77.
4. Chen AM, Jennelle RLS, Grady V, et al. Prospective study of psychosocial distress among patients undergoing radiotherapy for head and neck cancer. Int J Radiat Oncol Biol Phys 2009;73(1):187–93.
5. Zabora J, BrintzenhofeSzoc K, Curbow B, et al. The prevalence of psychological distress by cancer site. Psychooncology 2001;10(1):19–28.
6. Werner A, Stenner C, Schüz J. Patient versus clinician symptom reporting: how accurate is the detection of distress in the oncologic after-care? Psychooncology 2012;21(8):818–26.
7. Aarstad HJ, Osthus AA, Olofsson J, et al. Level of distress predicts subsequent survival in successfully treated head and neck cancer patients: a prospective cohort study. Acta Otolaryngol (Stockh) 2014;134(2):211–9.
8. American College of Surgeons Commission on Cancer. Cancer program standards 2012 edition version 1.2.1: ensuring patient-centered care. Chicago: American College of Surgeons; 2012.
9. National Comprehensive Cancer Network (NCCN): clinical practice guidelines in oncology: distress management version 3.2013. J Natl Compr Canc Netw 2013; 11:190–209.
10. Adler N, Page A, editors. Institute of Medicine Committee on Psychosocial Services to Cancer Patients/Families in a Community Setting. Cancer care for the whole patient: meeting psychosocial health needs. Washington, DC: National Academies Press; 2008.
11. Lazenby M, Tan H, Pasacreta N, et al. The five steps of comprehensive psychosocial distress screening. Curr Oncol Rep 2015;17(5):447.
12. Pirl WF, Fann JR, Greer JA, et al. Recommendations for the implementation of distress screening programs in cancer centers: report from the American Psychosocial Oncology Society (APOS), Association of Oncology Social Work (AOSW), and Oncology Nursing Society (ONS) joint task force. Cancer 2014; 120(19):2946–54.
13. Andersen BL, DeRubeis RJ, Berman BS, et al. Screening, assessment, and care of anxiety and depressive symptoms in adults with cancer: an American Society of Clinical Oncology Guideline Adaptation. J Clin Oncol 2014;32(15):1605–19.

14. National Comprehensive Cancer Network. Practice guidelines in oncology, version 1.2002: distress management. Fort Washington (PA): National Comprehensive Cancer Network; 2002.

15. Jensen MP. The validity and reliability of pain measures in adults with cancer. J Pain 2003;4(1):2–21.

16. Bultz BD, Johansen C. Screening for distress, the 6th vital sign: where are we, and where are we going? Psychooncology 2011;20(6):569–71.

17. Zigmond AS, Snaith RP. The hospital anxiety and depression scale. Acta Psychiatr Scand 1983;67(6):361–70.

18. Zabora J, Brintzenhofeszoc K, Jacobsen P, et al. A new psychosocial screening instrument for use with cancer patients. Psychosomatics 2001;42(3):241–6.

19. Vodermaier A, Linden W, Siu C. Screening for emotional distress in cancer patients: a systematic review of assessment instruments. J Natl Cancer Inst 2009; 101(21):1464–88.

20. Singer S, Krauß O, Keszte J, et al. Predictors of emotional distress in patients with head and neck cancer. Head Neck 2012;34(2):180–7.

21. Kugaya A, Akechi T, Okuyama T, et al. Prevalence, predictive factors, and screening for psychologic distress in patients with newly diagnosed head and neck cancer. Cancer 2000;88(12):2817–23.

22. Krebber A-MH, Jansen F, Cuijpers P, et al. Screening for psychological distress in follow-up care to identify head and neck cancer patients with untreated distress. Support Care Cancer 2016;24:2541–8.

23. Katz MR, Kopek N, Waldron J, et al. Screening for depression in head and neck cancer. Psychooncology 2004;13(4):269–80.

24. Nguyen NP, Frank C, Moltz CC, et al. Impact of dysphagia on quality of life after treatment of head-and-neck cancer. Int J Radiat Oncol Biol Phys 2005;61(3): 772–8.

25. Silveira MH, Dedivitis RA, Queija DS, et al. Quality of life in swallowing disorders after nonsurgical treatment for head and neck cancer. Int Arch Otorhinolaryngol 2015;19(1):46.

26. Perry A, Casey E, Cotton S. Quality of life after total laryngectomy: functioning, psychological well-being and self-efficacy. Int J Lang Commun Disord 2015; 50(4):467–75.

27. Lin B, Starmer HM, Gourin CG. The relationship between depressive symptoms, quality of life, and swallowing function in head and neck cancer patients 1 year after definitive therapy. Laryngoscope 2012;122(7):1518–25.

28. Gilony D, Gilboa D, Blumstein T, et al. Effects of tracheostomy on well-being and body-image perceptions. Otolaryngol Head Neck Surg 2005;133(3):366–71.

29. Wells M, Cunningham M, Lang H, et al. Distress, concerns and unmet needs in survivors of head and neck cancer: a cross-sectional survey. Eur J Cancer Care (Engl) 2015;24(5):748–60.

30. Gill SS, Frew J, Fry A, et al. Priorities for the head and neck cancer patient, their companion and members of the multidisciplinary team and decision regret. Clin Oncol 2011;23(8):518–24.

31. List MA, Rutherford JL, Stracks J, et al. Prioritizing treatment outcomes: head and neck cancer patients versus nonpatients. Head Neck 2004;26(2):163–70.

32. de Leeuw JRJ, de Graeff A, Ros WJG, et al. Prediction of depressive symptomatology after treatment of head and neck cancer: the influence of pre-treatment physical and depressive symptoms, coping, and social support. Head Neck 2000;22(8):799–807.

33. Adachi Y, Kimura H, Sato N, et al. Preoperative level of depression is a predictor of postoperative levels of depression in patients with head and neck cancer. Jpn J Clin Oncol 2014;44(4):311–7.

34. Holloway RL, Hellewell JL, Marbella AM, et al. Psychosocial effects in long-term head and neck cancer survivors. Head Neck 2005;27(4):281–8.

35. Karnell LH, Christensen AJ, Rosenthal EL, et al. Influence of social support on health-related quality of life outcomes in head and neck cancer. Head Neck 2007;29(2):143–6.

36. Howren MB, Christensen AJ, Karnell LH, et al. Psychological factors associated with head and neck cancer treatment and survivorship: evidence and opportunities for behavioral medicine. J Consult Clin Psychol 2013;81(2):299.

37. Tromp DM. Medical care-seeking and health-risk behavior in patients with head and neck cancer: the role of health value, control beliefs and psychological distress. Health Educ Res 2005;20(6):665–75.

38. Duffy SA, Ronis DL, Valenstein M, et al. A tailored smoking, alcohol, and depression intervention for head and neck cancer patients. Cancer Epidemiol Biomarkers Prev 2006;15(11):2203–8.

39. Duffy SA, Ronis DL, Valenstein M, et al. Depressive symptoms, smoking, drinking, and quality of life among head and neck cancer patients. Psychosomatics 2007;48(2):142–8.

40. Aarstad AKH, Beisland E, Osthus AA, et al. Distress, quality of life, neuroticism and psychological coping are related in head and neck cancer patients during follow-up. Acta Oncol 2011;50(3):390–8. Available at: http://www.tandfonline.com/doi/full/10.3109/0284186X.2010.504227. Accessed October 21, 2016.

41. Elani HW, Allison PJ. Coping and psychological distress among head and neck cancer patients. Support Care Cancer 2010;19(11):1735–41.

42. Horney DJ, Smith HE, McGurk M, et al. Associations between quality of life, coping styles, optimism, and anxiety and depression in pretreatment patients with head and neck cancer. Head Neck 2011;33(1):65–71.

43. Nipp RD, El-Jawahri A, Fishbein JN, et al. The relationship between coping strategies, quality of life, and mood in patients with incurable cancer. Cancer 2016; 122(13):2110–6.

44. Tromp DM, Brouha XDR, De Leeuw JRJ, et al. Psychological factors and patient delay in patients with head and neck cancer. Eur J Cancer 2004;40(10):1509–16.

45. Badr H, Gupta V, Sikora A, et al. Psychological distress in patients and caregivers over the course of radiotherapy for head and neck cancer. Oral Oncol 2014; 50(10):1005–11.

46. Buchmann L, Conlee J, Hunt J, et al. Psychosocial distress is prevalent in head and neck cancer patients. Laryngoscope 2013;123(6):1424–9.

47. Linden W, Vodermaier A, MacKenzie R, et al. Anxiety and depression after cancer diagnosis: prevalence rates by cancer type, gender, and age. J Affect Disord 2012;141(2–3):343–51.

48. Ichikura K, Yamashita A, Sugimoto T, et al. Persistence of psychological distress and correlated factors among patients with head and neck cancer. Palliat Support Care 2016;14(1):42–51.

49. Kam D, Salib A, Gorgy G, et al. Incidence of suicide in patients with head and neck cancer. JAMA Otolaryngol Neck Surg 2015;141(12):1075.

50. Misono S, Weiss NS, Fann JR, et al. Incidence of suicide in persons with cancer. J Clin Oncol 2008;26(29):4731–8.

51. Kendal W. Suicide and cancer: a gender-comparative study. Ann Oncol 2007; 18(2):381–7.

52. Zeller JL. High suicide risk found for patients with head and neck cancer. JAMA 2006;296(14):1716–7.

53. Ganzer H, Touger-Decker R, Byham-Gray L, et al. The eating experience after treatment for head and neck cancer: a review of the literature. Oral Oncol 2015;51(7):634–42.

54. Wu Y-S, Lin P-Y, Chien C-Y, et al. Anxiety and depression in patients with head and neck cancer: 6-month follow-up study. Neuropsychiatr Dis Treat 2016;12: 1029–36.

55. Neilson K, Pollard A, Boonzaier A, et al. Psychological distress (depression and anxiety) in people with head and neck cancers. Med J Aust 2010;193(5 Suppl): S48–51.

56. Neilson K, Pollard A, Boonzaier A, et al. A longitudinal study of distress (depression and anxiety) up to 18 months after radiotherapy for head and neck cancer. Psychooncology 2013;22(8):1843–8.

57. Suzuki M, Deno M, Myers M, et al. Anxiety and depression in patients after surgery for head and neck cancer in Japan. Palliat Support Care 2016;14(3):269–77. Available at: /core/journals/palliative-and-supportive-care/article/anxiety-and-depression-in-patients-after-surgery-for-head-and-neck-cancer-in-japan/B72D82E89924A4F4C065560E3034940C. Accessed October 30, 2016.

58. Dunne S, Mooney O, Coffey L, et al. Psychological variables associated with quality of life following primary treatment for head and neck cancer: a systematic review of the literature from 2004 to 2015. Psychooncology 2017;26(2):149–60.

59. de Graeff A, de Leeuw J, Ros W, et al. Pretreatment factors predicting quality of life after treatment for head and neck cancer. Head Neck 2000;22:399.

60. DiMatteo MR, Lepper HS, Croghan TW. Depression is a risk factor for noncompliance with medical treatment: meta-analysis of the effects of anxiety and depression on patient adherence. Arch Intern Med 2000;160(14):2101–7.

61. Østhus AA, Aarstad AK, Olofsson J, et al. Prediction of survival by pretreatment health-related quality-of-life scores in a prospective cohort of patients with head and neck squamous cell carcinoma. JAMA Otolaryngol Neck Surg 2013;139(1): 14–20.

62. Clark PG, Bolte S, Buzaglo J, et al. From distress guidelines to developing models of psychosocial care: current best practices. J Psychosoc Oncol 2012; 30(6):694–714.

63. Hollingworth W, Metcalfe C, Mancero S, et al. Are needs assessments cost effective in reducing distress among patients with cancer? A randomized controlled trial using the distress thermometer and problem list. J Clin Oncol 2013;31(29): 3631–8.

64. Howren MB, Christensen AJ, Hynds Karnell L, et al. Influence of pretreatment social support on health-related quality of life in head and neck cancer survivors: results from a prospective study. Head Neck 2013;35(6):779–87.

65. List MA, Lee Rutherford J, Stracks J, et al. An exploration of the pretreatment coping strategies of patients with carcinoma of the head and neck. Cancer 2002;95(1):98–104.

66. Jacobsen PB, Donovan KA, Trask PC, et al. Screening for psychologic distress in ambulatory cancer patients. Cancer 2005;103(7):1494–502.

67. Luckett T, Butow PN, King MT, et al. A review and recommendations for optimal outcome measures of anxiety, depression and general distress in studies evaluating psychosocial interventions for English-speaking adults with heterogeneous cancer diagnoses. Support Care Cancer 2010;18(10):1241–62.

68. Wagner LI, Spiegel D, Pearman T. Using the science of psychosocial care to implement the New American College of Surgeons Commission on cancer distress screening standard. J Natl Compr Canc Netw 2013;11(2):214–21.

69. Kroenke K, Spitzer RL, Williams JB, et al. An ultra-brief screening scale for anxiety and depression: the PHQ-4. Psychosomatics 2001;50(6):613–21.

70. Löwe B, Kroenke K, Gräfe K. Detecting and monitoring depression with a two-item questionnaire (PHQ-2). J Psychosom Res 2005;58(2):163–71.

71. Lazenby M, Dixon J, Bai M, et al. Comparing the distress thermometer (DT) with the patient health questionnaire (PHQ)-2 for screening for possible cases of depression among patients newly diagnosed with advanced cancer. Palliat Support Care 2014;12(1):63–8.

72. Verdonck-de Leeuw IM, de Bree R, Keizer AL, et al. Computerized prospective screening for high levels of emotional distress in head and neck cancer patients and referral rate to psychosocial care. Oral Oncol 2009;45(10):e129–33.

73. Kroenke K, Spitzer RL, Williams JBW. The PHQ-9: validity of a brief depression severity measure. J Gen Intern Med 2001;16(9):606.

74. Spitzer RL, Kroenke K, Williams JB, et al. A brief measure for assessing generalized anxiety disorder: the GAD-7. Arch Intern Med 2006;166(10):1092–7.

75. Luckett T, Britton B, Clover K, et al. Evidence for interventions to improve psychological outcomes in people with head and neck cancer: a systematic review of the literature. Support Care Cancer 2011;19(7):871–81.

76. Krebber AMH, Jansen F, Witte BI, et al. Stepped care targeting psychological distress in head and neck cancer and lung cancer patients: a randomized, controlled trial. Ann Oncol 2016;27(9):1754–60.

77. Kangas M, Milross C, Taylor A, et al. A pilot randomized controlled trial of a brief early intervention for reducing posttraumatic stress disorder, anxiety and depressive symptoms in newly diagnosed head and neck cancer patients: early CBT for PTSD, anxiety and depressive symptoms for HNC. Psychooncology 2013;22(7):1665–73.

78. Semple CJ, Dunwoody L, Kernohan WG, et al. Development and evaluation of a problem-focused psychosocial intervention for patients with head and neck cancer. Support Care Cancer 2009;17(4):379–88.

79. Rapkin DA, Straubing M, Holroyd JC. Guided imagery, hypnosis and recovery from head and neck cancer surgery: an exploratory study. Int J Clin Exp Hypn 1991;39(4):215–26.

80. Pollard A, Burchell JL, Castle D, et al. Individualised mindfulness-based stress reduction for head and neck cancer patients undergoing radiotherapy of curative intent: a descriptive pilot study. Eur J Cancer Care (Engl) 2016;26(2). http://dx.doi.org/10.1111/ecc.12474.

81. Meyers S, Ott MJ. Mindful eating as a clinical intervention for survivors of head and neck cancer: interdisciplinary collaboration and strategies to improve oral intake. Top Clin Nutr 2008;23(4):340–6.

82. Allison P, Nicolau B, Edgar L, et al. Teaching head and neck cancer patients coping strategies: results of a feasibility study. Oral Oncol 2004;40(5):538–44.

83. Linden W, Girgis A. Psychological treatment outcomes for cancer patients: what do meta-analyses tell us about distress reduction? Psychooncology 2012;21(4):343–50.

84. Montgomery GH, Schnur JB, Kravits K. Hypnosis for cancer care: over 200 years young. CA Cancer J Clin 2013;63(1):31–44.

85. Jensen MP, Patterson DR. Hypnotic approaches for chronic pain management: clinical implications of recent research findings. Am Psychol 2014;69(2):167.

86. Montgomery GH, David D, Kangas M, et al. Randomized controlled trial of a cognitive-behavioral therapy plus hypnosis intervention to control fatigue in patients undergoing radiotherapy for breast cancer. J Clin Oncol 2014;32(6):557.

87. Montgomery GH, David D, Winkel G, et al. The effectiveness of adjunctive hypnosis with surgical patients: a meta-analysis. Anesth Analg 2002;94(6):1639–45.

88. Potié A, Roelants F, Pospiech A, et al. Hypnosis in the perioperative management of breast cancer surgery: clinical benefits and potential implications. Anesthesiol Res Pract 2016;2016:1–8.

89. Mendoza ME, Capafons A, Gralow JR, et al. Randomized controlled trial of the Valencia model of waking hypnosis plus CBT for pain, fatigue, and sleep management in patients with cancer and cancer survivors: Valencia model of waking hypnosis for managing cancer-related symptoms. Psychooncology 2016. http://dx.doi.org/10.1002/pon.4232.

90. Schiff E, Mogilner JG, Sella E, et al. Hypnosis for postradiation xerostomia in head and neck cancer patients: a pilot study. J Pain Symptom Manage 2009;37(6):1086–92.e1.

91. Semple CJ, Dunwoody L, Sullivan K, et al. Patients with head and neck cancer prefer individualized cognitive behavioural therapy. Eur J Cancer Care (Engl) 2006;15(3):220–7.

92. Artherholt SB, Fann JR. Psychosocial care in cancer. Curr Psychiatry Rep 2011;14(1):23–9.

93. Katz MR, Irish JC, Devins GM. Development and pilot testing of a psychoeducational intervention for oral cancer patients. Psychooncology 2004;13(9):642–53.

94. Vilela L, Nicolau B, Mahmud S, et al. Comparison of psychosocial outcomes in head and neck cancer patients receiving a coping strategies intervention and control subjects receiving no intervention. J Otolaryngol 2006;35(2):88–96.

Changes at the Dinner Table and Beyond

Nourishing Our Patients Throughout the Trajectory of Their Cancer Journey

Amy Lewis Madnick, MSW, LCSW[a],*,
Elizabeth Grace Morasso, MSW, LCSW[b]

KEYWORDS

- Nutrition • Coping • Psychosocial • Patient-centered care • Decision-making
- Support system • Survivorship • End-of-life

KEY POINTS

- Viewing clinical roles as nourishing, as opposed to strictly focused on medical management, acknowledges patients' and families existing strengths that may assist themselves and the medical team in overcoming physiologic and psychosocial obstacles presented over the course of patient's illness.
- Patient-centered care practices involving all members of the HNC team assist in achieving the best possible outcomes given patients' health status.
- Concrete and psychosocial assessment and interventions should be considered when addressing patients' nutritional needs.
- There are significant psychosocial implications of diagnosis, treatment, and prognosis to be considered across the illness trajectory, including surveillance/survivorship and end-of-life.

INTRODUCTION

Patient-centered care involves accounting for what is meaningful and valuable to a patient to achieve the best possible outcome.[1] Medical oncology, especially, has led improvements in integrative care with the formation of multidisciplinary care teams, inclusion of ancillary assessments, and patient-centered interventions. It is now acknowledged that distress screening can help identify barriers to optimal care and recovery. Patients with head and neck cancer (HNC) may experience various

Disclosure Statement: The authors have nothing to disclose.
[a] Department of Care Coordination and Clinical Social Work, UCLA Health, 757 Westwood Plaza, B788, Los Angeles, CA 90095, USA; [b] Department of Radiation Oncology, UCLA Health, 200 Medical Plaza, B265, Los Angeles, CA 90095, USA
* Corresponding author.
E-mail address: amadnick@mednet.ucla.edu

functional impairments from diagnosis and treatment. Biopsychosocial functioning across the illness trajectory (ie, speaking, swallowing, breathing, taste, smell, and facial disfigurement) puts patients at higher risk of emotional distress, including symptoms of depression and anxiety, than other cancers, most likely associated with changes or loss of these functions.[2,3]

Although distress screening may identify patients who require thorough biopsychosocial assessment and intervention, all new patients with HNC deserve to receive support from allied health professionals to cope with practical and psychosocial issues presented from diagnosis through survivorship, such as management of nutritional needs and discharge planning following surgery. As noted by Marion F. Winkler, surgical nutrition specialist at Rhode Island Hospital and assistant professor at Brown University in a well-known lecture: "We learn so much from our patients and their families when we listen to their concerns, when we put aside our own biases and beliefs, and when we expand our focus."[4] Although referring to integrative nutritional practices, this concept is applicable to care provided by all members of a multidisciplinary HNC team and promotes nourishment of patients' whole selves.

OVERVIEW

Starting at diagnosis, it is of value to all members of the HNC team, including surgeons, radiation oncologists, medical oncologists, mental health professionals, swallowing/speech therapists, maxillofacial prosthodontics, and nurses, and chaplains, to encourage nourishment of patient and family medical, emotional, and spiritual needs. Thorough assessments enhance patient care, promoting optimal outcomes through increased understanding of the disease process and treatment options, healthy cognitive and emotional processing, informed decision-making, compliance to treatment plan, maintenance of nutritional and other basic needs, and perceived value in follow-up and surveillance. Viewing clinical roles as nourishing, as opposed to strictly focused on medical management, acknowledges patient and family strengths that may assist themselves and the medical team in overcoming obstacles presented over the course of a patient's illness.

NUTRITION

A vital piece of the HNC treatment plan is nourishment of patient nutritional needs because they are fundamental physiologic requirements and primary sources of motivation in any organism's lifespan. When unsatisfied, higher-level objectives, such as processing one's illness, decision-making, motivation, and maintenance of health needs, become more difficult to obtain. Nutrition is essential to life from birth. In addition, one's experience with nutrition, beginning in the womb, offers some of the first pleasurable experiences.

All patients present with existing schemas around food-related decision-making, such as what they like to eat, how much and when they like to eat, or a routine of what eating looks like in their everyday practices. Nutrition is an area where patients have previously practiced control. "Moreover, eating is a fundamentally rewarding behavior, and is thus intrinsically linked to mood and emotions."[5] When one's control over decision-making or routine is altered because of health status, it often serves as another loss.

Nutrition is a primary concern of all patients with cancer because it affects strength, ability, and psychological and emotional health. Despite considerable improvements in treatments for HNC, demands of treatment and disease state impact one's ability to maintain caloric and essential nutrient baselines, necessitating nutrition optimization. Insufficient intake and processing may be caused by changes in taste, xerostomia or increase in saliva production, mucositis or general mouth/throat discomfort, dysphagia, nausea/vomiting, poor appetite, and/or increase in metabolic rate. Assessment of these side effects should be performed across the illness trajectory because they affect physiologic health and overall enjoyment and motivation associated with eating and drinking.

Adjustments in nutritional intake can differ greatly from previously pleasurable experiences. Alternative methods to providing nourishment, such as enteral nutrition or adjustments to oral diet, may be needed. Whether patients require special food preparation, such as use of a blender, decrease in bite size, slower intake of food and drink, or bolus enteral feedings, these tasks are often labor intensive or triggers of emotions related to one's health status. Patients lacking energy, motivation, or caregiver support, for example, often are overwhelmed with these responsibilities.

Beyond individual and psychological factors affecting nutritional practices lay family, socioeconomic and cultural considerations. Many family and societal rituals and values are centered on eating and meaning of mealtimes. Culturally, individual foods and mealtime practices have incredible significance. When patients cannot eat "normally" and participate in these activities, there is considerable impact psychologically on the patient, and socially on the family and larger system. Just as an infant's first experience of attachment and bonding occurs at the breast or bottle, it is around the dinner table that patients develop relationships with others. Loss of pleasure and meaning in eating, added stress of a sometimes-complicated nutritional intake, and embarrassment and shame with drooling and/or difficulty eating are life changing and isolating for many patients and families. Wu and colleagues[3] report that trouble with social eating remained a primary factor related to depression at the 6-month interval of their study, demonstrating the significance of food, eating, and nutrition for these patients, despite cancer-related impairment of physical functions.

MIND, BODY, AND SPIRITUAL NEEDS ACROSS THE ILLNESS TRAJECTORY

Across the illness trajectory it is essential to acknowledge all aspects of the patient and their support system. There are many opportunities for patients to receive support from all members of the HNC team, optimizing curative or palliative treatment plans and allowing patients to cope with the challenges they face in a constructive way.

Presentation of Symptoms

From a physiologic perspective, it is important to consider such characteristics as severity and length of symptoms, prior health history and practices, how symptoms were identified, and genetic components/family history. Although these items assist the medical team in assessment, they also provide information on potential risk factors affecting patient's illness course. These items serve as triggers for involvement from ancillary staff, such as registered dietitian nutritionist (RDN) or mental health professionals. Inclusion of these staff members on presentation assists the team in understanding how patients are coping with indications of disease, underlying mental health or cognitive concerns, how patients understand the potential disease process, how patients learn best (ie, visually, small amounts of information at a time, through sound, or reading), and what it means to become a patient with cancer, all of which may affect engagement in care and clinical outcome. Socially, one may note who arrives with the patient for their first appointment, if anyone in patient's support system is aware of their experience and concerns, and what logistical and emotional support they can provide to the patient.

Nutrition management begins at presentation of symptoms. Ongoing assessment and discussion from providers and involvement of RDN reinforces the importance of patient and family understanding of biologic and emotional benefits of proper nutrition. Patient age, height, weight, ideal weight, weight loss history, and current psychosocial status should be considered when formulating goals of patient and medical team. Additional evaluation includes allergies; cultural preferences; usual diet; food preferences; financial abilities; existing tools, such as blenders or cutlery; and patient role and/or motivation in preparing food at home. Medical or RDN staff may also assess preference around special dietary needs or practices, such as vegetarianism or veganism, interest or need in gluten or dairy-free products, and/or desire for more natural foods. Of note, these products are often more expensive and rarely covered by insurance plans. Partnerships with proprietors have proved beneficial, because many are not well established in medical settings. Sales personnel may be open to providing financial assistance, samples, and more extensive information about their product for medical and RDN staff evaluation.

Assessment and support from the HNC team around techniques to improve control over intake may assist in improving fulfillment of nutritional needs. Some patients, for example, find solace in preparing foods themselves, whereas others may ask for assistance. Nourishing one's self with meaningful food items, such as homemade chicken soup prepared by a family member or friend, may fill a void emotionally and physiologically. Some patients even report positive sensations following behaviors like burping after a special enteral meal, such as pureed chicken soup, which, although not socially acceptable, may assist in reassociating with positive feelings around certain food or drink. Families may also create new rituals allowing for similar bonding opportunities, such as playing board games or a game of cards together. Such interventions achieve similar goals as mealtime and remove potentially negative emotional reactions. It is important to acknowledge variations in patient experiences, because some may desire to remain a part of the table to enjoy smells and other sensory experiences, whereas others may prefer distraction by activities that do not bring attention to the unattainable.

Involvement of the multidisciplinary team, including RDNs and mental health professionals, can assist in addressing logistical and emotional challenges surrounding maintenance of nutritional needs. One intervention that has shown promise is mindful eating, which can assist with transition to oral intake following completion of treatment.[6] In addition, motivational interviewing techniques can empower patients to implement realistic goals and better engage in their compliance.[7] Participation in support groups or engagement with other patients with HNC may offer concrete solutions to obstacles around mealtime and improve quality of life.[8]

Engagement in Care and Diagnosis

At this point in the trajectory, a fight or flight response is often observed. Fight or flight refers to the biologic response highly associated with psychological reactions of patients to information surrounding negative changes in their health status. Wu and colleagues[3] found that, when confronted with an HNC diagnosis, anticipatory anxiety, overwhelming information, distractibility, and poor sleep were commonly seen. When highly anxious at time of engagement, patients are often unable to process information in a meaningful way and apply it to such items as decision-making around treatment planning or consideration of logistical concerns, such as transportation, need for care giving, or employment. Patients who arrive with an attentive family member or friend to ensure processing of information, assist in documentation and scheduling of appointments, or ask questions for clarification have an opportunity to return to this information at a more cognitively appropriate time. Many patients require post-consultation follow-up, pretreatment appointments, or telephone consultation to ensure understanding and informed decision-making. Patients with intellectual impairments or psychiatric illnesses may have greater difficulty processing this information. Proper evaluation, with consideration of potential symptoms of underlying diagnosis, such as difficulty speaking or hearing, is a crucial element of assessment for all team members.

Thorough assessments should be performed to identify potential risk factors related to follow-up, such as housing, transportation, and childcare to provide optimal patient-centered care. Initial visits with newly diagnosed patients are also ideal times for the HNC team to engage around what gives patients joy and meaning to incorporate into treatment plans and overall engagement. Acknowledgment of patient's future goals, hobbies, interests, and passions can significantly affect a patient's experience while hospitalized or undergoing treatment, providing comfort and motivation to participate actively in their care. In the inpatient setting, this may include encouraging families to bring personal items to the bedside, such as a comfortable pillow or throw, or printing photographs to decorate a patient's room. Patients who enjoy the outdoors, for example, and experience claustrophobia may experience improved mood if arrangements are made for transport outdoors or incorporation of nature-related items in treatment spaces. These personalized and creative interventions remind patients that the HNC team recognizes their self-worth and is making efforts to incorporate this into a sometimes seemingly undignified treatment plan.

Treatment Plan and Decision-Making

As patients and families engage in decision-making regarding treatment, it is beneficial to understand their values and priorities around comfort and quality of life. Whether a patient is undergoing surgery or chemoradiation, there is opportunity to enhance autonomy and empowerment of the family unit. A patient's age, health and mental health, culture, history, strengths, vulnerabilities, family and support system, what they value, and their goals for their future should be considered as planning is initiated. An essential piece of preparing patients is acknowledging physiologic and emotional losses and general adjustments caused by diagnosis and treatment. The way patients and their support systems are educated and prepared for what comes next makes a difference in coping.[9] All team members can empower patients with thorough assessments, education, and resources related to their discipline for the best outcome possible given patient illness. Anticipating patient needs is indispensable to effective treatment planning and assists in preparing for potentially uncomfortable transitions. In the inpatient setting, this often requires preparation for transition home or to a facility that can best address patient safety and health needs. In the outpatient setting, this may mean longer consultation and treatment planning visits and involvement of ancillary staff to assist with the emotional impact of cancer and pros and cons of each treatment or palliative option. For many patients, logistical items are of primary concern and affect ability to make informed decisions around treatment planning.

Many interventions for patients with HNC present financial implications, which are important to address and incorporate at each stage of treatment planning and implementation. Patient education and acknowledgment from the medical team around importance of learning how to navigate insurance or knowing who can assist with this and other financial-related issues can prevent complications when patients and families are most vulnerable. Involvement of discharge planners, case managers, and/or social workers as soon as possible contributes greatly in decreasing anxiety and use of limited team resources. Ancillary staff can also assist the medical team in understanding parameters of patient benefits and financial status.

Treatment

Surgery

For patients undergoing surgery alone, or before radiation and/or chemotherapy/immunotherapy, there are many practical and emotional items that patients and their families/support system must consider. It is imperative that each member of the health care team assist the patient and family in understanding psychosocial and physiologic needs and ensuring appropriate self-care predischarge. For many patients receiving surgery, acceptance and negotiation of "a new reality" include stressors, such as unexpected nature of significant procedures, adjustment to dysphagia and other physical side effects, medical trauma, body image, compliance with postsurgery needs including nutrition, and coordination of discharge planning. It is important to acknowledge that not all patients have healthy support systems that provide assistance with these needs.

Discharge planning

Comprehensive discharge planning is essential for all patients receiving inpatient attention. This includes arrangements for safe travel home or to a facility; coordination of follow-up or consultation visits with specialties, such as medical oncology or radiation oncology; and assessment of ability to meet basic needs, such as housing, food, clean recovery area, and emotional support. Nutrition also plays a large role in discharge planning because many patients require arrangements for enteral feeding supplies, support around adjustments to oral diet, tracheostomy and laryngectomy care, and wound care. In addition, patients may have surgical wounds that are disfiguring and require proper attention. Scars may trigger emotional reactions and are a concrete reminder of patient diagnosis, present state, and prognosis. Patients may also look to reactions of family and friends to gauge extent of disfigurement, depending on them to provide emotional support and positive reinforcement for their rehabilitation.[10]

Skilled nursing and subacute facilities

Although returning home is desired by most patients, for some, the lack or loss of a home or insufficient support system may make this unrealistic after surgery or hospitalization for cancer symptoms. Accepting the reality of a caregiver, especially for those who identify as independent, and placement in an institutional setting can be difficult to accept. Ancillary staff, such as a discharge planner, care coordinator, case manager, or social worker in the hospital setting, can assist the patient and family in making realistic decisions following assessment of patient health and safety.

Insurance coverage for chemotherapy/immunotherapy and radiation while coordinating these placements often presents significant barriers. These facilities may be hesitant to admit patients receiving treatment or planning on receiving these interventions because of limitations in insurance billing structures. Medicare, for example, considers skilled nursing facility (SNF) placement a "carve out" benefit, resulting in little to no financial reimbursement for those receiving chemoradiation. Advocacy from medical and ancillary staff may be required to ensure patient postdischarge needs are fulfilled. Partnering with facilities that are affiliated with the HNC hospital system, building rapport with local facilities, and providing education around patient needs can assist with smoother transitions and assurance of commitment to care plans.

Enteral feedings

It is imperative to ensure discussion of medical and psychosocial considerations when deciding on nutritional interventions. Patients with Medicare coverage, for example, are held to strict guidelines surrounding approval of enteral feedings. Members of the medical, psychosocial, and nutrition teams must consider this when determining if patients are eligible for coverage. For all insurance types, clear documentation must be present because of risk for denial and delay.

Documentation should include RDN and medical assessment of presence of the following: permanent nonfunction or disease of structures that permit food to reach the small bowel, dysphagia caused by tumor obstruction of the esophagus or sore throat from radiation esophagitis or mucositis, risk of aspiration, whether a patient has permanent impairment or requires tube feeding greater than 90 days, elevated caloric requirements (>2000 calories daily), and functional impairment of the gastrointestinal tract. If necessary, documentation from speech language pathology, including results of a swallowing study, should be included.

For those whose insurance does not cover enteral feedings, options including involvement from community resources, hospital charity funds, pharmaceutical assistance programs, or discussions around alternative nutrition management should be explored. These complications can be frustrating and burdensome.

Tracheostomy and laryngectomy
Tracheostomy placement is anxiety provoking because of the high level of care needed. Some patients require ongoing reassessment to determine if a tracheostomy is long-term, causing anxiety for patients and families hoping for consistency or return to routines. Similarly, patients with laryngectomies must adjust to home-care and self-management, presenting logistical and emotional stressors. Patients and families faced with the prospect of such care vary in how they cope with these challenges. Although patients may understand the role and value of tracheostomy or laryngectomy care, some may become squeamish and/or intimidated by expectations placed on them by their team. When a realistic plan at home is unable to be established, short- or long-term placement in a subacute facility may be necessary.

Tracheostomy and laryngectomy supplies, including portable rechargeable suction machines (for safe transportation home), must be anticipated before discharge and insurance limitations considered. Allied health professionals, such as case managers and/or nurses, should assist the team and work with patients and support systems to ensure coverage of supplies, locate contracted vendors, coordinate equipment ordering and delivery to patients before discharge to lessen barriers in obtaining supplies, and ensure proper teaching on use and care of equipment.

Chemotherapy/immunotherapy and radiation
Some patients require radiation therapy alone, following surgery, and/or the addition of chemotherapy or immunotherapy. Both interventions add additional stressors, such as engagement with new medical teams; additional information to process around nature of treatment; decision-making; logistical considerations, such as transportation, child care, housing; employment-related items; and side effects. Medical oncology and radiation oncology teams should be available on initial consultation to provide education around services to decrease anxiety and improve long-term treatment planning. It is helpful for ancillary staff to be well versed in these interventions and potential obstacles, incorporating these items into assessments and better engaging with patients and families around the treatment plan, as a whole.

Many of the barriers related to engagement of care and treatment planning are relevant, once again, when initiating engagement with medical oncology and radiation oncology services. Of particular concern are logistical obstacles given the nature of these treatment options. Radiation, for example, may require patients to attend treatment daily. Although compliance to chemotherapy/immunotherapy treatments is important, effectiveness of radiation therapy is significantly compromised when treatment is missed or delayed. This should be communicated clearly with patients to ensure understanding of the value of compliance. Although initial assessments performed by HNC staff should be referenced, additional assessments around barriers to care and general patient education are essential in ensuring effective treatment. These assessments should include logistical emotional considerations, such as claustrophobia, concerns around aesthetics (discoloration of skin or loss of weight), perceptions around treatment, and fear of needles. Patients may benefit from touring treatment areas following patient education, allowing them to touch, see, and smell what is to come, clarify misconceptions, and decrease fear of the unknown. Ancillary staff should be available to deliver interventions, such as use of relaxation techniques, processing of feelings associated with these spaces, and validation of patient and family thoughts and concerns.

Engagement with radiation and/or chemotherapy also presents obstacles around nourishment of patient nutritional needs. Both interventions, and preradiation surgical and dental treatments, can affect patient intake and processing. RDN staff should be available to monitor weight and nutrient levels and present appropriate interventions for improvement. Many patients who have not required enteral feedings or adjustments to oral diet may now need assistance. Changes in oral diet may include transition to liquid or soft diet to assist with swallowing and decrease risk for aspiration or use of foods with healing properties, such as papaya. Patients with difficulty maintaining caloric or nutrient intake may require use of liquid supplements. Of particular concern are patients who have lost 10% or more of their body weight in which enteral feeding may be recommended to ensure optimal processing of treatment and recovery.

It is important to recognize and educate patients on psychosocial implications of these interventions and assist with navigation of systems affected by these treatment options. "Treatment for head and neck cancer may have a debilitating and lasting impact on a patient's functional status, limiting their ability to work during and after treatment."[11] Compared with other cancer diagnoses, patients with HNC have a greater chance of job loss, livelihood, and ability to pay for basic living expenses and additional expenditures related to treatment. Penner discusses how any cancer diagnosis affects employability and productivity of patients and families and how complex treatment regimens, which patients with HNC often require, may interfere with daily employment responsibilities and roles.[11] This may present not only significant financial burden but also emotional adjustment to changes in work-related identity. It is important to address patient concerns about financial wellbeing; acknowledge autonomy around employment-based decisions; and educate patients about rights in the workplace, private and state disability insurance, support for caregivers, such as Family Medical Leave Act (FMLA) and in-home support, and public assistance and/or community resources. Discomfort and poor health force some patients to adjust, lessen, or cease certain responsibilities in the workplace, potentially altering compensation, benefits, and other employer-based support mechanisms. These issues are of great importance to patients and families who worry about their ability to survive physically and maintain financial stability. It is important for the HNC team to acknowledge that financial implications, although logistical in nature, have an emotional impact even after completion of treatment, contributing to existing stress, anxiety, and sometimes depression. Use of resources, such as CaringBridge and MealTrain, allow patients to ask for help with logistical/financial items from the comfort and privacy of their home.

Surveillance and Survivorship

It is important for the HNC team to inform patients and families of expectations around surveillance and monitoring of recovery/disease status and convey the value in patient care, acknowledging efforts from engagement in care through treatment. Patients may feel burdened with need for follow-up, especially given logistical and emotional considerations. HNC team members should acknowledge that completion of treatment does not equate to lack of medical and psychosocial stressors.[12] Early education around role of HNC team, timeline, and plan following completion of treatment allows for preparation needed for appointments and processing of information provided during these visits. It is also important to acknowledge any anxiety related to follow-up, such as the return to unknowns and potential for bad news. In addition, patient anxiety around their status may result in frequent communication and scheduling attempts inconsistent with timeline and plan for evaluation. Assurance of engagement with specialists, such as pain/palliative services, and involvement of mental health professionals can assist with this transition, supporting patients with concrete and emotional adjustments to this piece of their illness trajectory.

Because time between follow-up appointments is often longer than what patients desire, engagement with community resources, such as cancer support centers, support groups, peer programs, or eHealth resources, may be helpful. Connection with these resources can assist patients by promoting social engagement, providing a sense of unconditional community, space to transition to self-management, and assistance with reflection on their identity as a survivor.[2,12] Gradually establishing identity with support from these mechanisms can promote healthy normalization of patient experiences, reflection on what diagnosis and treatment means to them, visualization of survivorship, and acquisition of tips on how to live a meaningful life after HNC. Patients seeking additional support or those residing in areas without quality support services may use online resources, such as blogs and forums, to obtain information and support.

A particular challenge seen across the illness trajectory is patients who are lost to follow-up. Often these patients have identified barriers, such as mental illness, substance abuse, and homelessness; however, some may also be struggling with emotional implications of diagnosis, treatment, and overall HNC experience. Logistical barriers, such as transportation, distance from facility, and difficulty navigating insurance, may also affect ability to maintain proper follow-up. Anecdotally, some of these patients return when the cancer has progressed, limiting treatment options. Reengagement should involve all members of the HNC team for reassessment of medical and psychosocial context, effective treatment planning, or discussion of palliative/end-of-life options.

ADDITIONAL AREAS TO BE CONSIDERED ACROSS THE ILLNESS TRAJECTORY
Communication

Many patients with HNC must cope with changes in communication abilities even on presentation of symptoms. Difficulty with speech is seen in patients with glossectomy or partial glossectomy, or other changes in their oral cavity, ear, nose, throat, and lips after surgery or chemoradiation. These challenges add additional obstacles to adjust to or overcome, especially because of the importance of communication with health care teams, support system, and general need for socialization. Patients may require someone to assist with communication throughout all stages of care, even if it is believed they will return to independence. Use of alternative communication techniques, such as notebooks, whiteboards, and tablets, in the inpatient and outpatient setting acknowledge the impact of communicative obstacles while empowering patients to express themselves and maintain their role in their care. These interventions should also be encouraged in the home to decrease isolation and allow for openness with family, friends, and other members of the patient's support network.

Social Isolation

Some patients experience or self-impose isolation from their support systems because of the physiologic and emotional effects of treatment. "The effects of disease and treatment often cannot be concealed by patients with HNC, making those who suffer from facial disfigurement vulnerable to distress, intimacy issues, social isolation, stigma, and untoward behavior from others."[2] Carlson[13] discusses a University of Chicago Pritzker School of Medicine study exploring social isolation in patients with HNC, described as having two components, loneliness and lack of social support. In this study, patients with high levels of perceived social isolation, as compared with those with adequate social support, exhibited decrease in medication compliance, increased missed appointments, and longer inpatient stays. Financial burdens were also greater. Penner[12] proposes that although a continuum of emotional reactions is normal in the coping process, some patients may exhibit unhealthy coping strategies that result in isolation and depression. Consistent with Carlson's study, Penner[12] also links isolation and loneliness with depression and financial burden.

Social isolation, identified early, can prevent or lessen many obstacles. Assistance with concrete services, such as transportation, linkage to support groups, and engagement with a social worker or psychologist on engagement in care, can serve as an improved social support system. Recommendations across various media types, such as the Mayo Clinic's "Living with Cancer" blog, include tips that can be applied on initial consultation. Suggestions, such as seeking support virtually, making plans when one has the most energy, and limiting engagement to activities with one or two friends instead of a large party, provide realistic ways to maintain connections with much needed support within realistic boundaries of patient health status.[14] Of particular concern are patients who present or become isolated because of diagnosis and treatment. Although the cause of isolation may vary from personality characteristics, to depression, dysfunctional family dynamics, and family estrangement, these patients present significant risk factors for treatment and recovery and require support of allied health professionals to assist with coordination of appointments, navigating resources, and ensuring basic needs, such as housing and adequate nutrition.

Smoking and Alcohol

It is known that smoking and drinking are risk factors for developing HNC. "Continued use of these substances beyond diagnosis complicates treatment, confers greater risk of recurrence or developing a second primary tumor, and ultimately impacts survival."[2] On diagnosis and mobilization to fight disease, it is an ideal time to engage and educate patients about the impact of these behaviors on their health, specifically cancer. Initial assessment of smoking and alcohol use presents a teachable moment when patients may be more receptive and motivated to change. Because these behaviors serve often as coping strategies, however dysfunctional, there may be increased reliance in the face of fear and distress.[11]

Cancer Care and Palliative Care

There is increasing recognition that separation of cancer care and palliative care, with palliative care offered only at the end of life, is no longer acceptable. This limited model fails to account for symptoms existing before diagnosis, through the trajectory of cancer, which can be addressed and palliated early on, regardless of whether a patient's cancer is considered curable. "Palliative care is a philosophy of care that has evolved into an integral part of the care of patients with cancer regardless of age, diagnosis, or life expectancy and engages actively in the management of patients with complex physical and psychological concerns to assist them with adopting effective coping strategies and live fulfilling lives."[11]

Advance Care Planning Along the Illness Continuum

Neil Wenger[15], Director of the UCLA Health System Ethics Center, suggests "...advance care planning conversations about what patients want at the end of life, and how they want to make choices to achieve their goals, need to occur for every seriously ill patient." Ahluwalia and colleagues[16] discuss the importance of initiating care-planning discussions as early as possible, particularly when patients are diagnosed with advanced cancer, demonstrating the value of multidisciplinary involvement in the earliest stages of patient care. Patients require time to process and accept their prognosis before considering the range of care options available to them at end of life.

Patients faced with HNC, like all patients with life-threatening illness, have an opportunity to explore their values and goals as they make health care decisions and reflect on situations when they might not be able to make decisions on their own behalf. Diagnosis presents an ideal opportunity for these discussions, addressing acceptable health care states, and what patients are willing to endure to continue living. All patients should be encouraged to partner with their HNC team to complete advance directives and POLST forms clarifying their wishes and communicating with loved ones. For patients without families or close support systems, this partnership can assist them in making decisions about who they could best trust to be their agent. Engaging patients early in the decision-making and treatment planning process provides an opportunity for discussion of goals of care and a foundation on which to have these dialogues when treatments are not working or a cancer recurs.

In providing patient-centered care, it is essential that one consider nourishment of patient autonomy and empowerment around end of life and what to offer patients when curative options are no longer viable. Patients deserve to know they will not be abandoned by the medical team in this stage of life, and that there are palliative care and hospice teams whose primary role is to relieve suffering.

REFERENCES

1. Epstein RM, Street RL. The values and value of patient-centered care. Ann Fam Med 2011;9(2):100–3.
2. Howren MB, Christensen AJ, Karnell LH, et al. Psychological factors associated with head and neck cancer treatment and survivorship: evidence and opportunities for behavioral medicine. J Consult Clin Psychol 2013;81(2): 299–317.
3. Wu Y-S, Lin P-Y, Chien C-Y, et al. Anxiety and depression in patients with head and neck cancer: 6-month follow-up study. Neuropsychiatr Dis Treat 2016;12: 1029–36.
4. Winkler MF. 2009 Lenna Frances Cooper Memorial Lecture: living with enteral and parenteral nutrition: how food and eating contribute to quality of life. J Am Diet Assoc 2010;110(2):169–77.
5. Meule A, Vögele C. The psychology of eating. Front Psychol 2013;4. http://dx.doi. org/10.3389/fpsyg.2013.00215.

6. Meyers S, Ott MJ. Mindful eating as a clinical intervention for survivors of head and neck cancer: interdisciplinary collaboration and strategies to improve oral intake. Top Clin Nutr 2008;23(4):340–6.

7. Britton B, McCarter K, Baker A, et al. Eating As Treatment (EAT) study protocol: a stepped-wedge, randomised controlled trial of a health behaviour change intervention provided by dietitians to improve nutrition in patients with head and neck cancer undergoing radiotherapy. BMJ Open 2015;5(7):e008921.

8. Vakharia KT, Ali MJ, Wang SJ. Quality-of-life impact of participation in a head and neck cancer support group. Otolaryngol Head Neck Surg 2007;136(3):405–10.

9. Richardson AE, Morton RP, Broadbent EA. Illness perceptions and coping predict post-traumatic stress in caregivers of patients with head and neck cancer. Support Care Cancer 2016;24(10):4443–50.

10. Aaronson NK, Mattioli V, Minton O, et al. Beyond treatment: psychosocial and behavioural issues in cancer survivorship research and practice. EJC Suppl 2014; 12(1):54–64.

11. Penner JL. Psychosocial care of patients with head and neck cancer. Semin Oncol Nurs 2009;25(3):231–41.

12. Ussher J, Kirsten L, Butow P, et al. What do cancer support groups provide which other supportive relationships do not? The experience of peer support groups for people with cancer. Soc Sci Med 2006;62(10):2565–76.

13. Carlson RH. Head & neck cancer patients face social isolation, financial burdens. Available at: http://journals.lww.com/oncologytimes/pages/articleviewer. aspxyear=2016&issue=04250&article=00009&type=Fulltext. Accessed May 5, 2017.

14. Cancer Expert Blog - Mayo Clinic. Available at: http://www.mayoclinic.org/ diseases-conditions/cancer/expert-blog/con-20032378. Accessed November 2, 2016.

15. UCLA Health. New law opens door to conversation about end-of-life issues. Available at: https://na01.safelinks.protection.outlook.com/?url=https%3A%2F%2Fwww. uclahealth.org%2FWorkfiles%2Fvitalsigns%2FVital-Signs_FA16.pdf&data=01% 7C01%7Camadnick%40mednet.ucla.edu%7Cc96086c5f6794ce3f8e108d493e8f6 a8%7C39c3716b64714fd5ac04a7dbaa32782b%7C0&sdata=llVYoYjestgshYNAD 2NAK4tT5K6UfpXjrmQE6FUP%2Bas%3D&reserved=0. Accessed March 30, 2017.

16. Ahluwalia SC, Tisnado DM, Walling AM, et al. Association of early patient-physician care planning discussions and end-of-life care intensity in advanced cancer. J Palliat Med 2015;18(10):834–41.

Maximizing Functional Outcomes in Head and Neck Cancer Survivors

Assessment and Rehabilitation

Nausheen Jamal, MD[a,b,*], Barbara Ebersole, MA, CCC-SLP[a,c],
Andrew Erman, MS, CCC-SLP[d], Dinesh Chhetri, MD[e]

KEYWORDS

- Head and neck cancer • Treatment • Complication • Morbidity • Dysphagia
- Dysphonia • Survivorship

KEY POINTS

- As survival from head and neck cancer (HNC) improves, quality-of-life (QOL) issues and functional preservation assume heightened relevance.
- The keys to successfully addressing the QOL issues and preserving function are threefold: (1) prevention, (2) timely assessment and treatment of QOL symptoms, and (3) regular, long-term follow-up of functional deficits.
- Dysphagia remains the most important factor for most long-term survivors, although issues of voice/speech, airway obstruction, neck and shoulder dysfunction, lymphedema, and pain control are also important to address.
- Central to providing comprehensive interdisciplinary care are the head and neck surgeon, laryngologist, and speech-language pathologist. Routine assessment, long-term follow-up, and regular communication and coordination among these specialists help maximize QOL in this challenging patient population.

Disclosure Statement: The authors have nothing to disclose.
[a] Department of Otolaryngology–Head & Neck Surgery, Lewis Katz School of Medicine, Temple University, 3440 North Broad Street, Kresge West #300, Philadelphia, PA 19140, USA; [b] Department of Surgical Oncology, Fox Chase Cancer Center, 333 Cottman Avenue, Philadelphia, PA 19119, USA; [c] Department of Speech Pathology, Fox Chase Cancer Center, 333 Cottman Avenue, Philadelphia, PA 19119, USA; [d] Department of Audiology & Speech, University of California, 200 UCLA Plaza, Suite 540, Los Angeles, CA 90095, USA; [e] Department of Head & Neck Surgery, University of California, 200 UCLA Plaza, Suite 550, Los Angeles, CA 90095, USA
* Corresponding author. Department of Otolaryngology–Head & Neck Surgery, Lewis Katz School of Medicine, Temple University, 3440 North Broad Street, Kresge West #300, Philadelphia, PA 19140.
E-mail address: nausheen.jamal@tuhs.temple.edu

Otolaryngol Clin N Am 50 (2017) 837–852
http://dx.doi.org/10.1016/j.otc.2017.04.004
0030-6665/17/© 2017 Elsevier Inc. All rights reserved.

oto.theclinics.com

INTRODUCTION

Until recently, the only goal in the care of patients with head and neck cancer (HNC) has been achieving a cure. As such, a 12% increase in the 5-year survival rate in HNC has been observed over the last decade.[1] However, the surgical and nonsurgical treatment options for HNC are fraught with significant morbidity affecting quality of life (QOL). As survival from cancer is improved, QOL issues and functional preservation assume heightened relevance.

The most common complaints in HNC survivors are QOL-related, including dysphagia, dysphonia, dysarthria, trismus, loss of salivation, dental caries, tracheostomy tube dependence, neck/shoulder dysfunction, chronic pain, feeding-tube dependence, and cosmetic deformity.[2–5] Many patients also suffer from morbidity related to neuropathy and lymphedema.[6,7]

The initial choice of cancer treatment (ie, surgery vs chemoradiation therapy [CRT], parallel beam vs intensity-modulated radiation therapy, and minimally invasive endoscopic cancer resection vs open procedures) often directly affects survivor QOL.[8,9] Other treatment-related factors known to increase the risk of dysfunction include multimodality treatment, high-dose or wide-field radiation therapy, and even a brief duration of nil per os.[10,11] For those patients who undergo radiation or multimodality treatment, dysfunction may be slowly progressive years after treatment.[12]

The keys to successfully addressing QOL issues and preserving function are threefold: (1) prevention; (2) timely assessment and treatment of QOL symptoms; and (3) regular, long-term follow-up of functional deficits. Thorough evaluation via comprehensive physical examination, and awareness of the breadth of complications and treatment options, enables the clinician to effectively prevent, recognize, and treat poor functional outcomes associated with treatment of HNC.

PATHOPHYSIOLOGY OF DYSFUNCTION

There are three primary modalities of cancer treatment: (1) surgery, (2) radiation therapy (RT), and (3) chemotherapy. Early stage cancers can often be treated with single-modality treatment, whereas advanced stage cancers require multimodality treatment.[13] These are associated with typical effects on functional outcomes (**Box 1**).

Dysphagia

Swallowing dysfunction is a well-recognized complication of HNC treatment. It is the number one QOL complaint in HNC survivors. With widespread adoption of CRT protocols for "organ preservation," the incidence of dysphagia seems to be rising.[4] The

---

Box 1
Typical dysfunctions that occur after head and neck cancer treatment

Soft tissue fibrosis

Dysphagia (with or without feeding tube dependence)

Oral cavity dysfunction (trismus, xerostomia)

Dysphonia and dysarthria

Tracheostomy-tube dependence

Hearing loss

Cosmetic deformity

Neck and shoulder dysfunction

incidence of dysphagia after treatment of HNC is likely underreported because of the lack of adequate and routine swallow assessment after cancer therapy. Presence of sensory deficits in HNC survivors also contributes to this.

All treatment modalities for HNC, alone or in combination, can lead to dysphagia.[2–5,10–12] The anatomic subsites with the greatest risk for posttreatment dysphagia are the larynx, oropharynx, and hypopharynx.[14–16] Other risk factors for dysphagia include advanced stage tumors, advanced age, female gender, and high-dose RT to surrounding structures.[15–17] Addition of chemotherapy to radiation increases dysphagia risk.[16,18–20] The prevalence of dysphagia in patients undergoing CRT for oropharyngeal and hypopharyngeal squamous cell carcinoma (SCCA) is between 36% and 81%.[21]

Signs and symptoms of dysphagia in the HNC patient population may vary and are listed in **Box 2**. Patients may report few or none of these symptoms if laryngopharyngeal sensation is impaired.

There is some variability in feeding tube placement protocols across institutions. Placement may occur at the beginning of treatment, during treatment (eg, with loss of 10% of body weight), or as needed when inadequate/unsafe per oral intake is observed. Feeding tubes maintain adequate nutrition, prevent unintended weight loss, and reduce pneumonia risk. However, exclusively using a feeding tube during RT/CRT without per oral intake or swallow exercises has been associated with worse dysphagia outcomes.[22] Feeding tubes may be left in place for supplemental purposes, such as for patients who may engage in per oral intake for pleasure but require augmented nutrition, or if a patient is unable to take medications safely by mouth.

Dysphonia and Dysarthria

Surgery or RT of the larynx may disrupt gross vocal fold motion, mucosal wave generation, lubrication, and voice projection. Dysarthria is a common side effect of oral

---

Box 2
Signs and symptoms of dysphagia in the head and neck cancer population

Aspiration

Coughing

Throat clearing during meals

Prolonged meal times

Avoidance/difficulty with certain consistencies

Oropharyngeal residue

Expectoration

Reduced pleasure with oral intake

Difficulty managing secretions/drooling

Difficulty chewing

Difficulty initiating a swallow

Nasal/pharyngeal regurgitation during eating

Sensation of food sticking in the throat or chest

History of pneumonia

Weight loss

Evidence of malnutrition

cavity cancer and its treatment. Xerostomia may impact consonant articulation. Glossectomy, particularly in cases of advanced stage tumors, leads to limited tongue mobility and reduced articulation. Free tissue reconstruction may mitigate these functional issues by reducing the likelihood of scar contracture and loss of bulk. Treatment of nasopharynx or oropharynx tumors can stiffen and scar the soft palate, leading to velopharyngeal incompetence, impaired speech resonance, and dysarthria.

Tracheostomy-Tube Dependence

Persistent upper airway obstruction may occur in patients with bulky free tissue reconstruction of the pharynx, and those with radiation-induced chronic laryngeal edema. In some cases, patients may suffer from bilateral vocal fold paralysis resulting from their cancer and/or treatment. In many cases, patients are ultimately decannulated.

Hearing Loss

Platinum-based chemotherapy agents are considered ototoxic because of the risks they pose to outer hair cells and subsequent high rate of sensorineural hearing loss.[23] Conductive hearing loss can also occur following surgery or radiation to the nasopharynx, oropharynx, or larynx. Obstruction or dysfunction of the eustachian tube can lead to fluid in the middle ear, leading to otitis media with or without effusion.[24]

Neck/Shoulder Dysfunction and Lymphedema

Neck and shoulder dysfunction are well-described consequences of radical neck dissection.[25] They are often the result of spinal accessory nerve palsy; however, it can occur in the absence of nerve injury because of adhesion of neck muscles to overlying platysma and skin.[26] Shoulder dysfunction can inhibit basic activities of living, such as dressing and bathing, and can prohibit return to work.

Secondary lymphedema of the head and neck is a common, although often unrecognized, side effect of HNC treatment with a reported incidence of greater than 50%.[7,27] Lymphedema is swelling that occurs 3 or more months after completion of treatment as a result of damage to the lymphatic system, leading to congestion or stasis of lymph fluid. It can occur internally or externally, although most patients experience both.[27] Lymphedema of the head and neck is a form of disfigurement that also may have significant functional consequences, including difficulty swallowing, difficulty breathing, and reduced cervical range of motion.

PATIENT EVALUATION OVERVIEW

A directed history and comprehensive head and neck evaluation are paramount in recognition of functional problems. Patients may not always volunteer information about functional problems, because they may assume that what they are experiencing is expected or normal. For example, when asked broadly about dysphagia, they may report that they are "swallowing fine." More directed questions may be revealing, such as inquiring about foods they avoid, coughing during meals, pneumonia episodes, weight loss, meal duration, social isolation, and any (supplemental) feeding tube use. Patients may have diminished sensation or have adjusted their lifestyles to their swallow dysfunction, and therefore fail to acknowledge some of these issues. The use of a validated patient-rated symptom questionnaire is another way of identifying areas of potential concern to explore further during the patient's visit.

Evaluation of Dysphagia

The most basic examination is that of the oral cavity. One must assess for degree of mouth opening (trismus), mucosal dryness, tongue mobility and strength, adequacy of dentition, and oral hygiene. A clinical swallow evaluation focusing on dysphonia, dysarthria, abnormal volitional cough, abnormal gag reflex, cough on trial swallow, and voice change on trial swallow may be predictive of the risk of aspiration.[28] However, an instrumental swallow examination is necessary to assess the severity of dysphagia and recommend a safe diet.

Flexible laryngoscopy plays a critical role in anatomic evaluation of the swallowing mechanism. By augmenting flexible laryngoscopy with an assessment of swallowing, a comprehensive anatomic and functional assessment of swallowing is performed.[29] Although flexible endoscopic evaluation of swallowing (FEES) has been invaluable for the otolaryngologist to connect anatomy with swallow function, it does have some minor limitations, such as inability to observe the oral phase of swallow, assess upper esophageal sphincter (UES) function, and observe events that occur during the swallow.

A videofluoroscopic procedure, the modified barium swallow study (MBSS), has traditionally served as the swallow evaluation procedure of choice in patients with HNC. Although it provides less anatomic information than FEES, it provides information on oral phases of swallowing, impression of pharyngeal strength, events during the swallow, UES opening, and the degree of aspiration and aspiration along the posterior tracheal wall.

FEES and MBSS have been found to have similar sensitivity with respect to detecting aspiration.[29] However, each test has unique strengths, and therefore, they should be considered complementary rather than interchangeable. In fact, many patients with HNC need both tests as a part of their dysphagia work-up to fully evaluate the anatomic and functional deficits and plan optimal treatment. In this regard, otolaryngologists should become facile at interpretation of both studies to develop a cohesive and effective treatment plan.

Screening for cervical esophageal stenosis is especially important in patients with HNC, especially if there is a history of gastric feeding tube placement during CRT and the patient senses obstruction and/or has solid food dysphagia. MBSS or a barium esophagram is often used to detect stenosis. A more specific test is esophagoscopy, which can now be performed transnasally with local anesthetic in the office setting.[30]

Evaluation of Dysphonia

Both surgical and nonsurgical treatment of HNC may lead to dysphonia. Ideally, patients with dysphonia should be assessed with laryngovideostroboscopic examination before referral for a voice evaluation to understand the anatomic and physiologic deficits present. Glottic insufficiency from vocal fold paralysis or tissue deficiency is managed with injection augmentation or thyroplasty. Referral for voice therapy is made for residual dysphonia and dysarthria. A speech-language pathologist's (SLP) clinical voice evaluation includes analyzing voice production, assessing stimulability to produce improved voice, and providing feedback to the patient on "what's wrong, why it's wrong, and what we are going to do about it."

Evaluation of Tracheostomy-Dependence

Patients may undergo tracheostomy placement for a variety of reasons, ranging from airway protection while undergoing cancer treatment, to alleviation of airway obstruction caused by bulky tumors, or because of laryngeal dysfunction that leads to airway obstruction or profound dysphagia. Evaluation of these patients begins with assessment of the patient's respiratory status with and without occlusion of an appropriately sized tracheostomy tube. Complete airway endoscopy is also critical. This begins with laryngoscopy to assess glottic and subglottic airway, followed by tracheoscopy through the established tracheostoma, performed after removal of the tracheostomy tube (if possible), so that the airway above and below the stoma is evaluated. In some cases, evaluation may need to be performed in the operating room setting. Sites of obstruction should be identified, with determination made as to whether they can be resolved. After sites of obstruction have been identified and addressed, the physician may proceed with his/her preferred capping and decannulation protocol.

Evaluation of Hearing Loss

The American Academy of Audiology recommends routine surveillance of hearing function before, during (before each dose), and after (several months) platinum-based chemotherapy treatment. For patients who also receive head and neck irradiation, 1 to 2 years of ongoing monitoring after treatment completion is recommended because of the potential for progressive decline in hearing function. The test battery should include basic audiologic assessment and, if able, high-frequency audiometry.[31] Predictors for hearing loss include baseline hearing levels, radiation dose to the cochlea, and cisplatin dose.[32] Medical oncologists and audiologists should work together to determine the ideal model of hearing monitoring based on the opportunities and constraints within their organizations.

Evaluation of Neck/Shoulder Dysfunction and Lymphedema

Patient-reported symptoms of neck and shoulder dysfunction may include report of pain, stiffness of the neck/shoulder, difficulty lifting arm, or difficulty turning the head. Patients often do not recognize or report mild dysfunction because of spontaneous compensatory techniques. Assessment of posture and neck/shoulder function should occur during the physical examination. It is important to assess these functions during follow-up visits to refer to physical therapy when the dysfunction is mild (before progression to moderate or severe). Automatic pretreatment and posttreatment evaluations by a physical therapist may be the most effective way of catching dysfunction early.[26]

Patient-reported symptoms of lymphedema may include a report of swelling or fullness, tightness, or heaviness in the affected area, and potential difficulty swallowing or breathing. External lymphedema typically presents in the neck and submental region.[7,27] Physical examination may identify neck edema with or without pitting. If lymphedema is identified, prompt referral to a lymphedema-certified rehabilitation therapist for decongestive therapy is recommended.

TREATMENT
Pharmacologic Treatment Options

Patients with HNC may experience pain before, during, and long after their treatment course because of somatic tissue or nerve injury.[33] The injury can be caused by the cancer itself or the cancer treatment (surgery, RT, or CRT). It is important that pain is routinely assessed and treated to the extent that it does not inhibit participation in rehabilitation activities. The inclusion of pain and palliative care within the treatment team is valuable, particularly for pain that persists beyond completion of active treatment. In addition to typical narcotic analgesics, botulinum toxin injections have been described as a potentially useful tool for pain associated with muscle spasms in the neck or jaw.[26,33] Gabapentin has been demonstrated in several small retrospective studies to be associated with reduction of narcotic use and mucositis-associated pain during RT, thereby facilitating oral intake and swallow function.[34–36] However, the only randomized controlled study to date found no significant benefit to its use when compared with standard care.[37] Further investigation is warranted.

Behavioral Treatment Options

Most patients with HNC benefit from rehabilitation services designed to address the sequelae associated with their disease and treatment. As such, rehabilitation clinicians (ie, SLP, physical and occupational therapists) and oncologists should have regular interface, to benefit from one another's respective expertise. Multidisciplinary clinics with speech pathology and head and neck surgery or laryngology offer benefits to providers and to patients.[38,39] Rehabilitation clinicians can also be valuable participants in the multidisciplinary tumor board, given that preservation of function is a treatment-planning consideration. In addition to rehabilitation therapists, social workers, psychologists, nutritionists, nurses, prosthodontists, and physiatrists are integral to the rehabilitation of patients with HNC.

Behavioral rehabilitation interventions should be considered for any patient with HNC experiencing oral motor dysfunction, dysarthria, dysphagia, dysphonia, aphonia, trismus, postural dysfunction, neck and/or shoulder dysfunction, or lymphedema. Rehabilitation approaches fall into four broad categories: (1) preventive, (2) restorative, (3) supportive, and (4) palliative. These approaches are not necessarily sequential, and are often used simultaneously as a part of the patient's individualized therapy plan. *Preventive approaches* aim to mitigate the risk of developing dysfunction. Notably, rehabilitation models have developed surrounding preservation of shoulder, jaw, and swallowing function during HNC treatment.[22,26,40–42] *Restorative approaches* aim to improve physical function via strengthening exercises, manual and myofascial techniques, passive and active stretching, neuromuscular re-education, compression, and/or lymphatic massage. Restorative approaches are typically used at the onset of dysfunction (ie, following surgery or RT/CRT), or if progressive dysfunction is identified following cancer treatment.[43] *Supportive approaches* aim to improve functionality by working around dysfunction. Compensatory strategies, education, and psychoeducational counseling are typically used. These may include postural or behavioral strategies to facilitate safe, timely oral intake with the least restrictive diet; techniques to improve speech intelligibility; use of communication devices; or strategies to ameliorate xerostomia.

Patients with recurrent or metastatic HNC experience significant physical impairment and may benefit from limited interventions to enhance QOL.[45] *Palliative approaches* focus on compensation and education to facilitate communication, eating, and other activities of daily living that are important to the patient. For example, swallowing strategies may make eating more comfortable or less time consuming. The use of an orthotic neck collar may diminish the functional impact of severe neck extensor weakness. Treatment goals are typically limited and target a specific QOL concern identified by the patient or family.

Distress is common in the HNC population and can negatively impact patient motivation and engagement in rehabilitation. Mental health professionals can facilitate improved functionality indirectly by addressing psychosocial barriers to rehabilitation. Therefore, mental health services and peer-based support groups are important elements of the rehabilitation process.[44]

Behavioral treatment challenges

Behavioral interventions present several challenges for patients with HNC. First, there is a paucity of therapists experienced and knowledgeable in HNC rehabilitation. It is difficult for patients to find or access therapists who are prepared to effectively evaluate and treat HNC survivors. Second, behavioral rehabilitation regimens typically involve long-term follow-up to maintain the highest level of function. Third, adherence to therapeutic exercises or recommendations is often difficult. This is especially true of patients with sensory deficits, who may not appreciate an intervention's value or benefit. Additional obstacles to compliance include pain, fatigue, lack of understanding regarding the importance of exercises, and forgetfulness.[46]

Surgical Treatment Options

Treatment of dysphagia

Although the bulk of effective swallow rehabilitation in this population depends on swallow therapy for prevention and treatment of swallow pathology, adjunctive surgical procedures also play a critical role. Surgical treatments are tailored to the sites of swallow dysfunction. In the experience of the authors, treatable swallow dysfunction often localizes to one or more of the following sites: pharynx, epiglottis, UES, and esophagus. Detailed information on the surgical techniques used at each subsite is available in the referenced studies. It should be emphasized that nearly all cases of surgical therapy are accompanied by swallow therapy.

Pharynx Pharyngeal structures may develop progressive fibrosis, and stenosis may develop.[47] These changes lead to decreased functional muscular contraction and pharyngeal scar band formation. Laryngoscopy may demonstrate scarring, reduced velopharyngeal closure, reduced medial pharyngeal contraction, and/or reduced base of tongue retraction (**Fig. 1**). FEES may show the presence of diffuse residual after the swallow (**Fig. 2**), and MBSS may reveal reduced laryngeal elevation, pharyngeal

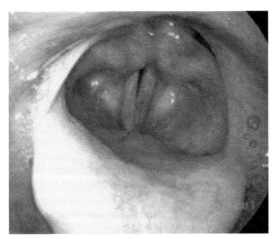

Fig. 1. Lateral pharyngeal scar bands between the epiglottis and posterior pharyngeal wall following radiation treatment. These impede normal bolus passage into the pyriform sinuses and upper esophageal sphincter.

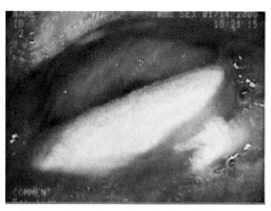

Fig. 2. Residual seen during endoscopic swallow testing in the presence of severe pharyngeal weakness, in part caused by pharyngeal fibrosis. Esophageal stenosis can lead to similar stasis in the pharynx.

weakness, and epiglottic dysfunction. Treatment consists of aggressive dysphagia therapy in conjunction with surgical laser dilation of scar bands. The carbon dioxide (CO_2) laser is typically used to create multiple radial incisions within each scar band. This is followed by balloon dilation to stretch the area of fibrosis and scar.[48]

Epiglottis CRT may also lead to fibrosis and thickening of the epiglottis. This may cause limited retroflexion during the swallow, accompanied by a "sticking" sensation in the pharynx. Laryngoscopy shows a typical thickened and stiff appearance of the epiglottis. FEES demonstrates presence of residual in the vallecula and lateral channels after the swallow (**Fig. 3**). MBSS shows absence of retroflexion with vallecular accumulation of residual, suggesting that the non-retroflexing epiglottis is obstructing bolus flow. In these cases, trimming of the suprahyoid epiglottis may improve swallow efficiency without increasing aspiration risk.[49] Surgery is performed endoscopically through a laryngoscope. A CO_2 laser is used to perform the partial resection (**Fig. 4**). Patients are discharged the same day on their preoperative diets, with follow-up swallow studies performed about a month thereafter to assess for possible diet advancement.

Upper esophageal sphincter and esophageal stenosis As with other parts of the pharynx and larynx, CRT may lead to progressive fibrosis of the cricopharyngeus and

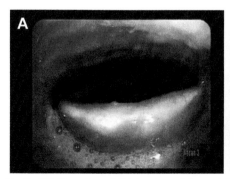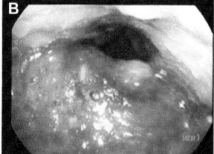

Fig. 3. (*A*) Fibrosis and thickening of the epiglottis as the result of chemoradiation. (*B*) This leads to vallecular residual, shown on endoscopic swallow evaluation.

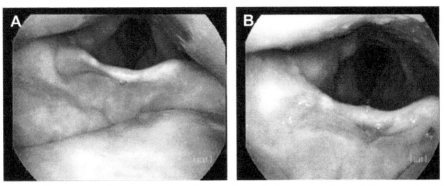

Fig. 4. (*A*) Postoperative appearance after endoscopic laser resection of the suprahyoid epiglottis. (*B*) There is reduced pharyngeal residual on the postoperative swallow evaluation.

cervical esophagus. FEES shows pooling of secretions and residue in the postcricoid region and pyriform sinuses. MBSS shows UES dysfunction (inadequate UES opening) with limited passage or obstruction of the food bolus at that level. In these cases, transnasal esophagoscopy is helpful in identifying the presence of a stenotic area or scar band (**Fig. 5**). Findings may be more subtle, such as the haptic feedback of increased resistance when passing the scope through the UES.

UES dysfunction is typically addressed effectively with endoscopic cricopharyngel myotomy. This is performed using a CO_2 laser, using an approach similar to that used for Zenker diverticulotomy (**Fig. 6**). Because of the fibrotic nature of the muscle fibers, it is helpful in the authors' experience to perform a dilation after myotomy to further improve the area of stenosis and dysfunction.

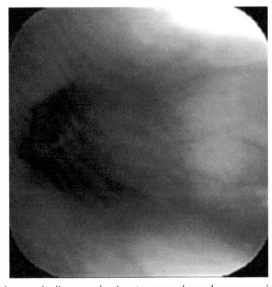

Fig. 5. Esophageal stenosis diagnosed using transnasal esophagoscopy in the office.

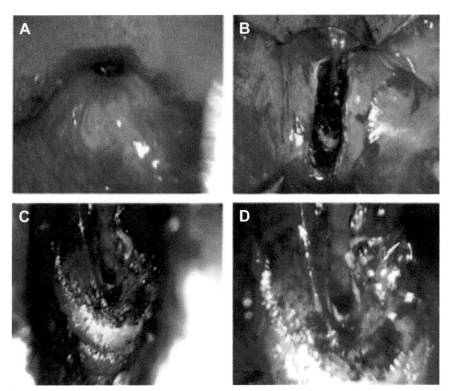

Fig. 6. Fibrotic cricopharyngeal muscle before (A) and after (B–D) endoscopic myotomy with a carbon dioxide laser. This step is followed by balloon dilation for optimal dilatory action at the level of the upper esophageal sphincter.

In cases of partial stenosis, dilation may be performed with a balloon catheter or over a guidewire to decrease likelihood of perforation or creation of a false passage, as compared with bougie dilation without guidewire use.[50] The authors recommend doing so under direct visualization with an ultraslim, flexible esophagoscope when possible. For more severe stenosis, the surgeon should plan to perform serial (and possibly staged) dilations every 2 to 4 weeks to assess for restenosis, or to sequentially increase the degree of dilation until a normal caliber is maintained. The number of dilations performed for these patients is variable, although typically at least three are needed in the authors' experience. Complete stenosis is technically more difficult to address. Simultaneous transoral and transgastric endoscopy, sometimes referred to as a transgastric retrograde esophagoscopy with antegrade dilation, may allow for a "rendezvous" procedure to re-establish an esophageal lumen.[51] Depending on experience and comfort level, this may be performed by the otolaryngologist alone or in conjunction with a gastroenterologist or general surgeon.

Treatment of dysphonia
As with swallow dysfunction, the bulk of effective voice and speech rehabilitation in this population depends on voice therapy for prevention and treatment of voice pathology, although adjunctive surgical procedures may play a critical role. Surgical treatments are tailored to the sites of voice and speech dysfunction.

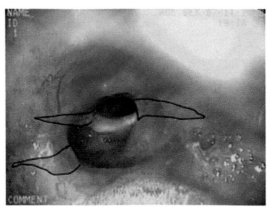

Fig. 7. A case of supraglottic stenosis where laser dilation might be helpful. The *shaded* areas show potential sites for radial laser incisions.

The primary subsystems of voice production relate to airflow from the lungs, appropriate laryngeal valving, and modification of fundamental tones by the vocal tract. Diminished pulmonary reserve and altered upper airway anatomy commonly affect vocal quality and are typically addressed by the nonsurgical techniques outlined in the previous section. Inadequate laryngeal valving is usually the result of vocal fold hypomobility or immobility. Vocal fold atrophy may contribute. In both cases, glottic closure is improved with injection augmentation in cases of temporary dysfunction, or in cases of permanent dysfunction or immobility, with medization thyroplasty, arytenoid adduction, and/or laryngeal reinnervation. These techniques have been well-described previously.[51–55]

Treatment of tracheostomy-dependence
Tracheostomy-dependence may be the result of one or more sites of airway obstruction. A full upper and lower airway endoscopic evaluation identifies these sites. Traditionally, supraglottic and tracheal stenoses have been managed via partial laryngectomy and tracheal resection, respectively. However, more conservative, endoscopic approaches are recommended in patients with HNC because of potential for complications caused by poor wound healing. For example, supraglottic laryngopharygneal stenosis can often be addressed using endoscopic laser dilation (**Fig. 7**).[48] Challenging subglottic and tracheal stenosis is addressed in a similar manner, even when the degree of stenosis or altered anatomy do not allow for orotracheal intubation or traditional neck extension.[56]

SUMMARY

With increases in survivorship for patients with HCN, attention is turning to QOL issues for survivors. Care for these patients is multifaceted. Dysphagia remains the most important factor for most long-term survivors, although issues of voice/speech, airway obstruction, neck and shoulder dysfunction, lymphedema, and pain control are important to address. Rehabilitation interventions are patient-specific and aim to prevent, restore, compensate, and palliate symptoms and sequelae of treatment for optimal functioning. Central to providing comprehensive interdisciplinary care are the head and neck surgeon, laryngologist, and SLP. Routine functional assessment, long-term follow-up, and regular communication and coordination among these specialists help maximize QOL in this challenging patient population.

REFERENCES

1. Pulte D, Brenner H. Changes in survival in head and neck cancer in the late 20th century and early 21st century: a period analysis. Oncologist 2010;15(9): 994–1001.
2. Rieger JM, Zalmanowitz JG, Wolfaardt JF. Functional outcomes after organ preservation treatment in head and neck cancer: a critical review of the literature. Int J Oral Maxillofac Surg 2006;35(7):581–7.
3. Connor NP, Cohen SB, Kammer RE, et al. Impact of conventional radiotherapy on health-related quality of life and critical functions of the head and neck. Int J Radiat Oncol Biol Phys 2006;65(4):1051–62.
4. Nguyen NP, Frank C, Moltz CC, et al. Impact of dysphagia on quality of life after treatment of head-and-neck cancer. Int J Radiat Oncol Biol Phys 2005;61(3): 772–8.
5. Duke RL, Campbell BH, Indresano AT, et al. Laryngoscope 2005;115(4):678–83.
6. Blanchard D, Bollet M, Dreyer C, et al. Management of somatic pain induced by head and neck cancer treatment: pain following radiation therapy and chemotherapy. Guidelines of the French Otorhinolaryngology Head and Neck Surgery Society (SFORL). Eur Ann Otorhinolaryngol Head Neck Dis 2014;131(4):253–6.
7. Smith BG, Hutcheson KA, Little LG, et al. Lymphedema outcomes in patients with head and neck cancer. Otolaryngol Head Neck Surg 2015;152(2):284–91.
8. Servagi-Vernat S, Ali D, Roubieu C, et al. Dysphagia after radiotherapy: state of the art and prevention. Eur Ann Otorhinolaryngol Head Neck Dis 2015;132(1): 25–9.
9. Lee S, Park Y, Byeon H, et al. Comparison of oncologic and functional outcomes after transoral robotic lateral oropharyngectomy versus conventional surgery for T1-T3 tonsillar cancer. Head Neck 2014;6(8):1138–45.
10. Rosenthal D, Lewin J, Eisbruch A. Prevention and treatment of dysphagia and aspiration after chemoradiation for head and neck cancer. J Clin Oncol 2006; 24(17):2636–43.
11. Caudell JJ, Schaner PE, Meredith RF, et al. Factors associated with long-term dysphagia after definitive radiotherapy for locally advanced head-and-neck cancer. Int J Radiat Oncol Biol Phys 2009;73(2):410–5.
12. Hutcheson KA, Lewin JS, Barringer DA, et al. Late dysphagia after radiotherapy-based treatment of head and neck cancer. Cancer 2012;118(23):5793–9.
13. Lango MN. Multimodal treatment for head and neck cancer. Surg Clin North Am 2009;89(1):43–52.
14. Locher JL, Bonner JA, Carroll WR, et al. Prophylactic percutaneous endoscopic gastrostomy tube placement in treatment of head and neck cancer: a comprehensive review and call for evidence-based medicine. JPEN J Parenter Enteral Nutr 2011;35(3):365–74.
15. Shune SE, Karnell LH, Karnell MP, et al. Association between severity of dysphagia and survival in patients with head and neck cancer. Head Neck 2012;34(6):776–84.
16. Jiang N, Zhang LJ, Li LY, et al. Risk factors for late dysphagia after (chemo)radiotherapy for head and neck cancer: a systematic methodological review. Head Neck 2016;38(5):792–800.
17. Pauloski BR, Rademaker AW, Logemann JA, et al. Comparison of swallowing function after intensity-modulated radiation therapy and conventional radiotherapy for head and neck cancer. Head Neck 2015;37(11):1575–82.

18. Koch WM, Lee DJ, Eisele DW, et al. Chemoradiotherapy for organ preservation in oral and pharyngeal carcinoma. Arch Otolaryngol Head Neck Surg 1995;121(9): 974–80.

19. Boscolo-Rizzo P, Maronato F, Marchiori C, et al. Long-term quality of life after total laryngectomy and postoperative radiotherapy versus concurrent chemoradiotheray for laryngeal preservation. Laryngoscope 2008;118(2):300–6.

20. Hanna E, Sherman A, Cash D, et al. Quality of life for patients following total laryngectomy vs chemoradiation for laryngeal preservation. Arch Otolaryngol Head Neck Surg 2004;130(7):875–9.

21. Nguyen NP, Frank C, Moltz CC, et al. Aspiration rate following chemoradiation for head and neck cancer: an underreported occurrence. Radiother Oncol 2006; 80(3):302–6.

22. Hutcheson K, Bhayani M, Beadle B, et al. Use it or lose it: eat and exercise during radiotherapy or chemoradiotherapy for pharyngeal cancers. JAMA Otolaryngol Head Neck Surg 2013;139(11):1127–34.

23. Rybak LP, Whitworth CA, Mukherjea D, et al. Mechanisms of cisplatin-induced ototoxicity and prevention. Hear Res 2007;226:157–67.

24. Jereczek-Fossa B, Zarowski A, Milani F, et al. Radiotherapy-induced ear toxicity. Cancer Treat Rev 2003;29(5):417–30.

25. Ahlberg A, Nikolaidis P, Engstrom T, et al. Morbidity of supraomohyoidal and modified radical neck dissection combined with radiotherapy for head and neck cancer. A prospective longitudinal study. Head Neck 2012;34(1):66–72.

26. Bradley PJ, Ferlito A, Silver C, et al. Neck treatment and shoulder morbidity: still a challenge. Head Neck 2011;33(7):1060–7.

27. Deng J, Ridner SH, Dietrich MS, et al. Prevalence of secondary lymphedema in patients with head and neck cancer. J Pain Symptom Manage 2012;43(2): 244–52.

28. Daniels SK, McAdam CP, Brailey K, et al. Clinical assessment of swallowing and prediction of dysphagia severity. Am J Speech Lang Pathol 1997;6:17–24.

29. Langmore SE, Schatz K, Olson N. Endoscopic and videofluoroscopic evaluations of swallowing and aspiration. Ann Otol Rhinol Laryngol 1991;100:678–81.

30. Aviv JE, Takoudes TG, Ma G, et al. Office-based esophagoscopy: a preliminary report. Otolaryngol Head Neck Surg 2001;125(3):170–5.

31. Durrant J, Campbell K, Fausti S, et al. American Academy of Audiology position statement and clinical practice guidelines: Ototoxicity monitoring. In: American Academy of Audiology Guidelines and Standards, 2009. Available at: http://www.audiology.org/publications-resources/document-library/ototoxicity-monitoring. Accessed October 1, 2016.

32. Theunissen E, Zuur C, Jozwiak K, et al. Prediction of hearing loss due to cisplatin chemotherapy. JAMA Otolaryngol Head Neck Surg 2015;141(9):810–5.

33. Epstein JB, Wilkie DJ, Fischer DJ, et al. Neuropathic and nociceptive pain in head and neck cancer patients receiving radiation therapy. Head Neck Oncol 2009;1: 26.

34. Bar Ad V, Weinstein G, Dutta PR, et al. Gabapentin for the treatment of pain syndrome related to radiation induced mucositis in patients with head and neck cancer treated with concurrent chemoradiotherapy. Cancer 2010;116:4206–13.

35. Bar Ad V, Weinstein G, Dutta PR, et al. Gabapentin for the treatment of pain related to radiation-induced mucositis in patients with head and neck tumors treated with intensity modulated radiation therapy. Head Neck 2010;32:173–7.

36. Starmer H, Yang W, Gourin C, et al. Effect of gabapentin on swallowing during and after chemoradiation for oropharyngeal squamous cancer. Dysphagia 2014;29:396–402.
37. Kataoka T, Kiyota N, Funakoshi Y, et al. Randomized trial of standard pain control with or without gabapentin for pain related to radiation-induced mucositis in head and neck cancer. Auris Nasus Larynx 2016;43(6):677–84.
38. Litts J, Gartner-Schmidt J, Clary M, et al. Impact of laryngologist and speech pathologist coassessment on outcomes, billing and revenue. Laryngoscope 2015;125:2139–42.
39. Starmer H, Sanquineti G, Marur S, et al. Multidisciplinary head and neck cancer clinic and adherence to speech pathology. Laryngoscope 2011;121(10):2131–5.
40. Carnaby-Mann G, Crary M, Schmafuss I, et al. "Pharyngocise": randomized controlled trial of preventative exercises to maintain muscle structure and swallowing function during head-and-neck chemoradiotherapy. Int J Radiat Oncol Biol Phys 2012;83(1):210–9.
41. van der Molen L, van Rossum MA, Burkhead LM, et al. A randomized preventive rehabilitation trial in advanced head and neck cancer patients treated with chemoradiotherapy: feasibility, compliance and short-term effects. Dysphagia 2011; 26:155–70.
42. Krisciunas GP, Golan H, Marinko LN, et al. A novel manual therapy program during radiation therapy for head and neck cancer: our clinical experience with 5 patients. Clin Otolaryngol 2016;41(4):425–31.
43. Hutcheson K, Lewin J, Barringer D, et al. Late dysphagia after radiation–based treatment of head and neck cancer. Cancer 2012;118(23):5793–9.
44. Vakharia KT, Ali MJ, Wang SJ. Quality-of-life impact of participation in a head and neck cancer support group. Otolaryngol Head Neck Surg 2007;136(3):405–10.
45. Schenker Y, Arnold R, Bauman J, et al. An enhanced role for palliative care in the multidisciplinary approach to high risk head and neck cancer. Cancer 2016; 122(3):340–3.
46. Shinn E, Basen-Engquist K, Baum G, et al. Adherence to preventive exercises and self-reported swallowing outcomes in post-radiated head and neck cancer patients. Head Neck 2013;35(12):1707–12.
47. Lazarus CL. Effects of chemoradiotherapy on voice and swallowing. Curr Opin Otolaryngol Head Neck Surg 2009;17(3):172–8.
48. Vira D, DeConde A, Chhetri DK. Endoscpoic management of supraglottic laryngopharyngeal stenosis. Otolaryngol Head Neck Surg 2012;146(4):611–3.
49. Jamal N, Erman A, Chhetri DK. Transoral partial epiglottidectomy to treat dysphagia in post-treatment head and neck cancer patients: a preliminary report. Laryngoscope 2014;124(3):665–71.
50. Peng KA, Feinstein AJ, Salinas JB, et al. Utility of the transnasal esophagoscope in the management of chemoradiation-induced esophageal stenosis. Ann Otol Rhinol Laryngol 2015;124(3):221–6.
51. Sullivan CA, Jaklitsch MT, Haddad R, et al. Endoscopic management of hypopharyngeal stenosis after organ sparing therapy for head and neck cancer. Laryngoscope 2004;114(11):1924–31.
52. Chhetri DK, Jamal N. Percutaneous injection laryngoplasty. Laryngoscope 2014; 124(3):742–5.
53. Isshiki N, Taira T, Kojima H, et al. Recent modifications in thyroplasty type I. Ann Otol Rhinol Laryngol 1989;98(10):777–9.
54. Isshiki N, Tanabe M, Sawada M. Arytenoid adduction for unilateral vocal cord paralysis. Arch Otolaryngol 1978;104(10):555–8.

55. Chhetri DK, Gerratt BR, Kreiman J, et al. Combined arytenoid adduction and laryngeal reinnervation in the treatment of vocal fold paralysis. Laryngoscope 1999;109(12):1928–36.
56. Vorasubin N, Vira D, Jamal N, et al. Airway management and endoscopic treatment of subglottic and tracheal stenosis: the laryngeal mask airway technique. Ann Otol Rhinol Laryngol 2014;123(4):293–8.

Survivorship
Morbidity, Mortality, Malignancy

Kelly M. Malloy, MD[a], Anna M. Pou, MD[b],*

KEYWORDS

- Survivorship • Palliative care • Guidelines • Surveillance • Morbidity

KEY POINTS

- A cancer survivor is someone who is "living with, through, and beyond a cancer diagnosis." This definition was expanded to include family and friends close to the survivor who also live through this period.
- Management of morbidity includes treating shoulder dysfunction, dysphagia, lymphedema, and anxiety and depression.
- Posttraumatic stress disorder occurs in 1 out of 3 patients with cancer; this has not been well studied in patients with head and neck cancer.
- Palliative care should begin at the time of diagnosis and continue to end of life.

PRINCIPLES OF SURVIVORSHIP

Survivorship encompasses the entire therapeutic, psychosocial, functional, and financial experience of living with and through a cancer diagnosis.[1] The period of survivorship starts on the day of the cancer diagnosis and lasts until the end of the survivor's life, regardless of the cause of death. The concept of survivorship essentially acknowledges that the survivor's life is forever changed as a result of being diagnosed, treated, and living through cancer. There is always a "new normal" that is the experience of the survivor after diagnosis.

The principles of survivorship include definitions of who a survivor is, as well as phases of survivorship.

- The National Coalition for Cancer Survivorship defines a cancer survivor as someone who is "living with, through, and beyond a cancer diagnosis."[2]
- The National Cancer Institute's Office of Cancer Survivorship expands the term "survivor" to include, importantly, caregivers, family, and friends close to the survivor who also live through this period.[3]

Disclosure Statement: There are no disclosures.
[a] Department of Otolaryngology–Head and Neck Surgery, University of Michigan, 1904 Taubman Center, 1500 East Medical Center Drive, Ann Arbor, MI 48019, USA; [b] Department of Otolaryngology–Head and Neck Surgery, Louisiana State University Health Sciences Center, New Orleans, 533 Bolivar Street, 5th Floor, New Orleans, LA 70112, USA
* Corresponding author.
E-mail address: apou@lsuhsc.edu

Otolaryngol Clin N Am 50 (2017) 853–866
http://dx.doi.org/10.1016/j.otc.2017.04.005
0030-6665/17/© 2017 Elsevier Inc. All rights reserved.

- Acute phase of survivorship
  - This phase commences at the time of diagnosis and persists through the completion of treatment. This is typically a period of great stress. The patient and caregivers are in crisis mode; however, attention is focused on diagnostics, treatment, learning new skills (speech and swallow therapy, tracheostomy care, feeding tube management, and so forth), and managing finances, work, and lifestyle to accommodate the acute phase of treatment. It is the time of greatest "action" for the survivor in the time course of survivorship, because the diagnosis is finalized and treatment is completed.[1]
- Extended phase of survivorship
  - This phase begins when treatment is completed. Surveillance commences, and the patient and their caregivers begin to resume "real life." For patients, this means less intensity of medical follow-up, but although doctors' appointments may be spaced further apart, there is often increased focus on functional recovery: physical therapy (PT), speech and swallow therapy, nutrition, and so forth. Surveillance visits and imaging typically provide an intermittent source of increased stress and anxiety, because these mark either continued progress toward long-term survival or dreaded relapse of disease.[1]
- Long-term or permanent phase of survivorship
  - This period coincides with the classic landmark of "cure," typically at the 5-year mark from the end of acute treatment. At this point, the patient is well into their experience of their "new normal"; they have likely come to terms with the long-term effects of their treatment, but may also be experiencing relatively new late effects of their cancer and its treatment.[1] *Long-term effects* are those that commenced during or shortly after treatment and persist to some degree on an ongoing basis, for example, xerostomia, lymphedema, shoulder dysfunction. *Late effects* are sequelae of cancer treatment that commence some time, even years, after the treatment is completed and the cancer is "cured." Examples of this would be esophageal or pharyngeal stricture, carotid arteriosclerosis, Lhermitte syndrome, and posttraumatic stress disorder (PTSD).

SURVIVORSHIP IN HEAD AND NECK CANCER: THE AMERICAN CANCER SOCIETY SURVIVORSHIP CARE GUIDELINE

This guideline was developed under the auspices of the National Cancer Survivorship Resource Center, a cooperative of the American Cancer Society (ACS), The George Washington University Cancer Institute, and the Centers for Disease Control and Prevention.[4]

The guideline defines head and neck cancer (HNC) as cancers of the *oral cavity, tongue, lip, larynx, and pharynx,* but recognizes that many of the same recommendations should apply to cancer of the salivary glands, nasal and paranasal sinuses, and nasopharynx.

- This guideline *does not apply* to cancers of the brain, thyroid, or esophagus; these cancers have markedly different symptoms, treatment, and long-term sequelae from the aforementioned HNCs.

Methods

- Published in the spring of 2016, this guideline is the collaborative effort of a multidisciplinary workgroup. Experts in head and neck surgical oncology, radiation

oncology, medical oncology, dentistry, speech language pathology, primary care, clinical psychology, physical medicine and rehabilitation, and nursing were members of the workgroup. Importantly, the patient's voice was represented by a head and neck cancer survivor member.
- An exhaustive literature search, including PubMed, and guidelines developed by other organizations (National Comprehensive Cancer Network [NCCN], American Society of Clinical Oncology [ASCO], as well as institutional and international resources), was performed and used to inform the guideline.
- Great emphasis was placed in evaluating the level of evidence (LOE) for each recommendation; the LOE for each element is specifically cited in the text of the guideline.
  - Greatest emphasis was given to publications from 2004 onward, randomized controlled trials, prospective cohort studies, and population-based case-control studies.
- The guideline was additionally vetted by internal and external stakeholders before publication. A commitment was made to revisit and update the guideline at least every 5 years.

Key Components of Head and Neck Cancer Survivorship

- The guideline defines 5 key areas to advise on best practices for HNC survivor care, with an *emphasis on primary care clinicians* who care for these survivors long term.
  1. Surveillance for HNC recurrence
  2. Screening for second primary cancers
  3. Assessment and management of physical and psychosocial long-term and late effects of HNC and its treatment
  4. Health promotion
  5. Care coordination and practice implications
- The Guideline provides a degree of education regarding each element of HNC survivorship care, which is critical. The guideline charges primary care providers with the responsibility of HNC survivorship care coordination. With HNC survivors representing only 3% of US cancer survivors, many, if not most, primary care clinicians will not have extensive experience with this survivor population and its unique survivorship needs. Education, *and support from HNC specialists in surgery, radiation, and medical oncology,* is vital to enable primary care clinicians to successfully coordinate HNC survivorship care.

SURVEILLANCE FOR HEAD AND NECK CANCER RECURRENCE

- The guideline recommends that primary care clinicians tailor follow-up care for HNC survivors based on their age, specific cancer diagnosis, and treatment protocol *as recommended by the treating oncology team.*
  - This implies that the treating oncology team has communicated a treatment summary and follow-up care plan, as recommended by the American Head and Neck Society's Survivorship Committee.[1]
- The primary care clinician should perform a cancer-related history and physical examination on the routine basis:
  - Every 1 to 3 months for the first year
  - Every 2 to 6 months for the second year
  - Every 4 to 8 months in years 3 to 5
  - Every 12 months ongoing.

- At these visits, the primary care clinician must confirm that the patient is following up for disease-specific surveillance with an otolaryngologist and/or other HNC specialist for a detailed head and neck–focused examination. *This examination should include nasopharyngolaryngoscopy and palpation of the neck.* Baseline posttreatment imaging should be performed as directed by the treating team and adhere to established NCCN disease-specific recommendations.
- Primary care providers are also charged with educating patients regarding the signs and symptoms of local and regional recurrence. The guideline provides some education regarding these warning signs and recommends the primary clinician screen for these symptoms and has a low threshold for referral to an HNC specialist.

SCREENING AND EARLY DETECTION OF SECOND PRIMARY CANCERS

- Primary care clinicians should ensure that the HNC survivor adheres to routine cancer screening, just as one would in the general population.
  - For example, mammography, colonoscopy, pap smear.
  - ACS Early Detection Recommendations are available at cancer.org/professionals.
- Primary care clinicians should also screen HNC survivors for lung cancer if they meet high-risk profile based on smoking history.
  - Annual low-dose computed tomography (LDCT) chest
  - The National Lung Screening Trial showed decreased mortality in current or former heavy smokers aged 55 to 74 when LDCT chest used for screening (endorsed by NCCN and ASCO).
    - Recommend annual LDCT chest for those aged 55 to 74 years with 30 plus pack-year history who are current smokers or quit within last 15 years.
    - Also recommend LDCT chest for those 50 years or older with 20 plus pack-year history and another risk factor for lung cancer, that is, history of HNC.
- Primary care clinicians should continue to monitor and screen for a second HNC or esophageal cancer; although no specific imaging is recommended, this does require close attention to symptoms, such as new onset dysphagia, odynophagia, and weight loss, all of which should prompt evaluation with endoscopy by an otolaryngologist or gastroenterologist.

ASSESSMENT AND MANAGEMENT OF PHYSICAL AND PSYCHOSOCIAL LONG-TERM AND LATE EFFECTS OF HEAD AND NECK CANCER TREATMENT

- The guideline recommends that primary care clinicians monitor HNC survivors for a long list of cancer and treatment sequelae, *at every visit.* Although a detailed description of these important long-term and late effects is beyond the scope of this article, the authors highlight a few interesting elements in later discussion.
- Neck and shoulder complaints:
  - The guideline provides some education for assessing SAN weakness, other cervical neuropathies, muscle dystonia and spasms, and shoulder dysfunction. Indeed, the primary care clinician is charged with performing a baseline posttreatment shoulder strength, range of motion, and impingement assessment and monitoring shoulder function on an ongoing basis.
- Swallowing and oral complaints:
  - Trismus, dysphagia, aspiration, stricture, and gastroesophageal reflux disease should also be assessed and monitored by the HNC survivor's primary care

provider, with a low threshold to refer to speech language pathology and/or HNC surgeon for assessment if stricture or recurrence is suspected.

○ The primary care clinician is further charged with ensuring the patient is following up for routine and specialized dental care as well as monitoring for taste disturbances and referring for dietician consultation for support for taste issues.

○ The guideline recommends that primary care clinicians assess, diagnose, and initiate treatment of osteoradionecrosis, lymphedema, and other head and neck–specific sequelae of HNC treatment; although all recommendations encourage appropriate referral, many of these are diagnoses that are not within the routine wheelhouse of most primary providers.

• Psychosocial and generalized complaints:

○ The guideline offers recommendations for assessing and supporting patients with body and self-image issues, depression and anxiety, fatigue, and issues of sexuality. Indeed, with many HNC survivors being human papillomavirus (HPV)-related malignancy survivors, issues of sexuality, intimacy, and self-image may take on additional complexity.

■ There are additional resources from ASCO to help address many of these issues, including symptom-based guidelines for cancer survivors with the following:

• Fatigue
• Chemotherapy-induced peripheral neuropathy
• Anxiety and depression

MORBIDITY/LONG-TERM EFFECTS/LATE EFFECTS
Shoulder Dysfunction

• Shoulder dysfunction and chronic pain following neck dissection are among the most common causes of decrease in quality of life (QOL).

○ These symptoms are due to dissection, injury, or sacrifice of the spinal accessory nerve (SAN), which causes diminished or absent function of the *sternocleidomastoid muscle* and upper part of the *trapezius muscle.*

○ Adjuvant radiation therapy can worsen dysfunction and increase pain due to fibrosis and muscle spasm.

• Rehabilitation of the shoulder girdle using PT results in improved/return of function and improvement in pain.[5,6]

○ The goal of PT is to promote wide passive range of motion and gradually active motion to stabilize the shoulder girdle and prevent "frozen" shoulder.

• Salerno and colleagues[5] studied the effects of PT on patients having undergone neck dissection with preservation of the SAN; one group underwent PT and the other study group did not.

○ In the PT group, there was a significant improvement in mobility, pain, QOL, and return to previous occupation. Approximately 63% of the PT group, as compared with 10% of the non-PT group, was able to achieve what is known as the zero position; achievement of this position is necessary for common daily activities.

○ The authors recommend that PT start within 1 month after surgery and continue for at least 3 months, although most significant results were noted after 6 months of aggressive therapy.

• However, obstacles to uninterrupted therapy do exist: pain; fatigue; depression; side effects of radiation/chemoradiation.

○ Neuropathic pain is one such obstacle. Pain in these patients was found to be more successfully treated with methadone than fentanyl; greater than 50% relief in pain was noted in 50% versus 15% of those treated with methadone versus fentanyl.[7]
- If patients can continue to perform any amount of PT, recovery following adjuvant therapy will be easier.
- Aggressive and long-term PT is recommended for long-term preservation of shoulder function and reduction of pain and should become a part of a survivor's daily routine indefinitely.

Dysphagia

About 50% of patients with HNC develop dysphagia resulting in about 10,000 to 20,000 new cases per year.

Dysphagia can become progressively worse over time; trismus, esophageal stricture, xerostomia, and cranial neuropathies can develop. Severe dysphagia often leads to psychosocial issues, health issues (aspiration), and isolation (patients would rather eat alone).

Emphasis has been placed on QOL as well as quantity of life following treatment. Tools for measuring QOL in relation to dysphagia include the following:

- SWAL-QOL
  ○ Outcomes tool measuring the impact of dysphagia on QOL
- SWAL-CARE
  ○ Addresses recommendations about food, liquid, dysphagia treatment, and satisfaction with treatment
- MD Anderson Dysphagia Inventory
  ○ First validated and reliable serf-administered questionnaire
  ○ Assesses dysphagia and QOL in patients with HNC
  ○ Can be paired with other QOL instruments to obtain different response/view points
- Head and Neck Cancer Quality of Life Questionnaire (HNQOL)
  ○ This instrument was developed in order to assess disease-specific health-related QOL
  ○ The HNQOL assesses eating, communication, pain, and emotion

Dysphagia therapy, similar to other rehabilitative therapies, should start as soon as possible and should continue throughout and following treatment to prevent hypopharyngeal/esophageal stenosis and weakness/fibrosis of tongue and pharyngeal muscles.

- Referral to speech pathology should be submitted preoperatively
  ○ Education regarding expected changes in speech and swallowing
  ○ Pretreatment swallow study
  ○ Pretreatment preventative exercises demonstrated and taught
  ○ Follow-up throughout and following treatment
- In a study by Wall and colleagues,[8] prophylactic swallowing therapy was initiated in patients with HNC receiving (chemo)radiotherapy. Only 27% adhered to the protocol over 6 weeks of treatment with a decline starting at week 4. However, clinician-directed face-to-face therapy yielded better compliance than did patient-directed therapy, which supports the value of regularly scheduled speech therapy appointments when possible.
- Virani and colleagues[9] demonstrated that formal dysphagia exercises performed throughout treatment compared with repetitive swallows only led to significantly less percutaneous endoscopic gastrostomy (PEG) tube dependence

immediately and at 3 months after treatment (35% and 10% compared with 69% and 50%) in patients undergoing chemoradiation.

Lymphedema

Lymphedema of the head and neck can result from surgical resection of cervical nodes (most common) or radiation to the head and neck and is compounded by dual treatment modality.

- Lymphedema occurs in about 50% to 75% of patients with HNC and can occur in the immediate postoperative period, following radiation or several months following completion of treatment.
  - It can develop in the face, submental area, larynx, and/or pharynx, causing physical deformity, tightness/fibrosis in the affected areas, dysarthria, dysphagia, and difficulty breathing.
  - It can cause distress because some think that the edema is tumor recurrence.
  - Complete decongestive therapy (CDT) is the gold standard of treatment and consists of the following:
    - Manual lymphatic drainage
    - Compression garments
    - Exercise program
    - Education regarding skin care and infection precautions
  - CDT can begin in the immediate postoperative period and should continue indefinitely.
- It is best for patients to meet with a therapist preemptively.
  - Preventative strategies, including exercise and self-massage, are taught to the patient, which may prevent or delay onset.
  - In many centers, speech therapists perform lymphedema therapy.
    - Lymphedema can cause trismus, poor mobility of tongue, and aspiration; this is part of dysphagia therapy.

Human Papilloma Virus

The role of HPV in oropharyngeal cancer has led to a younger group of patients developing HNC.

Although patients with HPV+ tumors have a better prognosis than patients with HPV− tumors, they currently face different challenges.

- Improved 5-year survival rate leads to a longer life during which they will endure posttreatment morbidities.
  - This highlights the need for ongoing clinical trials evaluating deescalation of therapy to decrease morbidity and improve QOL.
- Many patients who are told that their cancers were likely due the HPV experienced anxiety, and they as well as family members had unanswered questions regarding HPV.[10]
  - Many are concerned about infecting their spouse and how this diagnosis will affect their intimate relationships, and some wonder how they were infected, having only one sex partner, typically a spouse.
- In a study by D'Souza and colleagues,[10] almost half of patients with HPV+ oropharyngeal cancers thought that their health care provider did not adequately address the emotional effects of a having an HPV-related cancer.

Improving education and psychosocial support in this growing cohort of patients with HNC presents an opportunity for research.

DISTRESS/DEPRESSION/ANXIETY
Body and Self-Image

- Facial disfigurement is a major concern for those undergoing treatment of HNC, although not all are affected to the same degree. Because of altered facial appearance, speech, and swallowing, patients are prone to social and psychological problems, which may lead to self-isolation.
- Psychological distress can result from negative reactions by the public.
  - A study by Hagedoorn and Molleman[11] analyzed the effect of social self-efficacy (the ability to exercise control over social interactions) on the level of psychological distress. They found that in those patients who had the ability to master social self-efficacy the relationship between disfigurement and psychological distress was low; patients perceived little distress in reaction to negative behaviors of others and perceived little social isolation regardless of the degree of facial disfigurement.
- Social self-efficacy is an important skill to be learned by head and neck survivors.

Depression/Suicide

- The incidence of depression in patients with HNC is estimated to be as high as 40%. Depression in patients with HNC is often unrecognized and undertreated; it may even be present at initial presentation.
- Patients with cancer have a higher suicide rate than the general US population.[12] In a recent study by Kam and colleagues,[13] it was found that patients with HNC had 3 times the incidence of suicide than the general public.
- A retrospective review of Surveillance, Epidemiology, and End Results (SEER) data from 1973 to 2011 in patients with HNC was performed in 2014 looking for cause of death as "suicide and self-inflicted injury." Among 350,413 SEER registry patients, 875 suicides were identified with an age-, sex-, and race-adjusted suicide rate of 37.9/100,000 person-years. The suicide rate in the general US population was 11.8/100,000 person-years.[13]
  - Male patients and those with late stage disease had a statistically higher rate.
  - Those diagnosed between ages 60 and 79 years had the highest rate of suicide.
  - Patients treated with radiation alone had double the suicide rate than those who underwent surgery alone.
  - Patients with hypopharyngeal cancers had nearly a 12-fold higher incidence of suicide, and those with laryngeal cancer had a 5-fold higher incidence of suicide. These specific sites were at higher risk probably because of a decrease in QOL (PEG tube, tracheostomy, and change in speech).
  - Most suicides occurred within the first 5 years of diagnosis with a dramatic decline in the suicide rate thereafter.[13]

To prevent this outcome, newly diagnosed patients with HNC should be assessed for level of distress (anxiety and depression) in order to intervene early.

- In a study by Leung and colleagues,[14] the Distress Assessment and Response Tool was used to identify patients at risk for suicide. Of those patients completing the questionnaire, almost 6% admitted to suicidal ideation, and of these patients, more than 10% admitted to suicidal intentions as well.
  - This study impresses the importance of routine screening of patients with HNC for distress and referral to mental health specialist early.
  - If suicidal ideation is expressed, immediate referral to mental health specialists or Emergency Room is warranted.

- Because of depression/suicidal ideation, prophylactic counseling and/or antidepressant medication may prevent the effect of such stressors. Patients are adjusting to a "new normal" and likely grieving over the loss of self and life as they have known it.
  - Ostuzzi and colleagues[15] performed a Cochrane Database of Systematic Reviews regarding the treatment of patients with cancer with antidepressants. At the conclusion of his review, based on his findings, implications for use could not be determined due to few poor-quality studies.
  - At the University of Nebraska Medical Center, however, a study undertaken by Lydiatt and colleagues[16] determined that giving patients with HNC an antidepressant before starting treatment can reduce the incidence of depression by more than 50%.
    - In a randomized, double-blind trial, 148 newly diagnosed patients with HNC entered treatment that did not yet have a diagnosis of depression. Half the patients received escitalopram (Lexapro) and the other half received matching placebo pills.
    - Only 10% of patients taking the antidepressant developed depression compared with 24.6% of patients taking placebo.
    - Patients who took the antidepressant and completed the study without developing depression reported overall QOL as significantly better than those in the placebo group for 3 consecutive months after ending treatment.[16]

Patients with HNC, like many patients, benefit from a multidisciplinary approach to stress/anxiety/depression (antidepressants, psychotherapy, support groups).

- Unfortunately, there are many obstacles to treatment:
  - Lack of funding to pay for psychotherapy, counseling, or medications
  - Reluctance to admitting that there is a problem because of stigma
  - Reluctance to start treatment
  - Noncompliance with treatment plan and follow-up
  - Lack of recognition by health care providers may delay treatment.
- Nonetheless, patient's level of distress should be evaluated at every visit because it can fluctuate over time depending on the current circumstances and realization of life changes
  - A simple, helpful tool is the Patient Health Questionnaire 4, which can be given to patients to complete at each visit to help identify those who are getting worse over time and those who are in crisis.

POSTTRAUMATIC STRESS DISORDER IN CANCER SURVIVORS

PTSD has traditionally been associated with war Veterans; however, it can affect anyone who has experienced a serious threat of violence or death. Recently, there has been increased awareness of symptoms occurring after critical illness and injury.

- Beginning in 1994, PTSD was applied to patients with cancer when the Diagnostic and Statistical Manual of Mental Disorders (4th ed) redefined trauma criteria to include life-threatening illness such as cancer (American Psychiatric Association, 2000).
  - It has been found that as many as 1 in 3 patients with cancer suffer from PTSD,[17] and research has shown that PTSD sufferers are at high risk of suicide.
- Symptoms may present as flashbacks, nightmares, depression, hopelessness, irritability, anger, and feeling detached.

- Parker and colleagues[18] found that one-fourth of patients who survive a critical illness and an intensive care unit (ICU) stay experience PTSD.
  - Risk factors include preexisting depression and anxiety, large amounts of sedation, frightening memories in the ICU,[18] and the intensity of treatment, all which can apply to most of patients with HNC.
- Research done on patients with non-Hodgkin lymphoma showed that one-third had lasting symptoms of PTSD 10 years after completion of therapy.[19]
- Most clinicians do not make the link between PTSD and cancer so many patients are not diagnosed or treated. Screening for PTSD is not typically done.
- Patients with HNC are especially prone to endure emotional trauma because they are restrained with masks attached to the table for radiation therapy treatments (repeated trauma).

In 2011, the National Center for PTSD, part of the Department of Veterans Affairs, offered a free mobile app as a first line of support for Veterans. The app provides coping strategies, assesses symptoms, and directs Veterans to available mental health support.

- The National Center for PTSD has teamed up with researchers at Duke University to modify this app for cancer survivors; it is hoped this will be available in the near future.

Awareness and education regarding PTSD in cancer survivors present an opportunity to study PTSD in HNC survivors (screen specifically for PTSD) and their families because PTSD can also affect the patient's support system.

PALLIATIVE CARE

- Palliative care is also known as "comfort care," supportive care, and symptom management.
  - Many (physicians and patients alike) believe that it is reserved for the terminally ill and dying, but, in fact, palliative care should begin at the time of diagnosis and continue to end of life.
- The goal of palliative care is to provide the best QOL by preventing or treating the symptoms and side effects of the disease *as early as possible* as well as the related social, psychological, and spiritual challenges.
  - This is achieved through a multidisciplinary approach, and many cancer centers have both an outpatient palliative care clinic and inpatient services, which allows continuum of care.
- Benefits are many and include the ability to fully complete treatment; improved QOL during treatment; increased ability to perform daily activities; living longer[20]; improved ability to deal with emotions; increased connection to social support; and earlier referral to hospice with less resource use.[20–22]
- If cancer progresses and treatment is no longer a viable option, palliative care becomes the main focus of care. This does not mean that patients receive no care.
  - Physician's level of training, clinical experience, practice setting, personal and moral views, and personal bias may delay the end-of-life discussion.[21] Consultation with palliative care experts, when available, is recommended.
  - The role of the palliative care team at this juncture is to help the patient and his/her support system transition to end-of-life care.
    - Palliative care specialists provide an opportunity to discuss and document patients' wishes and provide support in a setting that is comfortable and not hurried.

- ■ Discussion of patient prognosis *early* in the disease course allows for better understanding regarding the seriousness of the illness at a time when emergent decisions regarding end-of-life care are not required.
  - • This allows patients to determine preferences regarding their treatment at this time, before the time comes, which has led to earlier hospice referrals and less intensive care at end of life.[20]

HEALTH PROMOTION

- • An important aspect of health promotion is continuous assessment of the information needs of HNC survivors and directing of patients to appropriate providers to obtain needed information and support. Beyond this general recommendation, the ACS guideline recommends the following for HNC survivor health promotion:
- • Patients should maintain a healthy weight, avoiding cachexia as well as obesity.
- • Survivors should be physically active, certainly to returning to pretreatment levels of activity and preferably performing at least 150 minutes of moderate exercise a week or 75 minutes of vigorous exercise a week. Strength training should also be emphasized and is recommended 2 times a week.
- • Survivors should maximize their nutritional status:
  - ○ Adhere to a plant-based, whole foods diet
  - ○ Minimize saturated fats, maximize dietary fiber
  - ○ Avoid alcohol
- • HNC survivors should be counseled and supported in their tobacco cessation efforts, with referrals to smoking cessation programs provided. Primary care clinicians should also continue to monitor tobacco abuse status, particularly for relapses, and provide additional support.
- • Primary care clinicians should also monitor patient follow-up with dentistry and encourage good oral hygiene, assess proper fit and maintenance of dentures, advise for oral hydration (humidifiers, nasal saline sprays, and so forth), and encourage self oral examinations.

CARE COORDINATION AND PRACTICE IMPLICATIONS

- • Here the ACS guideline addresses how best to transfer and/or share HNC survivor care. They do recommend a specific time point for transferal of care, but rather emphasize that both groups of providers need to be diligently involved throughout, and most importantly, establish clear communication from the end of treatment forward.
- • A *survivorship care plan* should be provided by the treatment team to the primary care clinician, and preferably, to the patient. If one is not immediately available, the primary provider should consult with the treatment team to obtain one.
- • The survivorship care plan includes both a treatment summary and a survivorship plan:
  - ○ The treatment summary includes tumor type, site, stage, and treatment (surgery, radiation fields and dose, systemic therapy and doses, and so forth).
  - ○ The survivorship plan should provide a schedule for follow-up visits, imaging, and laboratory tests. It should also include information on risks and expectations for late effects so that primary care clinicians can be guided in ongoing surveillance.
- • Primary care clinicians and HNC specialty providers should remain in consistent communication to assure well-coordinated, evidence-based survivorship care.

- Finally, although the HNC survivor is at the center of survivorship care, the guideline specifically calls for patient caregivers, spouses, and partners to be consistently included in survivorship care. The guideline also notes the need to acknowledge the stress and impact of HNC diagnosis and treatment on caregivers, and that part of survivorship care is support and collaboration with these important members of the survivorship team.

STRENGTHS

- A major strength of the ACS guideline is its effort to educate primary care clinicians in the complexities of surveillance care for HNC survivors. The details provided in the "clinical interpretation" of each recommendation of the guideline provide a nice primer on various aspects of HNC care and patient experience. As noted above, HNC survivors comprise a relatively small number of overall cancer survivors, and as such, primary care providers do not likely see many of these patients in their individual practices. The guideline alone is a big step toward involving primary care clinicians more comprehensively in the care of patients with HNC.
- As HNC survivors live longer and longer, reaching the milestones at which they only see their HNC specialists every 6 to 12 months for routine cancer follow-up, the primary care provider must recognize that their primary care providers become their major health provider resource, even for HNC survivorship issues. As such, shifting much of the care coordination and surveillance to the primary provider is appropriate, provided ongoing clear communication is maintained with the HNC treatment team.

OPPORTUNITIES

- The ACS guideline offers a new opportunity to form partnerships and collaborations with primary care colleagues that will not only improve HNC survivorship care but also provide for new opportunities to study survivorship.
  - To date, there is relatively sparse literature on HNC survivorship, as evidenced by the guideline itself; 64% of the evidence upon which the guideline is based is level 0, followed by 28% level III evidence. Thus, most of the guideline is based on expert opinion, observational studies, clinical practice, and literature reviews.[4] Clearly this is a field ripe for investigation.
  - Moreover, there is a need identified by patients and providers alike for improved information and educational materials regarding HNC survivorship.[22]
- Although many centers have established HNC survivor clinics, there is immense variability in the structure and scope of these clinics; this is another area ripe for investigation.
- Although the guideline is quite detailed, there are areas in which HNC specialists need to continue to contribute.
  - Late effects such as radiation-induced carotid atherosclerosis are not addressed in the current guideline, nor is HPV-related HNC information provided. Both of these topics are areas in which contributions to the first revision of the guideline are needed.
  - The guidelines may be onerous on primary providers in some respects. Asking a primary care clinician to assess and diagnose osteoradionecrosis and then start antibiotic therapy without the assistance and input of a head and neck surgeon would be burdensome and potentially harmful to the patient.

SUMMARY

As mentioned previously, survivorship encompasses the entire therapeutic, psycho-social, functional, and financial aspects of living with and through a cancer diagnosis. It begins at the time of diagnosis and continues to the end of life. HNC survivorship guideline is discussed in the text above.

The approach to care of patients with HNC is best achieved via a multidisciplinary approach. Due to a lack of resources, a multidisciplinary approach is particularly chal-lenging in the uninsured and indigent populations, leading to heath care disparities. Recommendations regarding targeted care of patients with HNC, particularly in the previously mentioned populations, are discussed below.

- The ideal situation is a multidisciplinary clinic where the major disciplines are rep-resented; head and neck surgery, radiation and medical oncology, dental oncology, speech therapy, palliative care, psychology, and social work are vital to the initial comprehensive patient evaluation and ongoing treatment.
  - "One-stop shopping" is especially helpful in the uninsured population because transportation to clinic visits is typically a problem and a cause for missed ap-pointments. Physical and occupational therapists can also be included to assist with rehabilitation.
- Psychosocial support at the time of diagnosis, throughout and following treat-ment, is necessary to help treat anxiety and depression to prevent suicide. In addition to the previously mentioned obstacles, there is a lack of mental health personnel who understand the issues facing this patient population and who are willing to counsel someone who has difficulty communicating (cannot speak or write).
  - If possible, the presence of a psychologist housed in the head and neck clinic allows evaluation of the level of patient distress at every appointment, identi-fying early those who are in need of a psychiatric referral or immediate inter-vention, and allowing for real-time counseling.
    - Medical schools with a Psychiatry residency or universities with a graduate program in Psychology are ideal for collaboration.
- Early referral to Palliative Care not only improves QOL and extends longevity but also assists with end-of-life decisions and decreased resource utilization during this time.
- Because many HNC survivors die from non–cancer causes because of long-term treatment toxicities and comorbidities, attention should be given to their diet, ex-ercise, and reduction in cardiovascular risks.
- Perhaps the most important issue in HNC survivorship is education of the HNC health care team regarding the life-long challenges facing these patients, the ne-cessity for early intervention regarding rehabilitation, and particularly, education in recognizing the signs and symptoms of emotional distress/stress and PTSD.

REFERENCES

1. Miller MC, Shuman AG. Survivorship in head and neck cancer: a primer. JAMA Otolaryngol Head Neck Surg 2016;142(10):1002–8.
2. National Coalition for Cancer Survivorship. Available at: http://www.canceradvocacy.org. Accessed February 15, 2017.
3. National Cancer Institute, Division of Cancer Control & Population Statistics. Available at: https://cancercontrol.cancer.gov/ocs/statistics/definitions.html. Ac-cessed February 15, 2017.

4. Cohen EE, LaMonte SJ, Erb NL, et al. American Cancer Society head and neck cancer survivorship care guideline. CA Cancer J Clin 2016;66(3):203–39.

5. Salerno G, Cavaliere M, Foglia A, et al. The 11th nerve syndrome in functional neck dissection. Laryngoscope 2002;112(7 pt 1):1299–307.

6. McGarvey AC, Hoffman GR, Osmotherly PG, et al. Maximizing shoulder function after accessory nerve injury and neck dissection surgery: a multicenter randomized controlled trial. Head Neck 2015;37(7):1022–31.

7. Haumann J, Geurrs JW, van Kuijk SM, et al. Methadone is superior to fentanyl in treating neuropathic pain in patients with head-and-neck cancer. Eur J Cancer 2016;65:121–9.

8. Wall LR, Ward EC, Cartmill B, et al. Adherence to a prophylactic swallowing therapy program during (chemo) radiotherapy: impact of service-delivery model and patient factors. Dysphagia 2017;32(2):279–92.

9. Virani A, Kundul M, Fink D, et al. Effect of 2 different swallowing exercise regiments during organ-preservation therapies for head and neck cancers on swallowing function. Head Neck 2015;37(2):162–70.

10. D'Souza G, Zhang Y, Merritt S, et al. Patient experience and anxiety during and after treatment for an HPV-related oropharyngeal cancer. Oral Oncol 2016;60: 90–5.

11. Hagedoorn M, Molleman E. Facial disfigurement in patients with head and neck cancer: the role of social self-efficacy. Health Psychol 2006;25(5):643–7.

12. Anguiano L, Mayer DK, Piven MI, et al. A literature review of suicide in cancer patients. Cancer Nurs 2012;35(4):E14–26.

13. Kam D, Salib A, Gorgy BA, et al. Incidence of suicide in patients with head and neck cancer. JAMA Otolaryngol Head Neck Surg 2015;141(12):1075–81.

14. Leung YW, Li M, Devins G, et al. Routine screening for suicidal ideation intention in patients with cancer. Psychooncology 2013;22(11):2537–45.

15. Ostuzzi G, Matcham F, Dauchy S, et al. Antidepressants for the treatment of depression in people with cancer. Cochrane Database Syst Rev 2015;(6):CD011006.

16. Lydiatt WM, Bessette D, Schmid KK, et al. Prevention of depression with escitalopram in patients undergoing treatment for head and neck cancer: randomized, double-blind, placebo-controlled clinical trial. JAMA Otolaryngol Head Neck Surg 2013. http://dx.doi.org/10.1001/jamaoto.2013.3371.

17. Scott C. Cancer treatment leaves survivors with PTSD scars. Healthline News 2015. Available at: http://www.healthline.com/health-news/cancer-treatment-leaves-survivors-with-ptsd-scars-031215#1.

18. Parker AM, Sricharoenchai T, Raparla S, et al. Posttraumatic stress disorder in critical illness survivors: a metaanalysis. Crit Care Med 2015;43(5):1121–9.

19. Smith SK, Zimmerman S, Willimas CS, et al. Post-traumatic stress symptoms in long-term non-Hodgkin's lymphoma survivors: does time heal? J Clin Oncol 2011;29(34):4526–33.

20. Teme JS, Greer JA, Muzikansky A, et al. Early palliative care for patients with metastatic non–small-cell lung cancer. N Engl J Med 2010;363:733–42.

21. Howie L, Peppercorn J. Early palliative care in cancer treatment: rationale, evidence and clinical implications. Ther Adv Med Oncol 2013;5(6):318–23.

22. Jabbour J, Milross C, Sundaresan P, et al. Education and support needs in patients with head and neck cancer: a multi-institutional survey. Cancer 2017; 123(11):1949–57.

Immunotherapy
Who Is Eligible?

Daniel Wang, MD[a], Jill Gilbert, MD[a], Young J. Kim, MD, PhD[a,b,*]

KEYWORDS

- Immunotherapy • Recurrent metastatic head & neck carcinoma
- Checkpoint inhibitors • PD-1/PD-L1 blocking antibodies • Nivolumab
- Pembrolizumab

KEY POINTS

- Immunotherapy with checkpoint inhibitors are now US Food and Drug Administration approved for recurrent and/or metastatic head and neck carcinoma.
- Cancer immunotherapy has distinct adverse events that are related to an induction of autoimmunity.
- Predictive biomarker analysis for head and neck immunotherapy is ongoing.
- Combinatorial trials for head and neck carcinoma are an active area of clinical research to improve the clinical efficacy of immunotherapy.

INTRODUCTION

An important paradigm shift in oncology in the past several years has been the adoption of immunotherapy for recurrent and/or metastatic cancer. Although cancer immunotherapy using antitumor T cells and interleukins has been used for melanoma previously, clinical trials for various forms of immunotherapy for epithelial cancers had not shown any clinical efficacy. Immune checkpoint inhibitors (ICIs; programmed death-1 [PD-1]/programmed death - ligand 1 (PD-L1)/cytotoxic T-lymphocyte–associated protein 4 [CTLA-4]), however, have altered the oncologic landscape such that many of the near future clinical trials may be based primarily on immuno-oncologic platforms. Head and neck carcinomas have not been immune from this revolution. In this article, the authors review the historical and immunologic basis of immunotherapy for head and neck squamous cell carcinoma (HNSCC).

[a] Department of Medicine, Division of Hematology and Oncology, Vanderbilt–Ingram Cancer Center, Vanderbilt University Medical Center, Nashville, TN 37232, USA; [b] Department Otolaryngology–Head & Neck Surgery, Vanderbilt-Ingram Cancer Center, Vanderbilt University Medical Center, Nashville, TN 37232, USA
* Corresponding author. Department Otolaryngology–Head & Neck Surgery, Vanderbilt-Ingram Cancer Center, Vanderbilt University Medical Center, Nashville, TN 37232.
E-mail address: young.j.kim@vanderbilt.edu

Otolaryngol Clin N Am 50 (2017) 867–874
http://dx.doi.org/10.1016/j.otc.2017.04.006
0030-6665/17/© 2017 Elsevier Inc. All rights reserved.
oto.theclinics.com

HISTORICAL PERSPECTIVE OF RECURRENT AND/OR METASTATIC HEAD AND NECK SQUAMOUS CELL CARCINOMA

Recurrent and/or metastatic (R/M) HNSCC remains a disease with poor morbidity and mortality. Traditional cytotoxic chemotherapy agents have been the only systemic treatment option until recently. Both single agents and 2 combination agents ("doublets") have demonstrated modest response rates with no survival advantage noted for combinations of drugs over single agents in the R/M setting.[1–8] The introduction of cetuximab (an immunoglobulin G [IgG1] chimeric monoclonal antibody to the epidermal growth factor receptor [EGFR]), to the armamentarium of agents for R/M HNSCC represented an important step away from dependence on traditional cytotoxic agents as the only systemic option for R/M disease. Clinical studies revealed that EGFR was overexpressed in greater than 90% of human HNSCC tissue samples and associated with poorer clinical outcomes.[9,10] In an Eastern Cooperative Oncology Group (ECOG) phase 3 randomized trial of cisplatin plus placebo compared with cisplatin plus cetuximab in R/M HNSCC, the combination of cisplatin plus cetuximab (26% vs 10%, $P = .03$) compared with cisplatin alone, with trends toward progression-free survival (PFS) and overall survival (OS), as the study was not powered for survival.[11] The landmark EXTREME phase 3 trial randomized patients to platinum- and fluorouracil-based therapy with or without cetuximab and demonstrated a survival benefit in R/M HNSCC since the approval of cisplatin in the 1980s.[12] The addition of cetuximab to a platinum doublet chemotherapy improved median OS to 10.1 months and median PFS to 5.6 months (hazard ratio [HR] 0.8, 95% confidence interval [CI] 0.64–0.99, $P = .04$). Currently, cetuximab is approved in first-line treatment (for nonsalvageable R/M settings) when combined with platinum/fluorouracil (5-FU) and in platinum-refractory treatment as monotherapy. Further investigations in other EGFR inhibitors such as monoclonal antibodies (panitumumab and zalutumumab) and tyrosine kinase inhibitors (gefitinib, erlotinib, and lapatinib) have not demonstrated any significant benefits. Afatinib, an irreversible pan-ErbB inhibitor to EGFR, HER2, and HER4, initially demonstrated comparable activity to cetuximab, especially in the setting of cetuximab failure. However, LUX-Head & Neck 1, a phase 3 trial in R/M HNSCC, which compared afatinib to methotrexate in the second-line setting, failed to demonstrate a significant OS benefit.[13] Thus, before immunotherapy, oncologists were presented with a therapeutic challenge for patients who failed first-line treatment because second-line regimens had no significant proven efficacy.

THE PROMISE OF IMMUNOTHERAPY

Cancer immunotherapy was first introduced in the 1890s by Dr William B. Coley,[14] who demonstrated antitumor responses in sarcoma patients who received "toxins" consisting of killed bacteria. Despite such anecdotal reports, immunotherapeutic modalities were not developed as a significant component of cancer therapy until more recently in the form of ICIs. From preclinical models and the infectious disease processes, T-cell responses were thought to be activated based on a "2-signal" model requiring engagement of T-cell receptor, major histocompatibility complex class molecules ("signal 1") and costimulatory molecules, B7 and CD28 ("signal 2"). However, the discovery of negative regulators of T-cell activation in the form of checkpoint inhibitors in the 1990s changed this paradigm. Cancer research shifted from enhancing antitumor T-cell response to removing the negative regulators of antitumor T-cell response. The scientific basis for these novel therapies originated from the discovery of the first checkpoint, CTLA-4, and the clinical development of ipilimumab (the monoclonal IgG1 antibody that blocks CTLA-4's activity), which showed remarkable improvements in survival for metastatic melanoma.[15] However, this success came with a unique and significant safety profile (up to 30% of patients with significant adverse events) defined by immune-related adverse events (irAEs). These irAEs are common among ICI and are characterized by various forms and degrees of autoimmunity-mediated damage by T cells to normal tissue. The clinical manifestations can range from manageable arthritis, dermatitis, and endocrinopathies to life-threatening colitis, pneumonitis, hepatitis, and endocrinopathies.

ANTI–PROGRAMMED DEATH-1 THERAPY

In parallel to the research and development of ipilimumab, Honjo and others who studied other regulators of T-cell activation discovered that PD-1 and ligand, PD-L1, can also inhibit this antitumor process through multiple, nonredundant regulatory pathways.[16–18] Preclinical models revealed that the blockade of this PD-1/PD-L1 interaction led to activation of T cells and development of antitumor responses.[16,19] These discoveries led to the development of nivolumab, a fully human IgG4 anti-PD-1 monoclonal antibody, and pembrolizumab, a humanized monoclonal IgG4-kappa isotype antibody against PD-1. Various trials found these anti-PD-1 therapies improved clinical outcomes in many epithelial cancers and had a significantly better tolerated safety profile as compared with ipilimumab.[20,21] As of 2016, anti-PD-1 therapies have been approved for melanoma, lung cancer, kidney cancer, and Hodgkin lymphoma[20–26] (Table 1).

Anti-PD-1 therapy has been investigated in R/M HNSCC with both pembrolizumab and nivolumab. Pembrolizumab was first investigated in a phase 1b trial (KEYNOTE-012) as second-line therapy in R/M HNSCC.[27] Patients with at least 1% of PD-L1 expression received pembrolizumab at 10 mg/kg intravenously every 2 weeks. Of the 60 patients treated, only 17% had any grade 3 to 4 drug-related adverse events. In terms of efficacy, 18% (8/45 evaluable patients) had an objective response among all patients. Notably, there was a higher response rate in human papillomavirus (HPV)-positive patients

Table 1
Summary of approved immune checkpoint inhibitors and combination therapies

Agent	Class	Tumor Types	Approval Date	Combo HNSCC Trials	NCT Trial No.
Ipilimumab	Anti-CTLA4	Melanoma	3/28/2011	Enoblituzumab	NCT02381314
				Cetuximab/radiation	NCT01860430
Nivolumab	Anti-PD-1	Melanoma	12/22/2014	Ipilimumab	NCT02741570
		NSCLC	3/4/2015	Varlilumab	NCT02335918
		RCC	11/23/2015	Epacadostat	NCT02327078
		Hodgkin	5/17/2016	Motolimod	NCT02124850
		HNSCC	11/10/2016	Radiation	NCT02684253
				Chemotherapy	NCT02764593
Pembrolizumab	Anti-PD-1	Melanoma	9/4/2014	Epacadostat	NCT02178722
		NSCLC	10/2/2015	Vorinostat	NCT02538510
		HNSCC	8/5/2016	Chemoradiation	Multiple
				T-VEC	NCT02626000
				Cetuximab/Chemo	NCT02358031
Nivolumab and Ipilimumab	Anti-PD-1 Anti-CTLA-4	Melanoma	1/23/2016		
Atezolizumab	Anti-PD-L1	Bladder	5/18/2016	Alone	NCT01375842
		NSCLC	10/18/2016	Varlilumab	NCT02543645

Abbreviations: NSCLC, non–small cell lung cancer; RCC, renal cell carcinoma.

(25%) as compared with the HPV-negative (14%) patients. An expansion cohort of 132 patients regardless of PD-L1 expression was also studied with pembrolizumab at 200 mg intravenously every 3 weeks.[28] Central imaging vendor review and investigator review revealed an objective response rate of 18% and 20%, respectively, and a median OS of 8 months. These results were encouraging because they were comparable to contemporary treatments, while maintaining a better tolerated safety profile.[12,13,29] The preliminary results from the nonrandomized phase 2 trial (KEYNOTE-055) with pembrolizumab confirmed these results with an ORR of 18%.[30] The phase 3 trial with pembrolizumab is ongoing. In CheckMate 141, a phase 3 clinical trial, nivolumab (3 mg/kg every 2 weeks) was compared with standard therapy (single-agent methotrexate, docetaxel, or cetuximab) in patients with platinum-refractory R/M HNSCC.[31] The study demonstrated superior efficacy in nivolumab based on OS (HR 0.70, 97.73% CI 0.51–0.96, $P = .01$), median OS (7.5 vs 5.1 months), and 1-year survival (36% vs 16.6%). In terms of safety, only 13.1% of patients developed serious grade 3 to 4 treatment-related adverse events with nivolumab as compared to 35.1% in those that received standard therapy. Based on the evidence from these clinical trials, pembrolizumab and nivolumab have been US Food and Drug Administration approved in 2016 for the use in second-line therapy in R/M HNSCC.

OTHER IMMUNE CHECKPOINT INHIBITORS

Other than nivolumab and pembrolizumab, other immune checkpoints that target the PD-1:PD-L1 pathway have been investigated in HNSCC clinical trials. These immune checkpoints include PDR001, PF-06801591, and REGN-2810 to name a few, which have been developed by other pharmaceutical companies. Most of these have gone into patients already, and their phase 1 clinical trials have either closed or are ongoing. There are also several anti-PD-L1 blocking antibodies, atezolizumab (Genentech) and durvalumab (AZ-Medimmune), which have treated HNSCC patients in various ongoing clinical trials as well. There is no clear consensus that one of these PD-1:PD-L1 blocking agents is better for HNSCC patients, and, unfortunately, there are no trials that will compare them in a head-to-head manner. Outside of these PD-1:PD-L1 targeting agents, CTLA-4 is the other ICI that has been used to treat HNSCC patients. Ipilimumab (Merck) and tremelimumab (AZ) are the 2 well-characterized CTLA-4 blocking agents, and there are ongoing clinical trials for these 2 agents in the HNSCC space. The immuno-oncologic field has rapidly expanded recently to develop other immunomodulatory agents that target other "druggable" cell surface molecules on the immune cells. Typically, these antibodies target other ICIs or coactivators that can either "release the brake" or "push the gas" on the cytolytic activity of the tumor specific T cells, respectively. Anti-LAG-3 (BMS-986916), anti-TIM-3 (TSR-022), and anti-KIR (BMS-986015) are examples of such other ICIs, while anti-4-1BB (PF-05082566) and anti-OX40 (PF-04518600, MEDI6469) are examples of the immune coactivators. Preliminary results from many of these agents are promising, and the investigators have been actively pursuing optimal combinations of these agents for recurrent and metastatic cancer.

CONSIDERATIONS BEFORE INSTITUTION OF ANTI–PROGRAMMED DEATH-1 THERAPY IN RECURRENT AND/OR METASTATIC HEAD AND NECK SQUAMOUS CELL CARCINOMA

There are many factors to consider when selecting candidates for ICI therapy in R/M HNSCC. In essence, ICIs induce some degree of autoimmunity in the context of R/M cancer. Attendant side effects that range from tolerable inflammation such as arthritis and dermatitis to life-threatening pulmonary pneumonitis are possible sequelae that must be discussed with the patient. First, patients and clinicians must both understand that because of their mechanism of action, the safety profile of ICIs differs significantly to traditional systemic chemotherapies, and the consequences of irAEs need to be thoroughly discussed with patients with preexisting comorbidities, including advanced age, autoimmune disease, and baseline organ dysfunction. Advanced age has been associated with immunosenescence, but retrospective studies have shown no significant difference with efficacy or safety profile with ICIs in the elderly population.[32,33] Conversely, a rare pattern of hyperprogression of the tumor has been observed retrospectively in patients on anti-PD-1/L-1 therapy that has been observed more frequently in elderly patients.[34] There are no clinical or molecular biomarkers to segregate these patients who can potentially hyperprogress. Although patients with preexisting autoimmune conditions were excluded from clinical trials, retrospective studies in patients with autoimmune conditions and melanoma have shown that irAEs were relatively more frequent, but mild and manageable, while still providing clinical responses.[35] In addition, a retrospective cohort study of patients with baseline organ dysfunction on anti-PD-1 therapy did not reveal significant worsening of organ function or irAEs, while still inducing clinical response in some patients.[36] All these findings were retrospective, and more research is needed to address some of these questions. Second, there are no available standardized biomarkers on tissue or blood now to predict response with anti-PD-1 therapy. Although there has been suggestions from clinical trials in other tumor types that higher PD-L1 expression on tumor correlates with improved response, even patients with no PD-L1 expression can achieve a clinical response.[37] In addition, issues with heterogeneity of samples, lack of standardization among PD-L1 assays, and an unclear definition of PD-L1 positivity limits the utility of PD-L1 expression. Further efforts are needed to evaluate other predictive biomarkers with anti-PD-1 therapy to select candidates for ICIs. Finally, although HPV status in oropharyngeal HNSCC predicts improved survival with chemotherapy, the role of HPV status with ICI is currently unknown.[38] Early studies have suggested a trend toward improved survival with HPV positivity, but larger prospective studies are needed.[31]

CANDIDACY FOR ANTI–PROGRAMMED DEATH-1 THERAPY

PD-1 blocking antibodies, either nivolumab or pembrolizumab, are approved as second-line agents for patients with R/M HNSCC that progress on or after a platinum-based therapy, based on the results from CheckMate 141 and KEYNOTE-012, respectively. As expected, study criteria for both trials included patients that were healthy with ECOG performance status of 0 to 1 and adequate organ function. Both studies excluded patients with brain metastasis, autoimmune diseases, or systemic immunosuppression. Unlike CheckMate 141, KEYNOTE-12 also required patients to have at least 1% of PD-L1 tumor expression. However, there are no predicative biomarkers, including PD-L1 expression, to assist in selecting patients currently. Future clinical and correlative studies will help to inform the generalizability of these results in other clinically relevant populations stratified by HPV status, bulky disease, or anatomic site as well as the development of clinical and molecular criteria to determine the appropriate candidates for therapy.

FUTURE DIRECTION WITH COMBINATION THERAPY

With the success with anti-PD-1 therapy in HNSCC, combination therapies with anti-PD-1 agents are currently being studied. These combinations include ICI, targeted therapy, chemotherapy, and radiation. Success with dual blockade of PD-1 and

CTLA-4, with nivolumab and ipilimumab, has already been shown in metastatic melanoma with a superior efficacy in the combination arm over both monotherapy arms (ORR 58% in combination vs 44% with nivolumab and 19% with ipilimumab).[39] This combination has been open in a clinical trial as first-line therapy for R/M HNSCC (CheckMate 651, NCT 027414570). Further combinations are being explored in other immunomodulatory agents such as anti-LAG3, anti-TIM3, anti-KIR, anti-41BB, and anti-OXO40 therapies as noted previously. Given the multimodal nature of HNSCC therapy, including targeted therapy, chemotherapy, and radiotherapy, multiple studies are exploring such modalities in various combinations with anti-PD-1 therapy. Current ongoing trials include studies with pembrolizumab, cetuximab, and chemotherapy (NCT 02358031), nivolumab, cetuximab, and motolomid (NCT 02124850), pembrolizumab and radiation (NCT 02318771), and nivolumab and SBRT (NCT 02684253) (see **Table 1**).

REFERENCES

1. Sullivan RD, Miller E, Sikes MP. Antimetabolite-metabolite combination cancer chemotherapy. Effects of intraarterial methotrexate-intramuscular Citrovorum factor therapy in human cancer. Cancer 1959;12:1248–62.
2. Wittes RE, Cvitkovic E, Shah J, et al. CIS-Dichlorodiammineplatinum(II) in the treatment of epidermoid carcinoma of the head and neck. Cancer Treat Rep 1977;61(3):359–66.
3. Jacobs C, Lyman G, Velez-Garcia E, et al. A phase III randomized study comparing cisplatin and fluorouracil as single agents and in combination for advanced squamous cell carcinoma of the head and neck. J Clin Oncol 1992; 10(2):257–63.
4. Forastiere AA, Metch B, Schuller DE, et al. Randomized comparison of cisplatin plus fluorouracil and carboplatin plus fluorouracil versus methotrexate in advanced squamous-cell carcinoma of the head and neck: a southwest oncology group study. J Clin Oncol 1992;10(8):1245–51.
5. Clavel M, Vermorken JB, Cognetti F, et al. Randomized comparison of cisplatin, methotrexate, bleomycin and vincristine (CABO) versus cisplatin and 5-fluorouracil (CF) versus cisplatin (C) in recurrent or metastatic squamous cell carcinoma of the head and neck. A phase III study of the EORTC head and neck cancer cooperative group. Ann Oncol 1994;5(6):521–6.
6. Gibson MK, Li Y, Murphy B, et al. Randomized phase III evaluation of cisplatin plus fluorouracil versus cisplatin plus paclitaxel in advanced head and neck cancer (E1395): an intergroup trial of the eastern cooperative oncology group. J Clin Oncol 2005;23(15):3562–7.
7. Posner MR, Hershock DM, Blajman CR, et al. Cisplatin and fluorouracil alone or with docetaxel in head and neck cancer. N Engl J Med 2007;357(17):1705–15.
8. Vermorken JB, Remenar E, van Herpen C, et al. Cisplatin, fluorouracil, and docetaxel in unresectable head and neck cancer. N Engl J Med 2007;357(17): 1695–704.
9. Dassonville O, Formento JL, Francoual M, et al. Expression of epidermal growth factor receptor and survival in upper aerodigestive tract cancer. J Clin Oncol 1993;11(10):1873–8.
10. Rubin Grandis J, Melhem MF, Gooding WE, et al. Levels of TGF-alpha and EGFR protein in head and neck squamous cell carcinoma and patient survival. J Natl Cancer Inst 1998;90(11):824–32.

11. Burtness B, Goldwasser MA, Flood W, et al, Eastern Cooperative Oncology Group. Phase III randomized trial of cisplatin plus placebo compared with cisplatin plus cetuximab in metastatic/recurrent head and neck cancer: an eastern cooperative oncology group study. J Clin Oncol 2005;23(34):8646–54.

12. Vermorken JB, Mesia R, Rivera F, et al. Platinum-based chemotherapy plus cetuximab in head and neck cancer. N Engl J Med 2008;359(11):1116–27.

13. Machiels JP, Haddad RI, Fayette J, et al. Afatinib versus methotrexate as second-line treatment in patients with recurrent or metastatic squamous-cell carcinoma of the head and neck progressing on or after platinum-based therapy (LUX-Head & Neck 1): an open-label, randomised phase 3 trial. Lancet Oncol 2015;16(5): 583–94.

14. Coley WB. The treatment of malignant tumors by repeated inoculations of erysipelas. With a report of ten original cases. 1893. Clin Orthop Relat Res 1991;(262): 3–11.

15. Leach DR, Krummel MF, Allison JP. Enhancement of antitumor immunity by CTLA-4 blockade. Science 1996;271(5256):1734–6.

16. Freeman GJ, Long AJ, Iwai Y, et al. Engagement of the PD-1 immunoinhibitory receptor by a novel B7 family member leads to negative regulation of lymphocyte activation. J Exp Med 2000;192(7):1027–34.

17. Strome SE, Dong H, Tamura H, et al. B7-H1 blockade augments adoptive T-cell immunotherapy for squamous cell carcinoma. Cancer Res 2003;63(19):6501–5.

18. Iwai Y, Ishida M, Tanaka Y, et al. Involvement of PD-L1 on tumor cells in the escape from host immune system and tumor immunotherapy by PD-L1 blockade. Proc Natl Acad Sci U S A 2002;99(19):12293–7.

19. Hirano F, Kaneko K, Tamura H, et al. Blockade of B7-H1 and PD-1 by monoclonal antibodies potentiates cancer therapeutic immunity. Cancer Res 2005;65(3): 1089–96.

20. Robert C, Long GV, Brady B, et al. Nivolumab in previously untreated melanoma without BRAF mutation. N Engl J Med 2015;372(4):320–30.

21. Robert C, Schachter J, Long GV, et al. Pembrolizumab versus ipilimumab in advanced melanoma. N Engl J Med 2015;372(26):2521–32.

22. Motzer RJ, Escudier B, McDermott DF, et al. Nivolumab versus everolimus in advanced renal-cell carcinoma. N Engl J Med 2015;373(19):1803–13.

23. Reck M, Rodriguez-Abreu D, Robinson AG, et al. Pembrolizumab versus chemotherapy for PD-L1-positive non-small-cell lung cancer. N Engl J Med 2016; 375(19):1823–33.

24. Borghaei H, Paz-Ares L, Horn L, et al. Nivolumab versus docetaxel in advanced nonsquamous non-small-cell lung cancer. N Engl J Med 2015;373(17):1627–39.

25. Brahmer J, Reckamp KL, Baas P, et al. Nivolumab versus docetaxel in advanced squamous-cell non-small-cell lung cancer. N Engl J Med 2015;373(2):123–35.

26. Ansell SM, Lesokhin AM, Borrello I, et al. PD-1 blockade with nivolumab in relapsed or refractory Hodgkin's lymphoma. N Engl J Med 2015;372(4):311–9.

27. Seiwert TY, Burtness B, Mehra R, et al. Safety and clinical activity of pembrolizumab for treatment of recurrent or metastatic squamous cell carcinoma of the head and neck (KEYNOTE-012): an open-label, multicentre, phase 1b trial. Lancet Oncol 2016;17(7):956–65.

28. Chow LQ, Haddad R, Gupta S, et al. Antitumor activity of pembrolizumab in biomarker-unselected patients with recurrent and/or metastatic head and neck squamous cell carcinoma: results from the phase Ib KEYNOTE-012 expansion cohort. J Clin Oncol 2016;34(32):3838–45.

29. Vermorken JB, Trigo J, Hitt R, et al. Open-label, uncontrolled, multicenter phase II study to evaluate the efficacy and toxicity of cetuximab as a single agent in patients with recurrent and/or metastatic squamous cell carcinoma of the head and neck who failed to respond to platinum-based therapy. J Clin Oncol 2007;25(16): 2171–7.

30. Bauml J, Seiwert TY, Pfister DG, et al. Preliminary results from KEYNOTE-055: pembrolizumab after platinum and cetuximab failure in head and neck squamous cell carcinoma (HNSCC). J Clin Oncol 2016;34(Suppl) [Abstract 6011].

31. Ferris RL, Blumenschein G Jr, Fayette J, et al. Nivolumab for recurrent squamous-cell carcinoma of the head and neck. N Engl J Med 2016;375(19):1856–67.

32. Tokarova B, Amirtaev KG, Krasavin EA, et al. [Role of the genotype in the mutagenic action of radiation with different LET on cells of Escherichia coli]. Radiobiologiia 1989;29(6):754–9 [in Russian].

33. Elias R, Morales J, Rehman Y, et al. Immune checkpoint inhibitors in older adults. Curr Oncol Rep 2016;18(8):47.

34. Champiat S, Dercle L, Ammari S, et al. Hyperprogressive disease (HPD) is a new pattern of progression in cancer patients treated by anti-PD-1/PD-L1. Clin Cancer Res 2016. [Epub ahead of print].

35. Menzies AM, Johnson DB, Ramanujam S, et al. Anti-PD-1 therapy in patients with advanced melanoma and preexisting autoimmune disorders or major toxicity with ipilimumab. Ann Oncol 2016. [Epub ahead of print].

36. Kanz BA, Pollack MH, Johnpulle R, et al. Safety and efficacy of anti-PD-1 in patients with baseline cardiac, renal, or hepatic dysfunction. J Immunother Cancer 2016;4:60.

37. Daud AI, Wolchok JD, Robert C, et al. Programmed death-ligand 1 expression and response to the anti-programmed death 1 antibody pembrolizumab in melanoma. J Clin Oncol 2016;34(34):4102–9.

38. Ang KK, Harris J, Wheeler R, et al. Human papillomavirus and survival of patients with oropharyngeal cancer. N Engl J Med 2010;363(1):24–35.

39. Larkin J, Chiarion-Sileni V, Gonzalez R, et al. Combined nivolumab and ipilimumab or monotherapy in untreated melanoma. N Engl J Med 2015;373(1):23–34.

Moving?

Make sure your subscription moves with you!

To notify us of your new address, find your **Clinics Account Number** (located on your mailing label above your name), and contact customer service at:

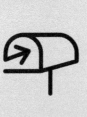

Email: **journalscustomerservice-usa@elsevier.com**

800-654-2452 (subscribers in the U.S. & Canada)
314-447-8871 (subscribers outside of the U.S. & Canada)

Fax number: **314-447-8029**

Elsevier Health Sciences Division
Subscription Customer Service
3251 Riverport Lane
Maryland Heights, MO 63043

Printed and bound by CPI Group (UK) Ltd, Croydon, CR0 4YY

03/10/2024

01040392-0002